Library of Congress Cataloging in Publication Data

Murty, A. S., 1943—
   Toxicity of pesticides to fish.

   Bibliography: p.
   Includes index.
   1. Fishes—Effect of water pollution on.
2. Pesticides—Toxicology. I. Title.
SH174.M87   1986   597'.024   85-4182
ISBN 0-8493-6058-7 (v.1)
ISBN 0-8493-6059-5 (v.2)

   Direct all inquiries to CRC Press, Inc., 2000 Corporate Blvd., N.W., Boca Raton, Florida, 33431.

© 1986 by CRC Press, Inc.
Second Printing, 1986
Third Printing, 1988

International Standard Book Number 0-8493-6058-7 (v.1)
International Standard Book Number 0-8493-6059-5 (v.2)

Library of Congress Card Number 85-4182
Printed in the United States

Dedicated
to my Parents and Mentors
especially Profs. K. Hanumantha Rao and K. V. Jagannadha Rao

FOREWORD

Ever since the increased use of synthetic pesticides during the past 40 years, it has become apparent that these highly toxic materials did not only affect target organisms but often harmed nontarget organisms like fish and other aquatic life. Some of these adverse effects were so subtle that they were not recognized until analytical and biological testing methods had been refined to discover heretofore unrecognized deleterious effects on fish. More recently, the attention of fish biologists has been turned towards nonpesticidal industrial pollutants, like polychlorinated biphenyls (PCBs) and dioxins, which in the past were often mistaken for DDT and related pesticides.

Although there are a number of books and reviews on the subject of pesticide toxicity on fish, the present treatise by Dr. A. S. Murty is the most comprehensive work on this subject. Dr. Murty, who has carried out basic research on the effect of pesticides on fish in his native land of India and Germany, has gathered the work of over 1800 papers published world-wide and critically placed them in the context of 12 chapters. This thorough coverage of the world literature attests to the fact that no part of the globe is too remote to obtain the current scientific literature on a particular technical subject, as for example the toxicity of pesticides to fish. This present work is a detailed treatment of the environmental fate of pesticides and their acute and chronic toxicological effect on fish. A shorter chapter on PCBs and related compounds enhances the coverage of the book. An interesting treatment on insecticide resistance in fish and the combined action of different pesticides, to the best of my knowledge, have not been discussed as thoroughly as in this book.

The fluent style and the comprehensive coverage of this book make it not only a pleasure to read but also a "must" on the shelf or desk of concerned scientists all over the world.

Gunter Zweig, Ph.D.
Washington, D.C.
March, 1985

PREFACE

The increasing awareness of the environmental problems during the last 2 decades kindled much interest on the environmental fate and behavior of the xenobiotic chemicals. This is evident from the fact that during the last 16 years or so, about 20 international journals have been launched to focus attention on environmental problems. Environmental disasters like the collapse of the coho salmon fishery in Lake Michigan and the mass mortality of fish elsewhere clearly established the toxicity of pesticides to fish and other aquatic organisms. Further, the realization that the aquatic environment is the ultimate sink for all pollutants stimulated studies on the toxicity of man-made chemicals to the aquatic organisms, especially pesticide toxicity to fish. Much of the information on the toxicity of pesticides to fish, however, lay scattered in diverse journals or in generalized summaries on the effect of pollutants on fish. The present work is the first major attempt at reviewing comprehensively all the available information on this fascinating subject.

I have attempted to trace the growth of this subject from the earliest toxicity tests that I could record, dating back to 1944, to the present day. In about 4 decades, the toxicity testing itself has undergone a conceptual change. In the early days, simple toxic effects with death as the end point were studied. At present the focus has shifted to hazard assessment and prediction to avert the environmental disasters caused by DDT-type compounds.

In dealing with the toxicity of pesticides to fish, one may feel that perhaps a discussion on polychlorinated biphenyls (PCBs) and other industrial organic chemicals is out of place. Although such chemicals have rarely been, if ever, used in combination with pesticides, their environmental behavior and uptake by fish are akin to those of the organochlorine pesticides. Hence, the similarity between the two groups of compounds is briefly pointed out and the methods of their separation are discussed.

This book is the result of the constant encouragement I received from Dr. Gunter Zweig of the U.S. Environmental Protection Agency, Washington, D.C. To him, I owe a deep debt of gratitude. I also thank him for readily agreeing to write the Foreword for this book.

The many discussions I had with the fellow scientists, during my tenure of work as a visiting scientist of the International Development Research Centre (IDRC), Canada, during 1980 to 1981 and as a Fellow of the Alexander Von Humboldt Foundation of West Germany during 1981 to 1983 helped me in planning and completing this work. Especially IDRC had funded my visit to a number of laboratories. I thank both these agencies for affording me an opportunity to meet my fellow scientists. I also thank my parent University for granting me leave to go abroad and work.

Mr. J. R. W. Miles and Dr. S. Sethunathan read critically Chapter 1, Volume I. Drs. Richard Addison and J. L. Hamelink commented upon Chapter 3, Volume I, and Dr. D. Desaiah, upon the part dealing with ATPase-inhibition studies in Chapter 6, Volume II. I am obliged to them for their comments and suggestions. I would like to thank Drs. D. V. Subba Rao, S. Pitchumani, Bhuwanesh Agrawal, and U. Schiecke, Ms. Seetha Murty, and the librarian of the Columbia National Fisheries Research Laboratory, Columbia, Missouri, for their help with the necessary reprints. I also wish to acknowledge the help extended by Messers K. Kondaiah, K. Krishna Prasad, M. V. Krishnaiah, and K. R. S. Sambasiva Rao, in the preparation, finalization, and typing of the manuscript. The excellent editorial help of the staff of CRC Press is also acknowledged.

The sources of the figures and tables have been mentioned at the appropriate place. Besides, I would like to acknowledge Drs. R. D. Wauchope, J. L. Hamelink, G. D. Veith, H. C. Alexander, W. B. Neely, and C. J. Schmitt for the original photographs of their graphs.

I am also indebted to my colleagues Dr. Y. Ranga Reddy and Prof. S. Krishna Sarma, who cheerfully read through the entire manuscript and commented upon style and syntax. The faults, if any, are mine.

This work would not have been possible but for the involvement of my wife, Ramani, who supervised the different stages of the preparation and typing of the draft, and patiently corrected the proofs. Lastly, it is indeed a pleasure to acknowledge the help of our children, Usha, Sudha, and Aditya in classifying the literature and organizing the references.

A. S. Murty

THE AUTHOR

Dr. Ayyagari S. Murty, Reader in Zoology at Nagarjuna University, Nagarjunana-gar, India is an environmental toxicologist interested in the toxicity of xenobiotic chemicals to nontarget organisms. He received his M.Sc. and Ph.D. in Zoology from Andhra University, India. As a teacher for postgraduate students for more than 20 years, Dr. Murty has taught diverse subjects ranging from systematic zoology to environmental biology.

Dr. Murty is presently engaged in research on environmental hazard evaluation of chemicals and also on the toxicity of pesticides and industrial organic chemicals to nontarget organisms, especially fish. During 1980 and 1981, he was one of the 18 scientists selected from the third-world countries in a world-wide competition by the International Development Research Centre and worked as a visiting scientist at London (Ontario) research station of Agriculture Canada. From 1981 to 1983, he worked as a Fellow of the Humboldt Foundation of West Germany, mostly at the Institute for Water, Soil, and Air Health of the Federal Health Office, West Berlin.

Dr. Murty presented several papers at national and international conferences. He is frequently invited to lecture at workshops and seminars on environmental toxicology. He published over 40 research papers and his work has brought to light certain lacunae in aquatic toxicity testing protocols with hydrophobic compounds.

TOXICITY OF PESTICIDES TO FISH

A. S. Murty

Volume I

Volume II

TABLE OF CONTENTS

Volume I

Chapter 1

PESTICIDES IN THE ENVIRONMENT

I. INTRODUCTION

During the brief period of man's existence on this planet, two things stand out prominently. First, human beings are not content to be just another species in the vast assemblage of organisms in nature. Second, although the attempts of human beings to alter nature to suit their needs have been successful in a limited way, their attempts to master nature and dominate all other organisms have led to disastrous consequences. Nowhere else are these undesirable consequences better illustrated than in man's endeavour to increase the food production and to reduce crop losses resulting from pest attack, by the application of pesticides. The problem of pests arose because the modern agricultural practices, while increasing our food production, also augmented the food supply for innumerable other organisms. It has been said that pests did not come into existence until intensive agriculture was attempted. It is now estimated that there are well over 68,000 species of pestilent and disease-causing insects, apart from a large number of species of ticks, mites, nematodes, and fungi whose existence and activities are in direct conflict with the interests of human beings.[1] The chemical warfare waged against pests during the last 40 years, under the euphoria generated following the discovery of the highly toxic action of synthetic organic chemicals — in the false hope of eradicating all pests — has damaged the environment much more than it has eased the pest menace.

This chapter attempts to focus attention on the various means through which pesticide residues reach the aquatic environment and the hazards to the aquatic organisms resulting from the excessive use of pesticides. It does not purport to be a review on the persistence of the pesticide residues in and their mobility from soils. Important contributions and reviews on various aspects discussed have been mentioned at the appropriate places.

A. History of Pesticide Use

The history of pesticide use and the development of modern pesticides has been well documented and discussed.[2] Extensive use of pesticides has facilitated an increase in agricultural productivity, despite a decrease in the total acreage of land under actual cultivation.[3] The 2 decades following World War II witnessed extensive use of organochlorine (OC) compounds — especially DDT in North America,[4] cyclodienes (aldrin and dieldrin in particular) and hexachlorocyclohexane (HCH) in Great Britain,[5] and HCH in Japan.[6] In particular, the use of DDT in North America was indiscriminate. While the rate of application of DDT to control the spruce budworm at 1 to 2 lb/acre[7,8]* was subsequently reduced to 0.5 lb and even to 0.25 lb/acre, its use for the control of mosquitoes was intense. For instance, in certain counties of New Jersey, between 1950 and 1966 the rate of DDT spraying ranged from 5 to 23 lb/acre.[9] Such an indiscriminate and heavy use of DDT and other pesticides invariably caused environmental disturbances. The disastrous implications of this were appreciated only after Rachel Carson[10] highlighted the environmental hazards of pesticides in her thought-provoking, though controversial, book, *Silent Spring*.

From 1950 onward, another group of pesticides, organophosphorus (OP) compounds, gained in importance. In the 1950s and 1960s, compounds like parathion and

_____

*   1 lb/acre = 1.12 kg/ha.

malathion partly replaced DDT and the cyclodienes. Fenitrothion was the most often-used compound in Canada and also in the U.S. for the control of spruce budworm. Subsequently another group, carbamates, was also introduced and carbaryl was the most extensively used compound on Maine forests between 1975 and 1980.[11] A number of other compounds like substituted ureas, substituted phenols, and nitro compounds have found diverse application as insecticides, fungicides, fumigants, herbicides, defoliants, desiccants, and the like. It is predicted that the world-wide crop losses due to pest attack may amount to 50% of the products;[12] even with the use of pesticides it is estimated that pests account for a 13% loss.[3] In the U.S., one of the countries where crop protection measures are vigorous, the estimated crop loss in 1970 amounted to $33 billion.[12]

Pesticides have found their use not only in agriculture, but also in man's fight against the spread of diseases like malaria, typhoid, plague, or sleeping sickness. Although in later years DDT has fallen into disrepute, the World Health Organization has estimated that until 1971, more than 1 billion people had been saved from the risk of malaria by the use of DDT alone.[13] Gold et al.[14] quoting from other sources, stated that until 1980, 4 billion lb of DDT had been used to control insect-borne diseases.

B. Adverse Effects of Pesticides

Extensive use of pesticides could have been the ultimate answer to the recurring problem of pests, as was hoped in the 1940s and 1950s but for a few unfortunate and unforeseen problems. First, prolonged exposure of a species to one and the same compound has led to the establishment of resistant populations, especially to cyclodienes.[3,15] Second, minor pests became major pests owing to the elimination of their natural predators as a result of intense pesticide application. For instance, Ware[16] pointed out that until 1972 to 1974, spider mites, cotton leaf-perforator, and tobacco budworm were classed as minor pests in Arizona. But, with the destruction of their predators following intense use of OP compounds, they became major pests. Similarly, at the time of introduction of OC compounds in Central America in 1950, there were only two cotton pests of economic importance. By 1955, subsequent to the use of DDT, HCH, and toxaphene, three more species emerged as major problems. By the mid-1960s, attempts to control the five species led to an increase in the number of pests of economic importance (ten species); pesticide use thus had the exact opposite effect to the desired one, i.e., instead of controlling pests, it brought new pests into being. Third, the ultimate effect of pesticides is seen on the nontarget organisms, especially those inhabiting the aquatic environment. After all, the aquatic environment is the ultimate sink for pollutants,[17] and any compound produced on an industrial scale is likely to reach there, sooner or later.[18]

One of the early works that helped us gain an insight into the possible environmental abuses caused by the excessive use of pesticides is the study on the effect of aerial application of DDT for the control of spruce budworm on the forests of New Brunswick, Canada, by Kerswill and Edwards[7] and Kerswill.[8] The spray program began in 1952 when DDT at the rate of 1 lb/acre was applied on 186,000 acres. In 1953, the sprayed area was ten times larger than in previous years, but was sprayed at the rate of 0.5 lb/acre. The spray operations continued annually and in 1957, 5.7 million acres were sprayed. The forests were initially sprayed with a low-flying aircraft from an altitude of about 15 to 75 m. Replacement of the smaller Stearman airplane by the larger American torpedo bomber, Medium, that was declared as surplus and hence became available for spray operations, resulted in greater fish kill; with the bigger aircraft it was not always possible to shut off the spray nozzles while crossing streams and rivers and while reversing directions. Subsequent studies indicated that effective control of spruce budworm could be achieved with DDT at as low as 0.25 lb/acre, if the spray was evenly distributed to deposit at least 10 drops per square centimeter over the target area. In the light of this finding, only in such well-organized investigations as the New Brunswick study was it possible to estimate how much excess DDT was used prior to 1958.

Kerswill and Edwards[7] studied the mortality of caged and free-living young salmon in the streams of forests sprayed with DDT. A single application of DDT at 0.5 lb/acre caused heavy loss of underyearling salmon and parr within 3 months. At 0.25 lb/acre, there was no apparent effect on parr, but all the underyearlings were killed. Further, two applications at 0.25 lb/acre each at 10-day intervals were as harmful as a single application of 0.5 lb/acre. They also noted delayed action of DDT: in the watersheds sprayed in June, wild young salmon were found dying in winter with the onset of very low water temperatures. Besides, DDD at 0.25 or 0.5 lb/acre or malathion at 0.125 lb/acre was as harmful as DDT at 0.25 lb/acre.

The forests of Maine were sprayed with DDT at 1 lb/acre, seven times between 1954 and 1967, with equally disastrous results as in New Brunswick.[19] Of the 680,000 acres sprayed, 306,000 acres were sprayed only once, but in different years; another 204,000 acres were treated twice with DDT, whereas 170,000 acres were sprayed thrice. Immediately after the application, there were high initial levels of DDT (all values in mg/kg; 0.83 in mud, 0.74 in plants, 8 to 21 in trout, and 9.84 in chubs). In the next 2 years, the residue levels dropped rapidly, but leveled off and persisted thereafter. Even 10 years after a single application, residues in all components of the streams (mud, plants, insects, fish, and birds) were higher than in the untreated areas. The prolonged persistence led to cumulative values in streams, adjoining the areas sprayed more than once.

The spraying of DDD on Clear Lake, Calif., is yet another classic instance of environmental mismanagement. On three occasions, in 1949, 1954, and 1957, DDD was sprayed directly onto the lake to control the Clear Lake gnats (*Chaoborus astictopus*). Following the last application, western grebes (*Aechmophorus occidentalis*) were found dying. Analysis of the samples in 1958 showed residues up to 1600 mg/kg DDD.[20] Reproductive failure of the birds was evident shortly after the first treatment. The residues persisted in the lake for over 19 years, and were recorded in 1976 in fish from the lake.[21]

Several instances of mass mortality of fish have been reported immediately following the massive application of pesticides. In 1950, simultaneous occurrence of fishkills in 15 tributaries of the Tennessee River in Alabama were reported. These fishkills were associated with rainfall runoff from agricultural fields, following the application of chlorinated hydrocarbon insecticides.[17] Repeated spraying of DDT around the lake, aerially twice a year, first in late June and a second application in late July, has been suggested to be the likely cause of drastic reduction in the population of landlocked salmon in Sebago Lake, Maine, and a decline in sport fishery and poor catches.[22] According to Holden,[23] many of the reported cases of mass mortality in Great Britain were attributable to accidental spillage of agricultural chemicals. The President's Science Advisory Committee[15] chronicled several instances of mass mortality of fish arising from pesticide use in the U.S. In 1967, it was estimated that about 13% of the fishkills in England and Wales was attributable to pesticides, particularly OC compounds.[24] In Scotland, dinoseb and 4-chloro-2-methylphenoxy acetic acid (MCPA), washed by rain from fields soon after application, have been thought to be responsible for fishkills in small streams. Elson et al.[25] reported that effluent from a wood-treatment plant using pentachlorophenol (PCP) flowed through a small brook in the Miramichi River area, Canada, into a tidal marsh and thence into the estuary. In one 8-week period of operation, about 500 kg of PCP was discharged. Because of 10 years of uninterrupted discharge of PCP and other wastes from this wood-treatment plant, the salmon caught in the vicinity had tainted flesh. Schmitt and Winger[26] cited several instances where sport and commercial fisheries had to be closed because of the occurrence of high pesticide residues in the fish. The discharge of about 90,700 kg of chlordecone into the James River estuary during the manufacture of this compound at Hopewell, Va., between 1966 and 1975, led to the closure of commercial and sport fishing in the estuary.[27]

In all the above instances, fishkills or harmful effects on fish populations have been the result of indiscriminate use, careless handling, accidental spillage, or discharge of untreated effluents into natural waterways. It is usually felt that pesticides, when used in recommended doses, should not pose environmental problems. Environmental disturbances, however, have been reported even when pesticides have been applied at recommended doses. For example, following the treatment of African rivers with Abate® for blackfly control, even in the absence of mortality of fish, behavioral changes (stressed swimming, altered behavior and preferences) appeared to have caused a change in population structure, with certain species being more prone to be captured.[28] Mass mortality of bluegills and bass, ducklings, and invertebrates was noted following the application of Dursban® to ponds, at rates recommended for mosquito control.[29,30]

Presence of pesticides has been reported, in human milk and canned baby food,[31] rainwater,[32,33] air,[34,35] the fauna of the Antarctic,[36] and many other unexpected places. HCH was detected in the paper of books published in Japan.[37] This ubiquitousness is evidently the ultimate result of excessive use of pesticides in various parts of the world. According to the estimates of the U.S. Environmental Protection Agency (USEPA), about 91% of all U.S. residents have detectable levels of polychlorinated biphenyls (PCBs)* in their fatty tissues.[38] PCBs have also been recorded in the indoor air of commercial, industrial, and residential buildings.[39] As early as 1945, the inadvisability of using DDT for mosquito control, in places where there was a possibility of contamination of municipal water supplies was emphasized; the possible health hazards as a consequence of the use of DDT to human beings and other nontarget organisms, were discussed.[40] The pervasive nature of DDT is reflected in the increasing concentration of DDT in the phytoplankton collected in Monterey Bay, Calif., between 1955 and 1969,[41] in the bioconcentration by algae and transfer to higher trophic levels.[42,43]

C. Other Sources of Pesticide Residues

With such widespread application, these pesticides are bound to enter the ecosystem. However, chlorinated hydrocarbons may have entered the environment, not necessarily through pest-control measures alone, but through other means as well. For instance, the possible production of chlorinated hydrocarbons in swimming pools as a result of reaction between chlorine and organic substances has been suggested.[44] The quantities of hexachlorobenzene (HCB) recorded in the environment and the biota indicate that there might be sources other than its limited use as a fungicide. According to Jansson and Bergman,[45] HCB has been reported as a contaminant in products like PCP and pentachloronitrobenzene, as a by-product in chlorine production by the electrolysis of brine and during the combustion of polyvinyl chloride. But the suggestion that DDE or DDT may act as a source of PCBs in the environment has been refuted by Harvey[46] and Metcalf et al.[47] Methylmercury is produced *in situ* in the environment, both biologically and nonbiologically.[48] Photoisomerization is known to be another means of production of some toxic compounds. It is reported that mirex is converted photolytically into chlordecone.[49] UV irradiation of DDT is known to produce DDE and to a

---

* Although PCBs are not pesticides, it becomes necessary to mention their environmental behavior because of their close similarity to DDT and, until 1967, the mistaken identity of certain PCB gas chromatographic peaks as belonging to the DDT group.

lesser extent DDD.[50] Sometimes, photo-oxidation leads to the formation of more toxic products.[51] Occasionally pesticides find their way into the environment when they are used for nonpesticidal purposes, such as the use of mirex as a flame retardant.[52]

II. PERSISTENCE OF PESTICIDES IN THE SOILS AND LONG-RANGE TRANSPORT IN THE ENVIRONMENT

Aquatic organisms are affected by pesticides, although often the aquatic environment is not the primary site of application of pesticides. Two factors ultimately contribute to the concentration of the pesticides in the aquatic ecosystem: persistence of pesticides in the soils and long-range transport of the pesticides in the atmosphere.

A. Persistence of Pesticide Residues in the Soil

Soils treated with pesticides act as traps releasing the residues to the atmosphere and also contributing to the residue load in the surface runoff. Hence, the longer the persistence of a compound, the greater the chances for its transport to the aquatic environment.

The persistence of DDT has been studied more often than that of any other compound since DDT is one of the most persistent pesticides and has caused many environmental problems because of its potential for bioconcentration. In soils treated with DDT at 10 and 100 lb/acre, respectively, 18 and 24% (expressed as total DDT or Σ DDT, i.e., DDT + DDE + DDD) of the initial quantity persisted even after 15 years.[53] Similarly, 15 years after the application of aldrin at 20 lb/acre, 5.8% of the initial quantity persisted as dieldrin. Lindane was, however, less persistent, with only 0.2% of the initial dose (10 or 100 lb/acre) remaining after 15 years. Among the different types of soils, orchard soils have perhaps received the maximum amount of DDT. It is estimated that an acre of orchard in the U.S. would have received about 250 to 400 lb of DDT between 1947 and 1960.[54] In a survey of orchard soils in the U.S., DDT residues in the range of 0.07 to 245.4 mg/kg were recorded.[55] Kuhr et al.[56] reported 357 mg/kg DDT in the top 15 cm of orchard soil that had not been sprayed with DDT for 15 years preceding that analysis. Likewise, up to 40 mg/kg DDT was found in the top 1.25 cm layer of orchard soil that had not been sprayed with DDT for several years.[57] Weber,[58] reviewing the published work, stated that the levels of DDT accumulated in the orchard soils in the U.S. were well over 100 lb/acre. The estimated half-life of DDT is 10 to 20 years. In an investigation, Harris et al.[59] reported 0.01 to 82.3 mg/kg DDT in 15 farm soils in southwestern Ontario, 4 to 5 years after the use of DDT was severely restricted. Even in an urban soil like that of West Berlin, high concentrations of Σ DDT (up to 1 mg/kg) were found.[60] Concentrations of mirex and mirex-related OC compounds, detected in soils, amounted to 50% of the initial quantity of mirex applied 12 years earlier.[61] The half-life of toxaphene, a chlorinated camphene product, was reported to be 11 years.[58]

In general, OC compounds are more persistent than the other types of compounds. The persistence of OC compounds has been discussed in detail.[62] It is the chemical structure of the pesticide molecule that primarily influences the extent of its degradability. Kawasaki[63] has discussed the biodegradability of chemicals, on the basis of their structure. Among the aliphatic compounds and their derivatives, main carbon bonding influences the extent of degradability of the substance. The compounds with a tertiary or quaternary carbon bonding (even if they are alcohols or carboxylic acids) are less degradable than those with primary or secondary carbon bondings. Halogenated aliphatic compounds, other than derivatives of monochloroacetic acid, are generally less susceptible to degradation. Among the aromatic compounds, biodegradability depends chiefly upon the atomic groups of the substituents.[63]

OP and carbamate compounds are less persistent than OCs, and hence have to be applied repeatedly. Repeated use of OP and carbamate compounds may lead to their accumulation in the environment, as has been reported in the organic soils used for vegetable production in Ontario.[64] Stewart et al.[65] reported that parathion persisted in the soil for over 16 years. Evaluation of the physicochemical properties of OP compounds indicates that some of them possess properties (poor water solubility, high octanol-water partition coefficient, and resistance to hydrolysis) that would favor at least limited environmental and biological transport and accumulation under certain conditions.[66] For instance, the more complex aryl-substituted OP compounds are more stable and hence have a longer residual life than the alkyl phosphates. Also, octanol-water partition coefficient (K_{ow}) tends to increase by halogen-substitution on the aryl groups. Compared with a log K_{ow} value of 5.69 of *p,p'*-DDE and 6.19 of *p,p'*-DDT, the log K_{ow} values of chlorpyrifos, dichlofenthion, and leptophos, according to Freed et al.[66] are 5.11, 5.14, and 6.31, respectively. OP compounds with sulfide or sulfoxide groups are degraded to sulfone and both sulfoxide and sulfone are persistent in the soils.[3]

Although not a separate class of compounds having a common chemical structure, herbicides need to be considered here because of the enormous increase in their use. In Canada, between 1947 and 1970, the sale of insecticides and fungicides increased three- to fourfold whereas that of the herbicides increased far more than 20 times during the same period.[3] In U.S., the production of herbicides exceeded that of insecticides in 1967 and since then continued to increase whereas that of chlorinated hydrocarbon insecticides decreased.[4] Although the toxicity of many herbicides to nontarget organisms is very low, the fact that they have to be used in large quantities for effective control may be a real threat to the nontarget organisms. For instance, dichlone, molinate, propanil, sodium arsenite, and dichlobenil may be employed at field rates that result in residue concentrations in excess of the median effective concentration (EC 50) for *Daphnia*.[67] Also, as in the case of OP compounds with substituted halogens, herbicides with halogen groups persist over extended periods in the soil. For instance, nitrofen, a pre- and postemergent, chlorine-containing herbicide used against broad-leaved weeds, accumulated in large quantities (up to 35 mg/kg) in organic muck soils of Ontario; occasionally residues as high as 15 mg/kg have been reported to persist until the next season.[68]

As soils receive the major part of the globally used pesticides and residues are transported eventually to the water bodies, persistence in the soils ultimately constitutes a threat to the aquatic environment. Ever since the imposition of severe restrictions on the use of OC compounds in the western countries,[69,70] there are indications that the overall DDT concentrations in the environment of these countries are steadily declining. No such restrictions have been imposed on the use of DDT and other OC compounds in the rest of the countries of Asia, Africa, and Latin America. There has been a steady increase in the use of such compounds in these countries, in an all out effort to raise the agricultural production. The extent of accumulation of DDT and other OC compounds in the soils of the Third World countries (similar to the work carried out in the west, as explained earlier in this section) is not yet known. Also, DDT is known to have spread far and wide in the global ecosystem within 20 years of the commencement of its use, as is evident from the finding of DDT in the Arctic and Antarctic environments in the early 1960s. To what extent the current use of DDT in the developing countries contributes to the global persistence of this compound, despite the restrictions imposed on its use by the industrialized nations, remains as yet unknown. Further research efforts have to be directed towards this study. Furthermore, the need to evaluate the extent of pollution by persistent compounds like toxaphene, that have been used in the western countries even after restricting the use of DDT, cannot be overemphasized.

B. Long-Range Transport of the Pesticides in the Environment

During application, pesticides are carried into the atmosphere by drift. Also, many of the pesticides, being volatile organic compounds, readily evaporate from plant surfaces and soils and may then either reside in the atmosphere, for longer periods or be brought down by precipitation or be slowly deposited as dry particulate matter.

1. Loss during Application

Considerable quantity of the sprayed pesticide fails to hit the target area and is thus lost as spray drift. Weather conditions influence the extent of drift, and application from an airplane has far more drastic consequences than application from ground. It has been reported that aerial application of dieldrin and endosulfan for controlling *Glossina* in Nigeria resulted in more deleterious effects on bird and other nontarget species than discriminative ground application.[71] During aerial spraying of DDT, about one third of the sprayed compound failed to contact the target area despite the fact that it was sprayed early in the morning when the wind velocity was minimal.[72] It was also found that while spraying forests aerially, about 95% of the aerosol droplets failed to reach the target plants and contaminated the forest canopy and the ground. In such instances, aerosol efficiency may be increased by using equipment that disperses finer and smaller particles, but such a move would increase drift-tendency. In another study, the average recovery of endosulfan at ground level was 47%[73] following aerial application to a delta in Botswana for the control of tsetse fly. The concentration of endosulfan in water, after spraying the delta, ranged from 0.5 to 4.2 $\mu g/\ell$, which is equal to or more than the 96-h LC 50 values for many species of fish. About 1% of the total fish population was estimated to have been killed by the spray drift. The percent mortality differed among different species and ranged from 0 to 60, although the very high percentage was one of rare occurrence.[73] On the basis of a 5-year study, Hindin and Bennett[74] concluded that 35% of DDT and 50% of ethion applied by airplanes did not reach the plant canopy and persisted in the treated area for as long as 2 weeks after application. After aerial spraying of fenitrothion, 77 $\mu g/\ell$ was recorded in rainwater in the vicinity of spraying; even at a site 85 km away, 0.16 $\mu g/\ell$ was recorded.[75] Following aerial application of 30% DDT on the Blue Nile to give an initial nominal concentration of 0.09 mg/ℓ to control the green chironomid, *Tanytarsus lewsii,* hundreds of fish were found dying the same day, about 13 km downstream of the point of application.[76] On the other hand, aerial spraying of fenitrothion at 2 or 3 oz/acre on New Brunswick forests has been reported to have no deleterious effect on fish in streams in the treated area.[77] Similarly, spraying forests with Roundup,® a herbicide, at recommended rates (4.85 lb/acre) or even at 10 times or 100 times the recommended rate, did not affect the rainbow trout in the field streams.[78]

2. Loss due to Volatilization

Volatilization is a major cause of loss of pesticides from crops and soils. Vapor pressure influences the extent of volatilization; the higher the vapor pressure, the higher the volatility of a compound and the greater the mobility in the gaseous phase.[79] Temperature increases the rate of volatilization. A temperature increase of 10°C increases volatilization fourfold.[80] Increased airflow over the surface also increases the rate of evaporation.[80] Further, the rate of evaporation of pesticides from the soils is related to the vapor pressure, water content of the soil, adsorption of the chemical by the soil, and soil characters.[81] The movement, volatilization, and bioactivity of pesticides depend on the partitioning between soil, water, and air. Volatilization from soil, water, and plant surfaces, is a significant means of loss, even for relatively nonvolatile compounds.[82] Acree et al.[83] postulated that pesticides escape from soils by codistillation with water. But, Spencer and Cliath[84] clearly established that pesticide volatilization was independent of water loss from soils. Also, Chiou and Manes[85] offered conclusive evidence for the evaporation of DDT while water is condensing into the system, disproving the codistillation theory of Acree et al.[83]

Vapor density is another factor controlling volatilization. Farmer et al.[80] found that the rate of volatilization of dieldrin from gila silt loam increased with increasing soil pesticide concentration. An earlier study by the same group[84] showed that soil water content had no effect on the vapor density until it was reduced to less than one molecular layer of water. Igue et al.[86] reported that dieldrin loss from gila silt loam was dependent on the soil water content, but not on the rate of water loss from the soil. The relative humidity of air indirectly influences the loss of pesticides from the soil by affecting the soil water content. The latter influences pesticide volatilization by competing for soil adsorption sites and thereby controls the vapor density of the pesticide. These authors emphasized that pesticide volatilization will occur regardless of whether water is volatilizing from the soil surface or not, as long as sufficient water (2.8%) is present to inhibit pesticide adsorption. According to these authors, pesticides are lost from the soils by the "wick effect" [water that is moving from the subsurface levels to the top (to replace water lost by evaporation) carries with it pesticide molecules to the surface] and not by codistillation. Pesticide volatilization rate is controlled by the diffusion of the compound and mass flow of water to the soil surface. Water loss from soils accelerates pesticide volatilization rate, but only after the soil surface had been depleted of the pesticide, indicating the operation of "wick effect". At low relative humidity of air, dieldrin accumulated at the soil surface and when the soil surface was again moistened, it evaporated rapidly.[87]

Among the different compounds studied, lindane was more volatile than dieldrin and the latter was more volatile than DDT.[80] Volatilization of dieldrin was more from moist fields rather than from those that were flooded or nonflooded. In general, compounds with a vapor pressure $> 1 \times 10^{-6}$ mmHg at 20°C are more volatile.[58] Volatilization has been reported to be a primary route of loss of HCB,[88] lindane,[89] and endrin[90] from soils. It has been suggested that part of the reason for the shorter persistence of many OP compounds in soils is their greater volatilization;[3] on the other hand, Weber[58] considered that OP compounds were not readily volatilized, despite their higher vapor pressure than that of the OC compounds, because of their greater solubility in water and relatively high adsorption by soil particulate matter. Volatilization accounted for 73.6% loss of S-ethyl *N,N′*-dipropylthiocarbamate from soils, whereas surface runoff accounted for only 7% loss.[91] On the other hand, volatilization of carbaryl from soils was not rapid.[58]

Lloyd-Jones[92] calculated the evaporation rates of DDT from aluminium planchets, sprayed with radioactive DDT. The observed evaporation rates agreed with theoretical values. The predicted evaporation losses amounted to 2 lb/acre/year in summer and 0.3 lb/acre/year in winter. Lloyd-Jones asserted that at this rate of evaporation, half of the applied DDT escapes into the atmosphere. In a subsequent study, Freed et al.,[93] on the basis of theoretical considerations and experimental observations, concluded that the loss of DDT from an inert surface like a glass or metal plate was high, while the rate of volatilization from soils was low, being 0.1 lb/acre/year, at 30°C. Further, evaporative loss is very much reduced in soils rich in organic matter. Hence, Freed et al. concluded that aerial contamination and atmospheric input of DDT by evaporation would be significant only near the sites of treatment. No satisfactory explanation could be offered for the observed world-wide distribution and occurrence of DDT. Erosion of sprayed soils by water and wind might be a more important factor in the mobility of DDT than vaporization. It was concluded that DDE, which vaporizes at least eight times faster than DDT, might be the principal means of loss of DDT from soils. Apparently, volatilization contributes to rapid dispersion of more volatile components in the environment away from the point of application while less volatile components accumulate in the soil.[94] Cliath and Spencer[95] reported that 66% of the total DDT (Σ DDT) over a field containing residual DDT was *p,p'*-DDE. This study suggested that most of the DDT present in well-aerated soils presumably volatilizes as *p,p'*-DDE. The rate of volatilization of *p,p'*-DDE is higher than that of *o,p'*-DDT which is higher than that of *p,p'*-DDT.[3] Likewise, the primary degradation product of lindane is more volatile than the parent compound.[95]

3. Pesticide Residues in the Atmosphere

Spray drift and volatilization apart, surface erosion of treated soils by wind appears to be another significant means of transport of pesticide residues to the atmosphere. The airborne residues are associated with dust or may exist mostly in the vapor phase, as indicated by recent studies. Depending on the local weather conditions and the patterns of wind movement, such residues may be carried over considerable distances or may be returned to earth through rain and snow. Dry deposition is now recognized as an important means of enrichment of residues in the aquatic environment.[96] Thus, the atmosphere can act both as a reservoir and a sink for pesticide residues. Bidleman and Olney[97] reported that toxaphene was carried through the atmosphere at least 1200 km away to the sea. Mean toxaphene levels ranged from 16 to 2520 ng/m³ which were twice those of PCB values and more than 10 times the levels of other pesticides, hitherto reported over the marine environment. Bidleman and Olney[98] observed that the major part of the collected chlorinated hydrocarbons was trapped on polyurethane foam plugs and not on glass fiber filters that were capable of removing 98% of the particles having a radius greater than 0.015 μm. Hence they concluded that most of the DDT, chlordane, and PCBs collected from the atmosphere resided mainly in the vapor phase and was not adsorbed to the particulate matter. The levels of atmospheric chlorinated hydrocarbons measured by Bidleman and Olney in this study were two orders of magnitude higher than the previously reported values. Representative levels of the compounds in Bermuda air were (all values in ng/m³): *p,p'*-DDT, 0.011 to 0.03; *o,p'*-DDT, 0.008 to 0.027; PCBs, 0.21 to 0.65; and chlordane, less than 0.005 to 0.12; comparable figures over the marine environment were 0.009 to 0.055 for *p,p'*-DDT and 0.72 to 1.6 for PCB. They also found that DDT and PCB were enriched in the surface 150 μm layer, relative to their concentration at 30 m depth. Risebrough et al.[99] reported the transport of chlorinated hydrocarbons by airborne dust from European-African land areas across the Atlantic to Barbados. But, on the basis of collected data and theoretical calculations, McClure[100] considered that PCBs introduced into the atmosphere would be confined to within 100 km of the source. Mirex has been identified in the fish of Lake Ontario[101] although it has not been used in any of the states having rivers draining into Lake Ontario. This suggests the possibility that mirex too is transported in the atmosphere. During 1971 to 1973, Σ DDT and PCB levels recorded in airborne fallout in Iceland were DDT — not detectable to 100 ng/m²/month and PCB — 45 to 1050 ng/m²/month.[102]

The annual atmospheric input of PCBs into Lake Superior has been estimated to be 3000 to 8000 kg.[96] The PCB contamination of soil at various distances from a manufacturing site suggests that aerial transport chiefly contributes to the residues found in the soil around the plant.[103] In a survey on the pesticide residues of the Mississippi atmosphere, *p,p'*-DDT, *o,p'*-DDT, toxaphene and parathion were detected.[104] The maximum values were recorded from June to September coinciding with the peak agricultural activity. Södergren[105] collected airborne fallout from different regions of Sweden, on a 30 × 30 cm nylon net impregnated with 0.9 g of SE 30 silicone oil. The average monthly values in Sweden ranged from 100 to 2075 ng/m²/month of Σ DDT and 550 to 10,510 ng/m²/month of PCB, from various collection sites from 1970 to

1971. In the atmosphere of the Gulf of Mexico in 1977, average concentration of p,p'-DDT, p,p'-DDE, and PCB recorded were 0.034, 0.049, and 0.35 ng/m^3.[106] In the same study, very high concentrations of phthalate esters 0.72 to 1.92 ng/m^3 of DEHP (di-2-ethylhexyl phthalate) and 0.16 to 3.71 ng/m^3 of DBP (di-*n*-butyl phthalate) were noticed in the atmosphere of the Gulf of Mexico. As in the study of Bidleman and Olney,[98] the OC residues were found primarily on foam plugs and not on glass fibers, indicating their existence mostly in the vapor phase.

That the residues of pesticides and industrial organic chemicals are transported in the atmosphere over long distances is now well established. Dieldrin, p,p'-DDT, and p,p'-DDE were detected in air samples collected over Bantry Bay in Southwest Ireland, a place remote from areas of use of OC compounds.[107] Similarly, the detection of low-level accumulation of DDT and its metabolites in demersal fish and benthic organisms collected from depths of 60 to 75 m in St. Margaret's Bay, Nova Scotia, Canada, an area far removed from the sites of pesticide use, indicates atmospheric transport.[108] The occurrence of a higher proportion of undegraded DDT than its metabolites in filter feeding animals, and snails that feed on epiphytic weeds, and plankton in St. Margaret's Bay, according to these authors, suggests that particulate matter is the main source of DDT. OC compounds, mainly HCH, DDT, and DDE have been detected in the West Berlin air, too.[35] Airborne permethrin and Rovral®, a fungicide, are reported from The Netherlands.[109] Long-range transport of DDT from the Pacific Northwest to Ithaca, N. Y., a distance of about 4000 km, has been reported by Peakall.[110] In general, the total DDT content of the atmosphere steadily declined, after its ban by most of the western countries.[111]

The enrichment of atmospheric residues, in recent years, especially those of industrial organic chemicals (HCB, PCBs) seems to be aided by the attempts at disposal of solid wastes by incineration. Veith and Lee[112] stated: "Stability of the more highly chlorinated mixtures to low temperature flames may result in aerial transport of the PCBs from industrial and municipal solid waste incinerators to natural waters". In a study on the optimal conditions of incineration which would ensure complete destruction of OC compounds, lindane was completely destroyed at 800°C in a transit time of 1.7 sec.[113] A temperature of 800°C and a transit time of 1.5 sec were required for the complete destruction of DDT. In about half this transit time and at the same temperature, 500 mg/kg of DDT was left uncombusted in the emission. In the pyrolytic destruction of PCBs, very high quantities of HCB were found in the emissions, higher amounts of HCB being formed at higher temperatures of combustion.[114]

4. Pesticide Residues in Rainwater and Snow

Pesticide residues in rainwater have been reported from different parts of the world. Wheatley and Hardman[115] reported the finding of γ-HCH, p,p'-DDT and dieldrin in central England. Weibel et al.[116] recorded the presence of chlordane, heptachlor epoxide, DDT, DDE, dieldrin, ronnel, and 2,4,5-T (2,4,5-trichlorophenoxy acetic acid) in the rainwater collected at Cincinnati, Ohio, in 1965. Tarrant and Tatton[117] reported the occurrence of OC residues in the rainwater collected at seven widely distributed sites in the British Isles. DDT group residues, principally p,p'-DDT, were detected in 76 out of 101 samples of rainwater collected in New Brunswick in 1967 and 1968, the levels ranging from less than 0.01 to 1.33 μg/kg. Pollen of four species of forest trees had a very high concentration of residues (0.54 to 1.0 mg/kg). Contaminated pollen was suggested to be the source of such high concentrations of DDT in rainwater. High levels of residues of α-HCH (45 to 830 ng/ℓ) and γ-HCH (29 to 398 ng/ℓ), were reported in the rainwater collected in Tokyo in 1968 and 1969.[119] OC residues were reported in the rainwater from Hawaii,[34,120] Scotland,[33] and Kiel Bight, West Germany.[121] Wells and Johnstone[122] used polyurethane foam coated with about 30 mg of

DC 200 silicone grease to collect residues from rainwater and calculated the annual OC residue input from the British mainland into the North Sea. From 1975 to 1976, the levels (ng/m²/100 days) of OC compounds found in the precipitation at various sites in UK were p,p'-DDT, 20 to 2100; o,p'-DDT, not detectable to 293; p,p'-DDE, 9 to 625; dieldrin, not detectable to 455; α-HCH, 29 to 1247; γ-HCH, 94 to 1539; and PCBs, 178 to 6010. These residue concentrations in 1975 to 1976 were one order of magnitude less than those reported earlier by Tarrant and Tatton[117] from 1966 to 1967. Following a special authorization by the Environmental Protection Agency in the summer of 1974, to spray DDT to control the Douglas fir Tussock moth over 426,560 acres in the Pacific Northwest, DDT was detected in the rain and snow samples collected 4000 km to the east, in Ithaca, N.Y.[110] Although there was no definite proof that the spray program in the Pacific Northwest was the source of DDT detected in Ithaca, the occurrence of DDT residues in the precipitation from August to November, but not in winter suggests that Tussock moth program was the source of these DDT residues.[110] Tanabe et al.[123] detected PCBs, DDT, and HCH isomers in Antarctic ice, snow, air, and lake water samples. Likewise, in 1978, α-HCH, γ-HCH, and low levels of aldrin and dieldrin were recorded in 31 snow samples collected in the Bavarian Alps.[124] From January to February 1983, I recorded high concentrations of γ-HCH and PCBs and traces of DDT and DDE, in snow samples collected in West Berlin.[125]

III. TRANSPORT OF PESTICIDE RESIDUES TO THE AQUATIC ENVIRONMENT

Pesticides that are transported to the aquatic environment are primarily of agricultural origin; they may also arise as effluents from manufacturing and formulating plants. The atmospheric transport of residues to the aquatic ecosystem has already been dealt with. Two sources of contamination of the aquatic ecosystem are recognized: point and nonpoint. The former refers to a single source of contamination like effluents from a pesticide-manufacturing or -formulating plant; the latter refers to contamination of widespread and diffuse nature as in the case of agricultural runoff. Significant quantities of pesticides are transported by sediment which constitutes an important nonpoint source.

A. Nonpoint Sources
1. Agricultural Lands
Cropland clearly is a major source of sediment and the sediment resulting from soil erosion is regarded as the largest pollutant that affects water quality.[126] Annually, 3.1 billion m³ of sediment reach the waterways in the U.S.[127] The load of suspended solids in runoff from urban areas and intensely cultivated agricultural lands is 10 to 100 times that of forested or uncultivated land. More than land use, land form characteristics like soil texture, soil type (mineral or organic), surface geology, slope and drainage density and also soil chemistry influence the degree of nonpoint source of pollution.[128] Overland runoff from finegrained clay soils is much more than that from coarse sandy soils. Clay particles are easily suspended and settle slowly. Pesticide molecules, adsorbed to clay particles, are transported to considerable distances. When land is exposed to erosive forces like rain and surface runoff, the hazard of aquatic pollution is greater. It must also be stressed that the lands that are eroded to the maximum extent (croplands, grasslands, and harvested forest as against undisturbed forests and uncultivated land) receive the highest application of pesticides. Agricultural practices like tilling also contribute significantly to the erosion of soils and hence to the transportation of pesticides to the aquatic environment.

Waterbodies closer to agricultural lands understandably have higher residue levels.

Often the period of maximum transportation of the residues to the aquatic environment coincides with the peak period of agricultural activity. In a study on the entry of residues into Lake Utah during 1970, definite surges of pesticides entering the lake at different times were recorded: aldrin and HCH from March to April; heptachlor, heptachlor epoxide, and methoxychlor from May to June; and aldrin, heptachlor, heptachlor epoxide, and methoxychlor from October to November.[129] These surges corresponded to the times of application of the respective pesticides in the Utah county. Sometimes loss of residues from arable lands may not be confined to the season of application alone. For instance, loss of sediment and its transport to the aquatic environment from 11 agricultural watersheds of southwestern Ontario reached the maximum in the January to April period, corresponding to the spring thaw and erosion.[130]

In an effort to evaluate the effect of nonpoint sources of water pollution, surface runoff from orchard soils and water of the receiving streams were analyzed. The results indicated the presence of conditions of severe stress downstream to orchards. Several species of invertebrates were highly susceptible to runoff from orchard soils. In Clear Creek-Cox Creek, that had a history of fish kills, mass mortality of fish occurred one day after spraying the orchard farms in their drainage basin with pesticides. In 1977, endrin was implicated in the fish kills.[131] Streams that drain orchard soils and residential areas are known occasionally to contain residue concentrations that might be toxic to fish.[132] For example, although the maximum concentration of pesticides was never found for more than $1/2$ hr, no macroinvertebrates or fish were found[57] in Latimore Creek, Pa. The very high concentrations of DDT residues usually recorded in orchard soils (see Section II.A), however, were not reflected in similar high concentrations in the streambed sediments or runoff. This suggests that DDT is fixed in the soil and is not easily leached.[57] Similarly, carbaryl is very soluble in water; but very little of it (5.77 g out of 4 kg applied) was lost through runoff. Of the small quantity that was lost with runoff, 75% was associated with runoff water and the rest with particulate matter. The concentration of carbaryl in water, 17 and 19 days after application was 248 and 160 $\mu g/\ell$, respectively, and came down to 8.4 and 3.7 $\mu g/\ell$, 29 and 37 days after spraying. The amount of carbaryl adsorbed to soil particles was 1.22 $\mu g/kg$ after 19 days and 0.08 $\mu g/kg$, 29 days after application.[133]

a. Mobility of Pesticide Residues in the Soil

Transport of pesticides to the aquatic environment is chiefly effected by volatilization, leaching, and surface erosion. The first of these has been considered already; leaching is governed by the solubility of the compound and, to a certain extent, by its adsorption to the soil particles. Surface erosion by wind and water carries the residues in the gaseous phase, solution, or as soil-pesticide complex. Compounds with a water solubility of 10 mg/ℓ or more are transported in solution in the runoff water, whereas those that are less soluble are mostly transported by adsorption to the particulate matter.[26] The greater the water solubility, the greater the mobility (Figure 1). For instance, lindane, which has a high solubility, is more mobile than many other OC compounds. Under identical soil water conditions, the soil adsorption coefficient of DDE is 20 times that of lindane, as the former is at least 1000 times less soluble than the latter.[134] Endrin, aldrin, and dieldrin are slightly more mobile than DDT as they are more soluble than DDT.[58] OP compounds, with higher solubilities and higher vapor pressure than the OC compounds, are also highly adsorbed to the soil particulate matter, and hence are not any more mobile than the OC compounds. Similarly, among the herbicides, substituted anilines are immobile. Of the phenyl ureas, compounds with smaller molecules are, as a rule, more soluble than those with larger molecules and hence more mobile.[58] Helling et al.,[135] in a study on the relative movement of 82 pesticides, reported that acidic compounds were highly mobile, phenyl ureas and triazines were less mobile, and OCs and large cations were the least mobile.

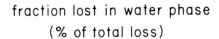

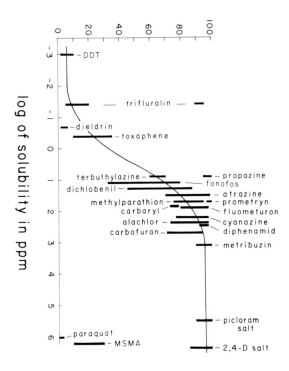

FIGURE 1. Partitioning of pesticides between water and sediment in runoff samples. (From Wauchope, R. O., *J. Environ. Qual.*, 7, 459, 1978. With permission.)

b. Adsorption

Adsorption to the soil particles is another important factor that determines the degree of mobility of a compound. Soil moisture and organic matter content decide the extent of adsorption.[136] Under conditions of high humidity and high water content, adsorption of pesticides to soil is low, because water molecules displace the pesticide molecules from adsorption sites. When water was added to soils containing adsorbed aldrin, dieldrin, or endrin, the compound was released.[58] The adsorption of pesticide molecules by organic peaty muck soils is reversed by increasing temperatures.[26] Adsorption to the soil is also inversely proportional to the soil grain size.[137]

Using the soil sorption coefficient (calculated on the basis of soil organic carbon content and octanol-water partition coefficient, K_{oc}), Kenaga[138] discussed the mobility of pesticides in soils, with water. He found good agreement between the experimentally obtained K_{oc} values and those calculated from water solubility. Compounds with a K_{oc} higher than 1000 are tightly bound to the soil and consequently immobile, compounds with a K_{oc} value of 100 or less are moderately-to-highly mobile. The former are likely to enter the aquatic environment mostly sorbed to the soil particles and the latter, with water in solution. Steep slope of the land will increase the runoff and aid the mobility of the pesticide both ways, i.e., in solution and via adsorption to soil particles. The predictions of Kenaga have been confirmed by many studies. Sharom et al.[139] studied the behavior of 12 insecticides (4 OCs, 6 OP compounds, and 2 carbamates) in soil and aqueous suspensions of soil and sediment. In general, insecticide adsorption to the soil or sediment was inversely related to the water solubility of that compound. DDT and leptophos, with very low solubility, were more strongly adsorbed than was dieldrin. Dieldrin, endrin, ethion, chlorpyrifos, lindane, parathion, diazinon, carbaryl, carbofuran, and mevinphos in that order were decreasingly adsorbed by the soils. In an experiment to determine the extent of desorption of these insecticides from the adsorbed state in the soil, Sharom et al. observed that the amount of a chemical desorbed was proportional to its water solubility. Little of the least soluble leptophos or DDT was desorbed from soil even with four water rinses (for each rinse 200 mℓ of distilled water was added to 1 or 5 g of mineral soil containing 2 mg/ℓ of each insecticide and the bottles were tumbled for 4 hr, centrifuged at 16,300 g for 1 hr and the supernatant was analyzed for its pesticide content). Carbofuran and mevinphos were almost completely removed by the very first rinse. Results of this study are shown in Figure 2. Sharom et al. also studied the extent of leaching and mobility of these compounds with water flow. They observed that the more strongly an insecticide was adsorbed to the soil, the less mobile it was. Leptophos and DDT which were strongly adsorbed to the soil were not leached by any of the 10 fractions of water (200 mℓ each) allowed to flow through the insecticide-adsorbed soil. Mevinphos which was miscible with water, in contrast, was almost totally leached from the treated soil by the first 200 mℓ flow. Sharom et al. also observed that adsorption, desorption and mobility were influenced by the soil properties. Organic soils, sediment, sandy loam, and sand — in that order — adsorbed decreasing quantities of insecticides. Adsorption correlated significantly (r^2 = >0.95) with the soil organic matter content. Sand, sandy loam, and sediment desorbed decreasing quantities of any compound. Similarly, the amount of the insecticide leached was inversely related to the organic matter content; of the total carbaryl present in the organic soil, 53% was leached by 10 fractions of distilled water, whereas 52% of the total carbaryl was leached from the sandy soil by the first fraction alone. The relationship between the water solubility and leachability of the 12 insecticides in organic and sandy soils is shown in Table 1.

c. *Runoff Losses*

Runoff, besides volatilization, constitutes the main pathway of transport of pesticides from arable soils. When a compound is strongly adsorbed to the soil particles, losses in runoff water, in solution, will be minimal, while loss will be maximum with eroded soil particles.[140] Dieldrin was mostly lost through erosion and carried by sediments. Transport of dieldrin in solution was negligible, the maximum amount in runoff water being 0.07% of the initial quantity applied. The dieldrin concentration in runoff water never exceeded 20 μg/ℓ, whereas loss through sediment was as high as 22% of the original application.[141] It has also been reported that less than 0.2% of the total endrin applied to a sugarcane plot was lost in solution in runoff.[142] On the other hand Ritter et al.[143] opined that although pesticide concentrations at any time may be higher in the sediment fraction, greater loss from soils is associated with the water because of the larger volumes involved. They found that the concentration of atrazine lost from agricultural soils was high with the sediment fraction and low with the water fraction of the runoff. More atrazine, however, was transported in solution than was adsorbed to sediment, owing to the greater quantities of the water that moves from and over the arable lands.

It is now well established that in the event of storms following application, runoff losses will be maximum soon after application for less persistent compounds, whereas for persistent compounds, significant runoff losses occur for several months after application.[26] The amount of atrazine that was transported from cultivated lands was directly proportional to the rainfall,[144] atrazine content in runoff being highest during the early stage of runoff. Also, the intensity of rainfall and the time that has lapsed since the application of a pesticide influence the extent of loss through runoff.

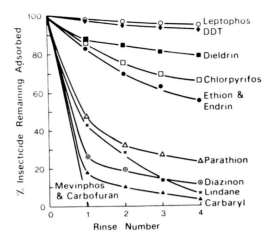

FIGURE 2. Desorption of 12 insecticides from Beverly sandy loam with four rinses of distilled water. (From Sharom, M. S., Miles, R. W., Harris, C. R., and McEwen, F. L., *Water Res.*, 14, 1095, 1980. With permission. Copyright 1980, Pergamon Press, Ltd.)

Table 1
WATER SOLUBILITY OF 12 INSECTICIDES
AND THEIR LEACHABILITY FROM ORGANIC
AND SANDY SOILS BY 10 SUCCESSIVE
FRACTIONS OF 200 mℓ DISTILLED WATER

Insecticide	Solubility	Insecticide leached by 10 fractions of water %	
		Organic soil	Sand
Mevinphos	Miscible with water	90.8	99.4
Carbofuran	320[a]	99.1	98.9
Carbaryl	40[a]	53	86.3
Diazinon	40[a]	49.9	94.6
Lindane	10[a]	34.2	92.6
Parathion	12.4[a]	23.2	63.4
Chlorpyrifos	700[b]	1.6	16.9
Ethion	600[b]	1.2	13.9
Endrin	230[b]	1.5	13.6
Dieldrin	186[b]	0.8	10.2
Leptophos	70[b]	0	0
p,p′-DDT	1.2[b]	0	0

[a] Solubility in ppm.
[b] Solubility in ppb.

Data from Sharom, M. S., Miles, J. R. W., Harris, C. R., and McEwen, F. L., *Water Res.*, 14, 1095, 1980.

The normal concentration of herbicides in runoff water in the U.S. is estimated as 1 μg/ℓ.[145] Benthiocarb, following application to rice paddies, was detected in river water, probably due to flooding and over-flowing of the rice paddies.[146] Likewise, CNP, a herbicide applied to paddy fields in Japan, was found in surface waters from June to September, indicating runoff from the treated rice paddies.[147]

Excellent reviews on the interaction of pesticides with soil-water systems can be found in Bailey and White,[136] Weber,[58] Pionke and Chesters,[148] Wauchope,[149] and Schmitt and Winger.[26]

2. Urbanland Source

Urban areas, which have construction sites with exposed soil contribute the highest amounts of nonpoint pollution loads.

Transportation corridors in urban areas are sources of high amounts of pesticide residues. Also, soil impermeability results in more runoff and hence greater pollutant levels in the hydrosphere. Contrary to widely held belief, concentration of pollutants in urban drainage does not vary much with flow. That diffuse sources like house building and urbanization lead to the contamination of the aquatic environment with anthropogenic chemicals is best illustrated by the condition in Lake Anne, a man-made recreational lake in Reston, Va. Although this lake received no industrial wastes or sewage discharges, PCB concentrations of 0.1 to 0.2 $\mu g/\ell$ in unfiltered water and less than 2.5 to 105 $\mu g/\ell$ in the sediments were recorded in this lake.[150]

3. Sewage

Urban sewage is yet another nonpoint source of pesticide residues to the aquatic environment. OC residues, particularly HCH, of domestic origin were present in the sewage effluents entering the rivers that discharged into Lough Neagh in the U.K.[151] The HCH residues of river water in the U.K. showed a high correlation with the urban population.[151] In a survey of sewage of three cities in the U.S., hexachlorophene (HCP) and PCP were present in the sewage and water samples. Sewage treatment removed only 60 to 70% of HCP and 4 to 28% of PCP in the three cities. In the Willamette River near Corvallis, Ore., 0.01 to 0.1 $\mu g/\ell$ HCP and 0.1 to 0.7 $\mu g/\ell$ PCP were recorded. Conventional processing of the river waters for purposes of supplying water to cities removed only 60% of the contaminants leaving the rest in the drinking water supplies.[152] It has been claimed that between 1950 and 1970, about 1.9 million kg of commercial DDT had passed through the sewers of Los Angeles into the offshore region of California,[153] though the validity of this claim has been questioned by Jukes.[154] Residues of dieldrin (0.03 to 0.44 mg/kg) and PCBs (less than 0.01 to 11.6 mg/kg) have been reported from the sewage in 16 cities in the U.S.[155] Fish exposed for 9 months to the treated effluents from the cities of Grandville and Wyoming in Michigan accumulated considerable quantities of tetra- and pentachlorophenols, PCBs, DDT, toxaphene, chlordane, and nonachlor.[156] In Britain, sewage sludge, containing less than 0.1 to 14 mg/kg PCBs, has been reported to be a major source of PCB in the aquatic environment.[157] Holden and Marsden[158] reported dieldrin (100×10^{-6} to $10,000 \times 10^{-6}$ mg/ℓ dieldrin) and DDT (100×10^{-6} to 500×10^{-6} mg/ℓ DDT) in the domestic sewage effluents in the U.K. Municipal sewage is thought to have contributed significantly to the huge amounts of PCBs (estimated at 76,000 kg) presently associated with the sediments of tidal Hudson.[159]

4. Used Pesticide Containers

Careless handling of the spraying equipment and used containers is another important means of transfer of pesticide residues to the aquatic ecosystem, as in the case of the washing and cleaning of spraying equipment in the rivers, reported from Iran.[160] In 1969, about 3.87 million pesticide containers were reported to have been used in California alone.[161] In the U.S. about 240 million containers of all types were used in 1968.[162] When the total number of containers used all over the world is considered, one can assess the total quantity of residues left in the environment after the completion of the spraying operations. In an experimental study to determine the quantity of parathion that adheres or gets adsorbed to the container walls, different types of containers (125 mℓ glass bottles, 1 gal glass bottles, and 1, 5, and 55 gal metal cans) were filled with a parathion EC formulation (4.76% active ingredient [a.i.]), in volumes normally used to fill the containers. The containers were closed, shaken, and swirled to wet the walls thoroughly and then inverted, opened, and allowed to drain until dripping stopped. The parathion residue remaining adsorbed to the walls, when quantified, ranged from 150 to 45,000 mg. The quantities of the formulation that remained inside the container depended largely on the shape of the container as well as the location of the spout. In general, metal drums retained greater quantities than glass containers.[161] The formulations could be effectively removed from the containers by repeated washings with small volume of water or alkaline detergent solution. In another study,[163] even after complete draining of the formulation-containing metal drums, approximately 0.12%, and 0.05 to 0.07% of the initial volume was retained, respectively, in the case of 5, and 30 or 55 gal metal drums. Eight washings with water followed by three washings with ethanol and acid or ethanol alone removed 95 to 99% of the retained formulations. In order to avoid contamination of the environment, these authors recommended disposal of the rinsings as in the case of the spray mixture. Lamberton et al.[164] estimated that an empty 55 gal drum can retain as much as 5 ℓ of the pesticide formulation. A few hundred such empty containers can add an amount of pesticide to the environment equivalent to a small spill or a minor accident, with its associated hazards. Lamberton et al. caution against the use of the larger drums for any other purpose, even after rinsing them several times with an appropriate detergent solution, as considerable quantities of pesticide residues can remain even after three washes.

B. Point Sources
1. Sheep Dips
Sheep dips have been listed as a source of pesticide residues to the aquatic environment. In the U.K., contaminations arising from sheep dips eventually reached a feeder station of the Chew Valley Lake, where the residues killed or caused reproductive failure of *Daphnia, Bosmina,* and some chironomids. Following the reduction in the number of crustaceans in the lake, algal blooms that made the lake waters unpotable, ensued.[165]

2. Effluents from Pesticide Formulating Plants
Among the point sources of pesticide residues in the aquatic environment, it has been estimated that the effluents of pesticide manufacturing plants contain a few to 100 lb/day.[166] In Lake Ørsjøen, Norway, at a point near a plant nursery school, the Σ DDT in the sediments was 25 mg/kg, the concentration attenuating as one moved from the source, until 5 km away, the concentration was 0.1 mg/kg in the sediments. Similarly, fish collected near the point of entry of the effluent from the plant nursery had a concentration of 14 mg/kg Σ DDT; fish collected 5 km away from the source had 0.16 mg/kg Σ DDT.[167] In water and hydrosoil samples collected from Ashley and Charleston Harbor in South Carolina, residues of *S,S,S*-tributyl phosphorotrithioite and *S,S,S*-tributyl phosphorotrithioate, an oxidation product of the former, were detected. The former was produced by a pesticide manufacturer and the untreated effluent was discharged into the Ashley River.[168] In the vicinity of a chlordecone manufacturing plant at Hopewell, Va. residue levels up to 60 mg/kg were observed following environmental contamination.[169]

3. Accidental Spillages
Accidents constitute another important point source of pesticide residues and contribute significantly to the residue load in the aquatic environment. After accidental

spillage of endosulfan, residue concentration of 0.7 $\mu g/\ell$ and fishkills were recorded in the Rhine River.[170] In Lake Tanganyika, in 1972, a boat accident resulted in the spillage of 6510 ℓ of pesticide solutions. Adult *Tilapia,* collected after the accident, had (values in mg/kg): 1.57, DDE; 7.54, DDD; 1.97, *o,p'*-DDT; 17.83, *p,p'*-DDT; 0.11, dieldrin; 0.18, lindane, and 3.55, endrin.[171] Nicholson[17] described how the breakdown of the waste treatment facility of a pesticide manufacturing plant in Alabama resulted in the discharge of parathion and methyl parathion into sewage. Approximately 60% of the combined untreated sewage with residues was diverted into a small stream, killing fish, turtles, and snakes in a stretch of 45 km downstream. Fishkills occurred even 144 km downstream to a lesser extent. In the effluent of a nematicide and defoliant manufacturer, levels of 6.5 and 300 mg/kg of the nematicide in water and sediment, and 1.5 mg/ℓ and 5000 mg/kg of the defoliant in water and sediment were recorded.[17] Extensive fishkills were reported in a Mississippi man-made lake when PCP-containing waters overflowed the wastewater holding pond of a plant that was treating poles with PCP.[172] Fishkills caused by accidental spillage of trifluralin have been reported in the Eden water, U.K.[173] Following the filling of the Teton dam in southwest Idaho (on the Teton River which is a tributary of the Upper Snake River), the dam broke on June 5, 1976 and released 29.6 billion m^3 of water.[174] The gushing waters swept clean at least three commercial units supplying pesticides to the farmers, as well as countless small pesticide containers. While it was impossible to assess the total quantity of pesticides washed away, a minimum 2000 lb of granular Disyston®, 200 gal of liquid Furadan®, and unknown quantities of DDT, Guthion®, 2,4-D (2,4-dichlorophenoxyacetic acid), Thimet®, Systox®, malathion, and PCBs were lost. Analysis of rainbow trout sampled in September and October 1976 from stations along the river showed (all values in $\mu g/kg$ and calculated on wet weight basis): 1432, Σ DDT, 66, dieldrin, and 1010, PCBs; Utah suckers had up to 1420, Σ DDT, 32, dieldrin, and 1800, PCBs; Rocky mountain whitefish had 2650, Σ DDT, 30, dieldrin, and 1400, PCBs.

C. Identification of the Source and Other Considerations

It is possible, though not always, to identify and distinguish the point and nonpoint source of contamination. *o,p'*-DDT which constitutes 20% of the technical DDT, is seldom recorded in natural samples and is presumably rapidly degraded. The presence of *o,p'*-DDT in environmental samples, especially water and sediment, is considered to indicate specific point source of contamination.[175] On the other hand, the presence of mirex residues in the environmental samples indicates nonpoint source of contamination.[176] In the marine environment, the ratio of PCB to the other OC residue concentration is useful in identifying the source of contamination. If this ratio is higher than 1, the source is more likely industrial than agricultural.[177]

When persistent and environmentally hazardous compounds have been replaced by less problematic compounds, even the latter started to appear in the environmental samples within a short time. This is best illustrated by Eulan WA Neu, a dieldrin replacement compound. In Sweden the use of dieldrin was banned in 1970 and Eulan WA Neu (a.i. — polychlorinated 2-aminodiphenyl ethers) was used for moth-proofing purpose. Within a year after the commencement of its use, Eulan WA Neu was recorded in fish samples.[178]

The aquatic environment is the ultimate sink for all anthropogenic chemicals and global pollutants. Any compound that has been used in large quantities ultimately reaches the aquatic ecosystem.[18] Generally, the residues are transported from the terrestrial environment to the aquatic environment; but the reverse can also take place. Menzie[179] considered that terrestrial insects with aquatic larval stages (dragonflies, may flies, and the like) may be a means of such a transfer. Larval insects, living in or on the sediments, bioconcentrate pesticide residues in their tissues and, at the time of their emergence as adults, transport the residues from the aquatic ecosystem to the terrestrial ecosystem. It was estimated that insects with a high level of production, i.e., 100 g/m²/year take only 1.2 years to transport 50% of the contaminants having a biconcentration potential of $\geq$ 10,000 and contained in a 30 cm-thick sediment layer. Insects with a moderate level of production (15 g/m²/year) require 8 to 80 years for a similar transport of compounds with a bioconcentration potential of 1000 to 10,000.

IV. PESTICIDE RESIDUES IN THE AQUATIC ENVIRONMENT

The residues that reach the hydrosphere are concentrated in certain parts of the aquatic ecosystem or remain in solution for extended periods, or are adsorbed to the particulate matter, and thereby deposited in the sediments. The last process may immobilize the residues permanently in the sediments, or it may be only a means of temporary removal of the residues from circulation until the particulate matter is resuspended or the pesticide molecules are desorbed from the sediment and once again are made available in the water column. Simultaneously, the residues are absorbed by the aquatic organisms, bioaccumulated in the trophic chain and deposited in the sediments along with the carcass. A detailed discussion of the factors that influence the level of pesticide residues in the aquatic environment follows.

A. Residue Levels in the Aquatic Environment
1. Concentration of Residues in the Surface Microlayers
The top few micrometers layer of the water column in any natural body of water constitutes a separate entity by itself, being characterized by its richness in hydrophobic organic substances. Ever since Seba and Corcoran[180] showed that surface slicks act as concentrators of pesticides in the marine environment, several authors have reported the occurrence of high concentrations of pesticide residues in the surface microlayers that act as a repository and a sink for anthropogenic chemicals. In the surface slicks collected off the Florida coast, Seba and Corcoran reported (all values in µg/ℓ): 0.049 to 3460, DDT; 0.061 to 9250, p,p'-DDE; 0.002 to 0.035, dieldrin; 0.002 to 0.081, o,p'-DDT, and 0.005 to 0.034, aldrin (PCBs were not differentiated from other OC compounds in this study). Enrichment of pesticides and organic pollutants in the top 100 to 150 µm layer of the sea in Narragansett Bay, in the U.S., was reported by Duce et al.[181] If the surface film is estimated as five molecular layers thick (10^{-2} µm) and all the chemical constitutents were in this layer, the actual concentration in this film, relative to the subsurface water, would be 1.5×10^4 times. Wind-generated lake foam and surface layers have been reported to be rich in fatty acids, esters, and alcohols, which are excellent concentrators of PCBs and other chlorinated hydrocarbons.[182] In Lake Mendota, Wis., the concentrations of the various pollutants observed in the foam were (all values in ng/ℓ): dieldrin, 44; p,p'-DDE, 175; p,p'-DDD, 204; and p,p'-DDT, 175, whereas in the lake water, the concentration of all these compounds was less than 1 ng/ℓ.[182] The foam acts as a scavenger and a trap for the organic pollutants. Following aerial spraying of fenitrothion in the surrounding area, 701 µg/ℓ of fenitrothion was recorded in a surface slick formed by wind action, as against 9.5 µg/ℓ in the subsurface water.[183] Södergren[184] reported that hydrophobic compounds were enriched a thousand to several hundred thousand times in the surface microlayer, relative to the subsurface water. A part of the hydrophobic compounds was transported to the atmosphere through the jet drops produced by the gas bubbles bursting at the surface. It is no surprise that the surface microlayers act as concentrators of the xenobiotic chemicals when one considers the report that lipid monolayers are much more efficient concentrators of hydrophobic compounds than pure solutions of lipids. For instance, the log of partition coefficient (log K_{ow}) of lindane between octanol and water (at different

concentrations of lindane) is 3.2 to 3.6; if octanol is in the form of a lens floating on water, log K_{ow} is 3.9 to 4.7, whereas between a monolayer of octanol and underlying water, the log K_{ow} is 4.5 to 5.[185] Similarly, the log molar partition coefficient of DDT and HCB between octanol and water are 5.1 ± 0.2 and 5.2 ± 0.2, respectively. If the alcohol is in the form of a thin surface layer, the log partition coefficient is 6 for DDT and 7 for HCB.[186] These two studies explain why surface films and slicks are rich in DDT-type compounds.

The air-water interface supports a separate community of organisms called neuston. These organisms, which alight on or live under the surface film, feed at the air-water interface and seasonally contribute significantly to the productivity of many freshwater bodies. The neustonic organisms actively feed on bacteria, protozoa, and small invertebrates at the air-water interface, and in turn, form an important source of food to many other organisms, both in aquatic and terrestrial ecosystems. Since aquatic organisms bioconcentrate lipophilic compounds several hundred to several hundred thousand times and the surface microlayers are rich in hydrophobic pollutants, it would be interesting to know the extent of bioconcentration of DDT-type compounds by the neuston. Hitherto, there have been few investigations into the role played by neuston in sequestering pesticide residues in the aquatic ecosystem.

2. Pesticide Residue Levels in Water

The level of pesticide residues in the open waters depends on many factors: the nature of the drainage basin, extent of flow, load of particulate matter, level of productivity, and depth of the water body. The size and nature of the water body and the extent of possible dilution, influence the level of accumulation of residues by organisms. The residue levels in organisms of various systems follow the order: closed ponds > free-flowing creeks > lakes > more contiguous bay-estuaries.[187] Streams that drain residential areas or orchards contain higher levels of residues than those that drain forest and farmlands.[57] Residues in lakes of residential areas in Ontario are reported to be higher than those in larger lakes like Lake Ontario and Lake Erie. According to Harris and Miles,[3] DDT is used more on agricultural lands and its application generally results in the incorporation of the residue in the soil; but spray application of pesticides in the recreational areas, either on or near water (for controlling nuisance insects like biting fly), results in a more rapid transfer of residues direct to the aquatic ecosystem. Likewise, urban waste water, even from small settlements, contributed significant amounts of OC contaminants to the Adriatic coastal waters.[177] Although residue input into the aquatic environment from farmlands is higher than that from noncultivated and forest lands, the extent of such an input from the cultivated lands is proportional to the extent of farming. For instance, in limited farming, lesser loads reached the aquatic environment.[129] Prior to the restriction or ban on the use of many OC pesticides, residues of the more commonly used compounds were detected even in drinking water supplies,[17,120,188] reflecting the higher levels usually present in natural freshwater bodies. It was not unusual to find more than 1 $\mu g/\ell$ of DDT and up to 0.5 $\mu g/\ell$ of dieldrin and γ-HCH.[24] Although the monitoring of OP residues in water is rare, according to Dupuy and Schulze,[189] OP insecticide residues are not uncommon in coastal waters. Miles and Harris[190] recorded high levels of OP residues in the water of Holland Marsh in southern Ontario. In the water in drainage ditches, diazinon concentration was 1 to 2 $\mu g/\ell$. Quoting earlier studies, Coppage et al.[191] emphasized that high malathion values (as high as 500 $\mu g/\ell$) were found in the waters in Texas. High levels of OP residues have been found in British waters as well.[192] Likewise, herbicide residues, although not reported as often as OCs, seem to be common in natural waters. In a study on the herbicide concentration in 11 agricultural watersheds in southern Ontario, Frank and Sirons[193] recorded 0.1 to 10 $\mu g/\ell$ of 2,4-D in 66 out of 949 water samples.

Although herbicide toxicity to fish is low, effective control of weeds can be achieved only at a concentration of the herbicide in water that exceeds, at least temporarily, the 96-h LC 50 value for many common species of fish.[194] For example, a concentration of 0.5 mg/ℓ of Hydrothal-191 (a salt of endothall) effects less than 10% control of the aquatic weed, *Hydrilla,* while the 96-h LC 50 of this compound, in hard water, to the golden shiners is 0.32 mg/ℓ. Although the general level of the herbicide concentration in natural waters in the U.S. is around 1 μg/ℓ,[145] higher initial residue concentrations are common in instances of direct application for the control of aquatic weeds.

Pesticide residues have been reported from many rivers around the world; α-HCH, γ-HCH, and PCB were present in all the samples of Rhine water analyzed; heptachlor, heptachlor epoxide, aldrin, dieldrin, endrin, and DDT were encountered occasionally in the Rhine.[195] PCBs in the range of 0.3 to 1.2 μg/ℓ were recorded from Göta river water in Sweden.[196] In Israel, α- and γ-HCH were the most common OC residues in natural waters.[197] Four years after the ban of its use, γ-HCH levels in river waters in Japan ranged from 46 to 307 μg/ℓ.[198] Herzel[199] reported less than 10 to 6350 μg/ℓ of endosulfan from 81 locations in Germany. High HCB levels, up to 2 μg/ℓ, were recorded from the Mississippi River.[200] In one instance, with a known source of contamination, HCB levels as high as 90 μg/ℓ were recorded. The OC residue levels recorded in the Danube River were (all values in ng/ℓ): 69, γ-HCH; 22, *p,p'*-DDE; and 42, *p,p'*-DDT.[201]

In a survey of 11 watersheds in southwestern Ontario,[202] DDT group compounds were present in 93% of the 949 stream water samples analyzed. DDE was the predominant component of DDT. The parent compound was frequently found in high concentration during high flow conditions and was almost absent in months of low stream flow. High flow rates, higher loads of suspended solids, and higher delivery of DDT to the stream were well correlated. Thus, with a 57 to 66% of the total annual water flow and 66 to 73% of the total suspended particle load from January to April, 58 to 84% of the annually transported DDT was carried in this period. No decline in the quantity of the Σ DDT transported from 1975 to 1977 was observed, in comparison with 1971, the year when DDT was deregistered in Canada. While soils were the main source of DDT and dieldrin, atmospheric precipitation appeared to be the main source of PCBs to these streams. Kellogg and Bulkely[203] studied the seasonal variation in the concentration of dieldrin in the Des Moines River, in Iowa, during 1971 to 1973. Dieldrin content of the water was low in early spring, increased rapidly thereafter and decreased in late summer, the average concentration ranging from 10 to 50 ng/ℓ in 1971, 10 to 40 ng/ℓ in 1972, and 1 to 31 ng/ℓ in 1973. Highest concentrations in any year were recorded in June and July. About two thirds of the dieldrin was carried in solution and the rest via adsorption to suspended particulate matter. The seasonal trends of accumulation of dieldrin by the biota corresponded to that in water.

The imposition of restrictions on the use of many OC compounds in the industrialized nations led to a definite decline in the OC residues in natural water as with soil residues in these countries. The picture in the developing countries, however, is unclear. Judging by the present trend of increased use of persistent pesticides in these countries, one would expect an increase in the overall levels of OC residues in the aquatic environment, despite the fact that degradation of pesticides in soils of these countries is supposed to be higher, owing to the higher temperatures in tropical and subtropical climates. This is an area of research that demands urgent attention in the less developed countries.

3. Residue Levels in the Sediments

The residues that enter the hydrosphere are partly lost to the atmosphere because of volatilization, partly degraded, partly incorporated in the biota, and partly moved into the sediments. They also remain in dynamic equilibrium either in solution or adsorbed to the particulate matter for subsequent incorporation into the sediments. Deep ocean sediments are supposed to be the ultimate sink for environmental pollutants.[204] But as pointed out by Halter and Johnson,[205] incorporation into sediments is only a first step before many complex processes of redistribution that recycle the materials back into water take place. Recycling of materials is normally desirable, but in the case of pollutants such a redistribution will prolong the availability of the toxicants for absorption by the aquatic organisms. Commenting on the report that benthic invertebrates can effectively concentrate OC compounds in their bodies, Zitko[206] stated "sediments may be reservoirs rather than ultimate sinks and may slowly release absorbed chemicals, thus maintaining the contamination of aquatic biota for prolonged periods of time . . . " In shallow water bodies, higher residue concentration has been reported on windy days, perhaps as a result of mixing.[207]

The behavior and persistence of DDT and PCBs in bottom sediments have been studied extensively. As with the transport of pesticide residues to the aquatic ecosystem, lowest concentrations of Σ DDT in streambeds were observed in those streams draining forest and farming lands, whereas highest concentrations were encountered in streams draining residential areas and orchard lands.[57]

DDT and its metabolites accumulate in the organic detritus at the bottom of lakes, estuaries, and coastal waters where they not only persist for many years, but also can form a potential source for their redistribution in the aquatic ecosystem, as a variety of organisms including fish use the detritus as a source of food. For instance, in 11 days, fiddler crabs, exposed to 10 mg/kg DDT in detritus, not only accumulated considerable amounts of DDT in their tissues, but showed altered behavior and impaired coordination of movement.[208]

The degradation of pesticides in the sediments is both aerobic and anaerobic. A major part of the DDT that enters the sediment is converted aerobically into DDE or anaerobically into DDD. Frank et al.[209] reported that of the Σ DDT recorded in the sediments of Lake St. Clair, Ontario, DDD constituted 54.5 and 62.5%, p,p'-DDE constituted 30.3 and 29.2%, and p,p'-DDT constituted 13.6 and 8.3%, respectively, in 1970 and 1974.[209] They reported a 64% decline in the total DDT concentration in the sediments of the lake betwen 1970 and 1974. The slight increase in the p,p'-DDD component of total DDT residues in 1974 indicates possible *in situ* degradation. In the surface sediments, representing newly laid material, the concentration of DDD was 53 μg/kg and that of DDE was 19 μg/kg. No parent material was encountered in the deeper, core samples.

In the sediments of Lake Michigan, Choi and Chen[210] reported that p,p'-DDE constituted 61 to 71%, and p,p'-DDD formed only 10 to 16.6% of the total DDT, contrary to the findings of Frank et al.[209] in Lake St. Clair. Other constituents of the sediments were 6.1 to 9.1%, o,p'-DDE; 3.4 to 7.8%, o,p'-DDD; 2.8 to 7.7%, p,p'-DDT; and 2.6 to 4.6%, o,p'-DDT. The OC concentration was related to the organic matter content of the sediments and the residues were adsorbed mostly on particles of 8 μm or less. The authors suggested an association between the OC compounds and humic substances. Adsorption of lindane to the lake sediments was shown to depend on the load of particulate matter in water, organic matter content, lindane concentration, clay content, and lindane-to-sediment ratio in that order.[211] The concentration of chlordecone in the sediments was significantly correlated with its concentration in water.[27] On the other hand, Fay and Newland[212] reported that no such relationship existed betw__a the insecticides present in water and those in the sediments. Heptachlor, endrin, and p,p'-DDT were detected in water whereas dieldrin and p,p'-DDD were detected in sediments.

Among the OPs, high concentration of parathion (up to 1.9 mg/kg) was reported from pond mud.[213] The concentration of parathion in the sediment increased with the progress of the agricultural season. Parathion was present in water, even months after the last application. Apart from the measurement of residues in nature, the distribution of residues in the sediment and water has been sought to be clarified on the basis of theoretical approach and modeling. Employing kinetic studies, Wolfe et al.[214] concluded that despite higher concentrations of DDT and methoxychlor normally found in the sediments than in water, in instances of low sediment-to-water ratio, a large fraction of the total compound would be found in the water column. Di Toro and Horzempa[215] developed a computational method to predict the two fractions of the pollutants associated with the sediment particles, i.e., those bound reversibly and nonreversibly.

a. Adsorption-Desorption Studies on Residues in the Sediments

As has been discussed previously, incorporation of pesticide residues into the sediments does not always immobilize pesticides permanently. Often, the pesticide molecules may undergo slow desorption into the overlying water or may get resuspended and redistributed through turbulence. Several factors control the degree of adsorption to, and desorption of pesticide molecules from, particulate matter. The degree of PCB sorption on to particles was reported to be inversely proportional to the size of the particles.[216] The smaller the size of the particle, i.e., the greater the surface area, the higher the adsorption of the pesticide molecules to the suspended particles.[217] The inverse relationship between particle size and adsorptive capacity seems to hold good only with inert particles, whereas with plankters, the reverse is true, i.e., DDT content is highest in the larger size fraction.[218] Further, the extent of sorption is directly related to the organic matter content.[137,219] When 1 $\mu g/\ell$ of ^{14}C-PCB was added to sea water, the chemical was partitioned between the suspended solids, water, and container surfaces. More than 50% of the added chemical was associated with the particulate matter when the organic matter content was less than 10%; about 10% of the chemical remained in water and 15% was sorbed to the surfaces. With increase in the organic matter content of the system, more of the compound was adsorbed on to the suspended particles. On the other hand desorption was not dependent on the size of the suspended particles or on the organic matter content of the water. When the ^{14}C-PCB contaminated particles were resuspended in PCB-free water, there was rapid desorption irrespective of the size of the particles and organic matter content of the system. The latter assumed importance, however, during the sorption of PCB once again on to the particles after 3 hr.[219]

The organic matter content of the natural waters, especially when present in higher quantities, is reported to decrease the extent of adsorption of polybrominated biphenyls (PBB) on to the sediment[220] and to keep the chemical in water. The amount of PBB sorbed on to sediments, in the experiments of Simmons and Kotz,[220] was always less in natural water than in experiments with distilled water. In lake water with a total organic matter content of 3 to 8 mg/ℓ, the adsorption by sediment was 12% less than when the same amount of suspended matter was present in distilled water. The adsorption by sediment was 33 to 43% less in river water with organic matter content of 12 mg/ℓ than in distilled water. Steen et al.[221] also concluded that the particle size and organic carbon were important factors in determining the extent of partitioning of PCB isomers between sediment and lake water; adsorption by sediments increased with increasing organic matter content of the sediments.

While the extent of sorption of pesticides and such other chemicals in the water column is inversely related to particle size, in organic matter-rich detritus, sorption seems to be directly related to particle size. Odum et al.[208] observed that 500- to 1000-μm-sized detritus particles contained the highest concentration of DDT, the average being 50 mg/kg; 250- to 500-μm-sized fraction contained about 45 mg/kg DDT and the smaller sized particles contained 30 to 35 mg/kg.

Rapid adsorption was noticed in the first 4 or 5 hr upon bringing natural aquifer sand in contact with lindane or dieldrin in water (100 g sand and 55 mℓ pesticide-containing water were shaken together for 24 hr, in a 125 mℓ ground glass, stoppered flask). The adsorption was in the nanogram range at aqueous concentrations of 5 to 500 μg/ℓ. Temperature and pH little influenced the extent of adsorption, but when the aqueous solutions were prepared using water from Lake Mendota or Lake Mary, Wis., a distinct reduction in the adsorption of dieldrin by the sand occurred. Hence, Boucher and Lee[217] concluded that the dissolved organics present in the Wisconsin lakes influenced the extent of adsorption of pesticides by sediments. In desorption studies, it was noted that the pesticide adsorbed on a natural aquifer sand or silica, was desorbed less by Lake Mendota water than by distilled water. When the pesticide-adsorbed sand was washed with water, only 17% of the adsorbed dieldrin was leached by three successive washes with distilled water. But 70% of the initially adsorbed lindane was leached. On the basis of these observations, the authors concluded that lindane would be immediately adsorbed and effectively removed if it enters the aquatic ecosystem as a single slug. On the other hand, if there is the possibility of repeated lindane contamination of the aquatic ecosystem, little reduction through adsorption to the sediment could be expected. Under such conditions, the adsorbed lindane may readily be desorbed in the aquatic environment, leading to harmful effects and chronic low-level exposures. With dieldrin, considerable reduction in its availability in water can be expected, because, once it is adsorbed to the suspended particles, little desorption takes place and the particles eventually get deposited as sediment.

Desorption of residues from contaminated sediments into clean water has been established clearly under experimental conditions. Hamelink et al.[222] found that in instances where the bottom sediments were contaminated intentionally with DDT, and clean water was introduced into the tank along with fish and other organisms, the biota readily concentrated DDT in their tissues. Clearly, sediments can act both as a reservior, and a source of contamination in the aquatic ecosystem. Desorption from sediments poor in organic matter was high. Evidently, pesticides pose less of a problem in eutrophic (highly productive) lakes than in oligotrophic (poorly productive) lakes. It was suggested that the level of contamination of the lake waters and hence of the biota, could be reduced if the binding capacity of the sediments could be increased.

B. Persistence and Degradation of Pesticide Residues in the Aquatic Environment
1. Persistence

As in the terrestrial environment, the persistence and degradation of pesticide molecules in the aquatic environment are influenced by many factors, primarily the chemistry of the molecule itself, the prevailing physicochemical conditions, the organic matter content, the physiography, and the productivity of the water body.

In deep lakes, the ratio of suspended matter to water is less than that in shallower and productive lakes, which would mean that the pesticide molecules have less chance to get adsorbed on particulate matter, and hence persist longer in the water column.[134] Thus, the metabolism and degradation of DDT in Lake Ontario appear to be slower than in Lake Erie, because of the greater depth, cooler water, and lower productivity of the former.[223]

In a study on the persistence of DDE and lindane, Hamelink and Waybrant[134] added identical quantities of DDE and lindane to an oligotrophic lime quarry. At the time of spraying, the quarry pond was thermally stratified,* with little mixing of the epilimnion with the other two layers. DDE was rapidly distributed all through the water column, whereas 70% of lindane remained only in the top 6 m of water, even 81 days after spraying. The remaining quantity of lindane was equally distributed between metalimnion and hypolimnion. Lindane, because of its greater solubility, was mostly present in solution and in the absence of circulation, remained in the top layer. DDE, which was poorly soluble in water, was associated with the suspended particulate matter and hence was distributed throughout the water column. The highest concentration of both the compounds, was initially present near the thermocline. Only after the fall turnover and mixing of the surface and subsurface layers (on the 144th day) was the concentration of lindane uniform all through the column, whereas the concentration of DDE became nearly uniform on day 5 itself. The concentration of lindane, once it attained homogeneity in the water column, started declining. Both insecticides were detectable in water even 358 days after spraying, but the concentration of lindane in water was higher (13 ng/ℓ lindane and 2.2 ng/ℓ DDE). On the other hand, very little lindane was present on the suspended particles, whereas DDE was mostly sorbed on to the particulate matter from day 21 onwards (0.1 μg/kg lindane and 1427 μg/kg DDE, dry weight basis, in association with freshly sedimented material). The authors calculated that 82% of the applied DDE was lost to the suspended sediments after 21 days, whereas 95% of lindane was still in water, 193 days after application to the pond. Furthermore, DDE did not penetrate deeper than 1.5 cm in the bottom mud, which made its redistribution into water possible. This is reflected by the higher DDE content of water recorded on day 358 than between days 102 and 242, and is attributable to the release of DDE to the water following the decomposition of organic matter plus an adsorption shift associated with higher water temperature in summer. In contrast to DDE, when and if lindane finally reaches the sediment, it would move deeper into the sediment through the interstitial water, because of its greater water solubility.

Of all the OC compounds studied, chlordecone and mirex are among the most stable pesticides in the aquatic environment. After 56 days of incubation under both aerobic and anaerobic conditions, there was no evidence of degradation of these two compounds. OP compounds have been reported to have negligible persistence in water. After the application of ^{14}C-diazinon and ethyl parathion, at a rate of 5 and 1 lb/acre, respectively, to a cranberry bog under conditions that simulated natural flooding (undertaken as a protective measure against frost), both pesticides disappeared from water within 144 hr.[225] Among other types of compounds, terbutryn was reported to persist in experimentally treated ponds, for over 420 days.[226] Although the lampricide TFM persisted in the aquatic environment under sediment-free conditions for extended periods of time, the levels at which it persisted in the Great Lakes were not hazardous to any other form of aquatic life in the Great Lakes.[227] Herbicides, like dichlobenil and terbutryn, are reported to persist in water and bottom sediments from a few months up to 1 year.[228]

Ever since Metcalf and associates[229] described a model ecosystem to study the persistence, biodegradability, eventual contamination of the aquatic ecosystem, and bioconcentration and bioaccumulation, several researchers studied the persistence of different types of compounds in model ecosystems or experimental ponds. These studies will be reviewed in a later chapter, in the context of bioconcentration and bioaccumulation of residues by aquatic organisms.

---

* Thermal stratification denotes a condition in the aquatic environment where a density gradient is established because of temperature differences between surface and subsurface layers. At the time of stratification three layers can be distinguished viz., a top epilimnion that is comparatively warmer and less dense, a middle metalimnion that has transitional conditions, and a deeper hypoliminon, that is comparatively cooler and hence denser.[224]

2. Degradation

Degradation of pesticides in the hydrosphere is mostly mediated by microbial activity and in certain instances chemical degradation also assumes importance. Sharom et al.[230] reported that p,p'-DDT rapidly disappeared in aqueous media and about 36% of the degradation product was p,p'-DDD. The remainder of the degradation products in natural waters were presumably too polar to be extracted by the polar-nonpolar solvent combination employed. The fact that DDT was stable in sterilized natural water and distilled water indicates that DDT degradation in nature, to the extent it exists, is promoted by microbes. In general, in the studies conducted by Sharom et al. there was little indication of chemical degradation of OCs in natural waters. Degradation of OP compounds can proceed chemically in natural waters. Degradation of carbaryl was mostly chemical, as is evident from its rapid degradation even in distilled water. In the case of both OP compounds and carbamates, microbial degradation in natural waters, complements chemical degradation and hastens the breakdown of the compound. Of the 12 compounds studied by Sharom et al. (4 OCs, 6 OPs, and 2 carbamates), dieldrin, endrin, ethion, and leptophos in that order were persistent in natural waters, during an 8-week study; parathion, carbaryl, p,p'-DDT, carbofuran, mevinphos, and diazinon in that order were less persistent. According to Sharom et al. residues of less persistent OP and carbamate compounds, if detected in water, will be more in solution rather than in association with particulate matter. Residues of the more persistent compounds will be found adsorbed to suspended particles or in bed materials where eventually they are likely to be immobilized to a considerable extent. These conclusions are in accordance with the earlier observations of Hamelink and Waybrant [134] discussed in the previous section.

In contrast to the finding of Sharom et al. on the degradation of OP compounds under experimental conditions, Sethunathan et al.[231] concluded that microorganisms, rather than chemical agents, are exclusively involved in the degradation of parathion in nature. In sea water, degradation of parathion has been reported to be mostly chemical through dearylation and dealkylation.[232] Hydrolysis and photolysis have been reported as the chief pathways of carbaryl degradation.[233] Dialkyl carbamates (pyrolan and dimetilen) are more stable to alkaline hydrolysis than monoalkyl carbamates like Baygon® and carbaryl.[234] These four carbamates are more stable to hydrolysis under acidic conditions. In the case of the two monoalkyl carbamates, from pH 7 onward, the rate of hydrolysis increases with pH. In natural waters, pH and temperature are important factors governing the persistence and degradation of carbamates.[234] Likewise, pH influenced the degradation of the insect growth regulator, diflubenzuron in water; at pH 10 the half-life was less than 3 days, but at pH 4, no appreciable degradation occurred even after 56 days.[235] At the ambient pH in natural waters, phenylamide pesticides were fairly stable, and hence chemical degradation of these compounds in natural waters was limited.[236] The role of suspended particles in the removal of phenylamide pesticides from water also seems negligible.[237] Phenylamide compounds have been reported to be resistant to the action of mixed culture of microorganisms,[238] which suggests that they are fairly stable compounds in natural waters.

In a study on the persistence of 28 common pesticides in natural river water,[239] no measurable change was detected in the concentration of HCH, heptachlor expoxide, dieldrin, DDE, DDD, DDT, and endrin in 8 weeks; telodrin, endosulfan, chlordane, and aldrin were degraded. Out of nine OP compounds (parathion, methyl parathion, malathion, ethion, trithion, fenthion, dimethoate, merphos, and azodrin), only azodrin was stable over an 8-week period. All the seven carbamates studied were completely degraded in 8 weeks. Lee et al.[240] reported that toxaphene rapidly loses its toxic action in lake sediments. Three months after spraying toxaphene, lake sediments were extracted and to test the toxicity of the extracts, bioassay tests were conducted with bluegills. Results indicate some detoxification of the sediment-incorporated toxaphene, compared with a commercial formulation aged for the same length of time. Rapid metabolism or promotion of degradation of pesticides in the aquatic system under natural conditions is a very interesting phenomenon. The fact that laboratory studies employing deionized or distilled or reconstituted water (especially used in fish toxicity tests) could be misleading is confirmed by the report that the half-life of methoxychlor in distilled water is 270 days, as compared with 8 days in aged Ann Arbor, Mich. tap water that had held fish earlier.[241]

Seasonal variation in the degradation of pesticides, reflecting the changes in both biotic and abiotic factors, has also been reported. Degradation of toxaphene was high during the high summer temperatures, and it remained negligible during freezing, winter conditions in Midway Lake, Saskatchewan.[242] Seasonal variation in the biodegradation of 2,4-D in river waters in Australia was attributed to the peculiar drainage patterns that obtained in those waters.[243]

Biodegradation of pesticides is both aerobic and anaerobic depending on their chemical structure. In the case of toxaphene, the former process is reported to be more important than the latter.[244] In the marine environment, degradation of pesticides in the open water column is negligible, most of the degradative activity is associated with biological materials in the surface film or plankters or algae, etc.[245] Mixtures of formulations were found more readily biodegradable than single pesticide compounds, especially when at least one of the components of the mixtures was readily biodegradable.[246]

Lastly, the role of certain organic molecules in association with naturally occurring inorganic compounds in the degradation of DDT has been examined. Quirke et al.[247] reported that degradation of DDT takes place in vitro in the presence of hematin and ammonia. While it is not known whether such a degradation takes place in nature too, the authors suggested that in nature, in anoxic water bodies rich in ammonia and decaying animal debris, release of iron porphyrins, and the presence of reduced iron salts may accelerate the degradation of DDT. H_2S, evolved from sulfate in anoxic environments was implicated in the dealkylation of amino parathion formed from parathion.[248] Likewise, H_2S interacted with amino analogs of methyl parathion and fenitrothion to form the desamino methylparathion and desamino fenitrothion.[249]

V. CONCLUSIONS

It must be emphasized that the chemistry of the molecule decides the environmental fate of pesticides in general. Poorly water-soluble compounds are more persistent in soils and the aquatic environment. Rapid disappearance of some compounds from soils need not necessarily mean that they do not pose any more environmental problems. Owing to a higher vapor pressure, or poor solubility or both, pesticides may readily volatilize and exist in the atmosphere in the vapor phase, in which state they may be transported to greater distances. Such compounds will ultimately contaminate the aquatic environment through wet and dry deposition. Besides atmospheric deposition, pesticide residues reach the aquatic environment through surface runoff, groundwater contamination, or because of deliberate application for the control of aquatic pests. In water, residues are present in solution or are adsorbed on to particulate matter, water solubility of the compound being the deciding factor. Poorly soluble compounds are readily adsorbed on to particulate matter and are eventually incorporated in the sediments. Pesticide residues pose a greater hazard in the aquatic ecosystems than in the terrestrial systems because of the longer distances they are carried through water and also because of the larger number of organisms that are likely to be exposed and the closer contact that is possible within the aquatic ecosystem.

REFERENCES

1. Melnikov, N. N., Chemistry of pesticides, *Residue Rev.,* 36, 480, 1971.
2. Edwards, C. A., Persistent pesticides in the environment, *CRC Crit. Rev. Environ. Control,* 1, 7, 1970.
3. Harris, C. R. and Miles, J. R. W., Pesticide residues in the Great Lakes region of Canada, *Residue Rev.,* 57, 27, 1975.
4. Matsumura, F., Current pesticide situation in the United States, in *Environmental Toxicology of Pesticides,* Matsumura, F., Boush, G. M., and Misato, T., Eds., Academic Press, New York, 1972, chap. 2.
5. Brooks, G. T., Pesticides in Britain, in *Environmental Toxicology of Pesticides,* Matsumura, F., Boush, G. M., and Misato, T., Eds., Academic Press, New York, 1972, chap. 3.
6. Ishikura, H., Impact of pesticide use on the Japanese environment, in *Environmental Toxicology of Pesticides,* Matsumura, F., Boush, G. M., and Misato, T., Eds., Academic Press, New York, 1972, chap. 1.
7. Kerswill, C. J. and Edwards, H. E., Fish losses after forest sprayings with insecticides in New Brunswick, 1952—62, as shown by caged specimens and other observations, *J. Fish. Res. Board Can.,* 24, 709, 1967.
8. Kerswill, C. J., Studies on effects of forest sprayings with insecticides, 1952—63, on fish and aquatic invertebrates in New Brunswick streams: introduction and summary, *J. Fish. Res. Board Can.,* 24, 701, 1967.
9. Klaas, E. E. and Belisle, A. A., Organochlorine pesticide and polychlorinated biphenyl residues in selected fauna from a New Jersey Salt marsh — 1967 vs. 1973, *Pestic. Monit. J.,* 10, 149, 1977.
10. Carson, R., *Silent Spring,* Houghton Mifflin, Boston, 1962, 360.
11. Haines, T. A., Effect of an aerial application of carbaryl on brook trout *(Salvelinus fontinalis),* *Bull. Environ. Contam. Toxicol.,* 27, 534, 1981.
12. Anon., The plant protection arsenal, *Environ. Sci. Technol.,* 13, 1335, 1979.
13. Devlin, R. M., DDT: a renaissance?, *Environ. Sci. Technol.,* 8, 322, 1974.
14. Gold, B., Leuschen, T., Brunk, G., and Gingell, R., Metabolism of a DDT metabolite via a chloroepoxide, *Chem. Biol. Interact.,* 35, 159, 1981.
15. The President's Science Advisory Committee, Use of pesticides: a report, *Residue Rev.,* 6, 1, 1964.
16. Ware, G. W., Effects of pesticides on nontarget organisms, *Residue Rev.,* 76, 173, 1980.
17. Nicholson, H. P., Pesticide pollution control, *Science,* 158, 871, 1967.
18. Zitko, V., Potentially persistent industrial organic chemicals other than PCB, in *Ecological Toxicology Research,* McIntyre, A. D. and Mills, C. F., Eds., Plenum Press, New York, 1975, 197.
19. Dimond, J. B., Getchell, A. S., and Blease, J. A., Accumulation and persistence of DDT in a lotic ecosystem, *J. Fish. Res. Board Can.,* 28, 1877, 1971.
20. Rudd, R. L. and Herman, S. G., Ecosystem transferal of pesticide residues in an aquatic environment, in *Environmental Toxicology of Pesticides,* Part VII, Matsumura, F., Boush, G. M., and Misato, T., Eds., Academic Press, New York, 1972, chap. 1.
21. Cairns, T. and Parfitt, C. H., Persistence and metabolism of TDE in California Clear Lake fish, *Bull. Environ. Contam. Toxicol.,* 24, 504, 1980.
22. Anderson, R. B. and Everhart, W. H., Concentrations of DDT in landlocked salmon (*Salmo salar*) at Sebago Lake, Maine, *Trans. Am. Fish. Soc.,* 95, 160, 1966.
23. Holden, A. V., The possible effects on fish of chemicals used in agriculture, *J. Proc. Inst. Sew. Purif.,* 4, 361, 1964.
24. Holden, A. V., The effects of pesticides on life in fresh waters, *Proc. R. Soc. London, Ser. B.,* 180, 383, 1972.
25. Elson, P. F., Meister, A. L., Saunders, J. W., Saunders, R. L., Sprague, J. B., and Zitko, V., Impact of chemical pollution on Atlantic salmon in North America, in Int. Atlantic Salmon Symp., International Atlantic Salmon Foundation, St Andrew's, New Brunswick, Canada, 1973, 83.
26. Schmitt, C. J. and Winger, P. V., Factors controlling the fate of pesticides in rural watersheds of the lower Mississippi River alluvial valley, *Trans. 45th N. Am. Wildl. Nat. Res. Conf.,* Washington, D.C., Wildlife Management Institute, Washington, D.C., 1980, 354.
27. Lunsford, C. A., Kepone distribution in the water column of the James River estuary — 1976—78, *Pestic. Monit. J.,* 14, 119, 1981.
28. Abban, E. K. and Samman, J., Further observations on the effect of Abate on fish catches, *Environ. Pollut., Ser. A.,* 27, 245, 1982.
29. Macek, K. J., Walsh, D. F., Hogan, J. W., and Holz, D. D., Toxicity of the insecticide Dursban® to fish and aquatic invertebrates in ponds, *Trans. Am. Fish. Soc.,* 101, 420, 1972.
30. Hurlbert, S. H., Mulla, M. S., Keith, J. O., Westlake, W. E., and Dusch, M. E., Biological effects and persistence of Dursban® in freshwater ponds, *J. Econ. Entomol.,* 63, 43, 1970.

31. Bradt, P. T. and Herrenkohl, R. C., DDT in human milk — what determines the levels?, *Sci. Total Environ.*, 6, 161, 1976.
32. Holden, A. V., Monitoring PCB in water and wildlife, PCB conference II, *Natl. Swedish Environ. Protect. Board Publ.*, 4E, 23, 1973.
33. Bevenue, A., Ogata, J. N., and Hylin, J. W., Organochlorine pesticides in rainwater, Oahu, Hawaii, 1971—1972, *Bull. Environ. Contam. Toxicol.*, 8, 238, 1972.
34. Södergren, A., Monitoring DDT and PCB in airborne fallout, in *Environmental Quality and Safety*, Suppl. Vol. III, Coulston, F. and Korte, F., Eds., Georg Thieme, Stuttgart, 1975, 880.
35. Herzel, F. and Lahmann, E., Insektizid-Bestimmungen in atmosphärischer Luftmittels der Filter-methode, *Gesund. Ing.*, 93, 202, 1972.
36. George, J. L. and Frear, D. E. H., Pesticides in the Antarctic, *J. Appl. Ecol.*, 3 (Suppl.), 155, 1966.
37. Ochiai, M., Ohotomi, M., Ambe, Y., Shinohara, H., and Hanya, T., Secular variation of BHC in the paper of books, *Sci. Total Environ.*, 5, 273, 1976.
38. Garvey, C., Controlling PCB's — a new approach, *EPA J.* July/August, 1981, 25.
39. Macleod, K. E., Polychlorinated biphenyls in indoor air, *Environ. Sci. Technol.*, 15, 926, 1981.
40. Carollo, J. A., The removal of DDT from water supplies, *J. Am. Water Works Assoc.*, 37, 1310, 1945.
41. Cox, J. L., DDT residues in marine phytoplankton: increase from 1955 to 1969, *Science*, 170, 71, 1970.
42. Glooschenko, W. A., The effect of DDT and dieldrin upon ^{14}C uptake by *in situ* phytoplankton in lakes Erie and Ontario, in *Proc. 14th Conf. Great Lakes Res.*, International Association for Great Lakes Research, Ann Arbor, Mich., 1971, 219.
43. Giam, C. S., Wong, M. K., Hanks, A. R., Sackett, W. M., and Richardson, R. L., Chlorinated hydrocarbons in plankton from the Gulf of Mexico and Northern Caribbean, *Bull. Environ. Contam. Toxicol.*, 9, 376, 1973.
44. Jeltis, R., On the possibility of the production of chlorinated hydrocarbons in swimming water, *Water Res.*, 13, 687, 1979.
45. Jansson, B. and Bergman, Å., Sulfur-containing derivatives of hexachlorobenzene (HCB)—metabolites in the rat, *Chemosphere*, 7, 257, 1978.
46. Harvey, G. R., Source of PCB's, *Science*, 180, 1122, 1976.
47. Metcalf, R. L., Sanborn, J. R., Lu, P.-Y., and Nye, D., Laboratory model ecosystem studies of the degradation and fate of radiolabeled tri-, tetra-, and pentachlorobiphenyl compared with DDE, *Arch. Environ. Contam. Toxicol.*, 3, 151, 1975.
48. Ramamoorthy, S., Cheng, T. C., and Kushner, D. J., Effect of microbial life stages on the fate of methylmercury in natural waters, *Bull. Environ. Contam. Toxicol.*, 29, 167, 1982.
49. Iwie, G. W., Dorough, H. W., and Alley, E. G., Photodecomposition of mirex on silica gel chromatoplates exposed to natural and artificial light, *J. Agric. Food Chem.*, 22, 933, 1974.
50. Crosby, D. G. and Moilanen, K. W., Vapor-phase photodecomposition of DDT, *Chemosphere*, 6, 167, 1977.
51. Khan, M. A. Q., Stanton, R. H., Sutherland, D. J., Rosen, J. D., and Maitra, N., Toxicity-metabolism relationship of the photoisomers of certain chlorinated cyclodiene insecticide chemicals, *Arch. Environ. Contam. Toxicol.*, 1, 159, 1973.
52. Kaiser, K. L. E., The rise and fall of mirex, *Environ Sci. Technol.*, 12, 520, 1978.
53. Lichtenstein, E. P., Fuhremann, T. W., and Schulz, K. R., Persistence and vertical distribution of DDT, lindane, and aldrin residues, 10 and 15 years after a single soil application, *J. Agric. Food Chem.*, 19, 718, 1971.
54. Kuhr, R. J., Davis, A. C., and Bourke, J. B., DDT residues in soil, water, and fauna from New York apple orchards, *Pestic. Monit. J.*, 7, 200, 1974.
55. Stevens, L. J., Colier, C. W., and Woodham, D. W., Monitoring pesticides in soils from areas of regular, limited and no pesticide use, *Pestic. Monit. J.*, 4, 145, 1970.
56. Kuhr, R. J., Davis, A. C., and Bourke, J. B., *New York Food Life Sci.*, 10, 18, 1977, in Boileau, S., Basil, M., and Alary, J. G., DDT in Northern pike (*Esox lucius*) from the Richelieu River, Quebec, Canada, 1974—1975, *Pestic. Monit. J.*, 13, 109, 1979.
57. Truhlar, J. F. and Reed, L. A., Occurrence of pesticide residues in four streams draining different land-use areas in Pennsylvania, 1969—71, *Pestic. Monit. J.*, 10, 101, 1976.
58. Weber, J. B., Interaction of organic pesticides with particulate matter in aquatic and soil systems, in *Fate of Organic Pesticides in the Aquatic Environment*, Faust, S. D., Ed., Advances in Chemistry Series 111, American Chemical Society, Washington D.C., 1972, 55.
59. Harris, C. R., Chapman, R. A., and Miles, J. R. W., Insecticide residues in soils on fifteen farms in southwestern Ontario, 1964—1974, *J. Environ. Sci. Health*, B12, 163, 1977.
60. Herzel, F., DDT and andere Insektizide in Berliner Böden, *Z. Kulturtech. Flurbereinig.*, 12, 306, 1971.

61. Carlson, D. A., Konyha, K. D., Wheeler, W. B., Marshall, G. P., and Zaylskie, R. G., Mirex in the environment: its degradation to Kepone and related compounds, *Science,* 194, 939, 1976.
62. Brooks, G. T., *Chlorinated Insecticides,* Vols. 1 and 2, CRC Press, Boca Raton, Fla., 1974.
63. Kawasaki, M., Experiences with the test scheme under the chemical control law of Japan: an approach to structure-activity correlations, *Ecotoxicol. Environ. Saf.,* 4, 444, 1980.
64. Miles, J. R. W., Harris, C. R., and Moy, P., Insecticide residues in organic soil of the Holland Marsh, Ontario, Canada, 1972—75, *J. Econ. Entomol.,* 71, 97, 1978.
65. Stewart, D. K. R., Chisholm, D., and Ragab, M. T. H., Long term persistence of parathion in soil, *Nature,* 229, 47, 1971.
66. Freed, V. H., Schmedding, D., Kohnert, R., and Haque, R., Physical chemical properties of several organophosphates: some implication in environmental and biological behavior, *Pestic. Biochem. Physiol.,* 10, 203, 1979.
67. Crosby, D. G. and Tucker, R. K., Toxicity of aquatic herbicides to *Daphnia magna, Science,* 154, 289, 1966.
68. Murty, A. S., Miles, J. R. W., and Tu, C. M., Persistence and mobility of nitrofen (niclofen, Tok®) in mineral and organic soils, *J. Environ. Sci. Health,* B17, 143, 1982.
69. Anon., EPA bans most DDT uses, readies lead action, *Environ. Sci. Technol.,* 6, 675, 1972.
70. Glass, G. E., Strachan, W. M. I., Willford, W. A., Armstrong, F. A. I., Kaiser, K. L. E., and Lutz, A., Organic contaminants. In the waters of Lake Huron and Lake Superior, Vol. III (Part B), *Report to the International Joint Commission by the Upper Great Lakes Reference Group.* Windsor, Ontario, 1977, 417.
71. Koeman, J. H., den Boer, W. M. J., Feith, A. F., De Iongh, H. H., and Spliethoff, P. C., Three years observation on side effects of helicopter applications of insecticides used to exterminate *Glossina* species in Nigeria, *Environ. Pollut.,* 15, 31, 1978.
72. Butler, P. A., Pesticides in the estuary, in *Proc. Marsh and Estuary Management Symp.,* Louisiana State University, Newsom, D., Ed., Thos. J. Horon's Sons, Baton Rouge, La., 1968, 120.
73. Fox, P. J. and Matthiessen, P., Acute toxicity to fish of low-dose aerosol applications of endosulfan to control tsetse fly in the Okavango Delta, Botswana, *Environ. Pollut., Ser. A,* 27, 129, 1982.
74. Hindin, E. and Bennett, P. J., Occurrence of pesticides in aquatic environments. I. Insecticide distribution on an agricultural plot, Wash. State Univ. Tech. Ext. Service, Pullman, 1970, in Gerakis, P. A. and Sficas, A. G., The presence and cycling of pesticides in the ecosphere, *Residue Rev.,* 52, 69, 1974.
75. Pearce, P. A., Brun, G. L., and Witteman, J., Off-target fallout of fenitrothion during 1978 forest spraying operations in New Brunswick, *Bull. Environ. Contam. Toxicol.,* 25, 503, 1979.
76. Burden, E. H. W. J., A case of DDT poisoning in fish, *Nature,* 178, 546, 1956.
77. Hatfield, C. T. and Riche, L. G., Effect of aerial Sumithion® spraying on juvenile Atlantic salmon (*Salmo salar* L.) and brook trout (*Salvelinus fontinalis* Mitchill) in Newfoundland, *Bull. Environ. Contam. Toxicol.,* 5, 440, 1970.
78. Hildebrand, L. D., Sullivan, D. S., and Sullivan, T. P., Experimental studies of rainbow trout populations exposed to field applications of Roundup® herbicide, *Arch. Environ. Contam. Toxicol.,* 11, 93, 1982.
79. Weber, J. B., The pesticide scorecard, *Environ. Sci. Technol.,* 11, 756, 1977.
80. Farmer, W. J., Igue, K., Spencer, W. F., and Martin, J. P., Volatility of organochlorine insecticides from soil. I. Effect of concentration, temperature, air flow rate, and vapor pressure, *Soil Sci. Soc. Am. Proc.,* 36, 443, 1972.
81. Howard, P. H., Saxena, J., and Sikka, H., Determining the fate of chemicals, *Environ. Sci. Technol.,* 12, 398, 1978.
82. Spencer, W. F., Distribution of pesticides between soil, water and air, *Pesticides in the Soil, Ecology, Degradation, and Movement,* Guyer, G. E., Ed., Michigan State University, East Lansing, Mich., 1970, 120.
83. Acree, F., Jr., Beroza, M., and Bowman, M. C., Codistillation of DDT with water, *J. Agric. Food Chem.,* 11, 278, 1963.
84. Spencer, W. F. and Cliath, M. M., Desorption of lindane from soil as related to vapor density, *Soil Sci. Soc. Am. Proc.,* 34, 574, 1970.
85. Chiou, C. T. and Manes, M., On the validity of the codistillation model for the evaporation of pesticides and other solutes from water solution, *Environ. Sci. Technol.,* 14, 1253, 1980.
86. Igue, K., Farmer, K. J., Spencer, W. F., and Martin, J. P., Volatility of organochlorine insecticides from soil. II. Effect of relative humidity and soil water content on dieldrin volatility, *Soil Sci. Soc. Am. Proc.,* 36, 447, 1972.
87. Spencer, W. F. and Cliath, M. M., Pesticide volatilization as related to water loss from soil, *J. Environ. Qual.,* 2, 284, 1973.
88. Isensee, A. R., Holden, E. R., Woolston, E. A., and Jones, G. E., Soil persistence and aquatic bioaccumulation potential of hexachlorobenzene (HCB), *J. Agric. Food Chem.,* 24, 1210, 1976.

89. Cliath, M. M. and Spencer, W. F., Movement and persistence of dieldrin and lindane in soil as influenced by placement and irrigation, *Soil Sci. Soc. Am. Proc.,* 35, 791, 1971.
90. Willis, G. H., Parr, J. F., Papendick, R. I., and Smith, S., A system for monitoring atmospheric concentrations of field-applied pesticides, *Pestic. Monit. J.,* 3, 172, 1969.
91. Cliath, M. M., Spencer, W. F., Farmer, W. J., Shoup, T. D., and Grover, R., Volatilization of S-ethyl N, N-dipropylthiocarbamate from water and wet soil during and after flood irrigation of an alfalfa field, *J. Agric. Food Chem.,* 28, 610, 1980.
92. Lloyd-Jones, C. P., Evaporation of DDT, *Nature,* 229, 65, 1971.
93. Freed, V. H., Haque, R., and Schmedding, D., Vaporization and environmental contamination by DDT, *Chemosphere,* 1, 61, 1972.
94. Spencer, W. F. and Cliath, M. M., Volatility of DDT and related compounds, *J. Agric. Food Chem.,* 20, 645, 1972.
95. Cliath, M. M. and Spencer, W. F., Dissipation of pesticides from soil by volatilization of degradation products. I. Lindane and DDT, *Environ. Sci. Technol.,* 6, 910, 1972.
96. Eisenreich, S. J., Hollod, G. J., and Johnson, T. C., Accumulation of polychlorinated biphenyls (PCBs) in surficial Lake Superior sediments. Atmospheric deposition, *Environ. Sci. Technol.,* 13, 569, 1979.
97. Bidleman, T. F., and Olney, C. E., Long range transport of toxaphene insecticide in the atmosphere of the Western North Atlantic, *Nature,* 257, 475, 1975.
98. Bidleman, T. F. and Olney, C. E., Chlorinated hydrocarbons in the Sargasso Sea atmosphere and surface water, *Science,* 183, 516, 1974.
99. Risebrough, R. W., Hugget, R. J., Griffin, J. J., and Goldberg, E. D., Pesticides: transatlantic movements in the Northeast Trades, *Science,* 159, 1233, 1968.
100. McClure, V. E., Transport of heavy chlorinated hydrocarbons in the atmosphere, *Environ. Sci. Technol.,* 10, 1223, 1976.
101. Kaiser, K. L. E., Mirex: an unrecognized contaminant of fishes from Lake Ontario, *Science,* 185, 523, 1974.
102. Bengtson, S.-A. and Södergren, A., DDT and PCB residues in airborne fallout and animals in Iceland, *Ambio,* 3, 84, 1974.
103. Stratton, C. L. and Sosebee, J. B., Jr., PCB and PCT contamination of the environment near sites of manufacture and use, *Environ. Sci. Technol.,* 10, 1229, 1976.
104. Arthur, R. D., Cain, J. D., and Barrentine, B., Atmospheric levels of pesticides in the Mississippi delta, *Bull. Environ. Contam. Toxicol.,* 15, 129, 1976.
105. Södergren, A., Chlorinated hydrocarbon residues in airborne fallout, *Nature,* 236, 395, 1972.
106. Giam, C. S., Atlas, E., Chan, H. S., and Neff, G. S., Phthalate esters, PCB and DDT residues in the Gulf of Mexico atmosphere, *Atm. Environ.,* 14, 65, 1980.
107. Baldwin, M. K., Bennett, D., and Beynon, K. T., The concentrations of aldrin and dieldrin and their photoisomers in the atmosphere, *Pestic. Sci.,* 8, 431, 1977.
108. Hargrave, B. T. and Phillips, G. A., DDT residues in benthic invertebrates and demersal fish in St. Margaret's Bay, Nova Scotia, *J. Fish. Res. Board Can.,* 33, 1692, 1976.
109. Wils, E. R. J., Hulst, A. G., and den Hartog, J. C., The occurrence of Rovral and permethrin in airborne particulate matter, *Chemosphere,* 11, 585, 1982.
110. Peakall, D. B., DDT in rainwater in New York following application in the Pacific North-West, *Atm. Environ.,* 10, 899, 1976.
111. Arthur, R. D., Cain, J. D., and Barrentine, B., DDT residues in air in the Mississippi Delta, 1975, *Pestic. Monit. J.,* 11, 168, 1977.
112. Veith, G. D. and Lee, G. F., Chlorobiphenyl (PCBs) in the Milwaukee River, *Water Res.,* 5, 1107, 1971.
113. Ahling, B., The combustion of waste containing DDT and Lindane, *Sci. Total Environ.,* 9, 117, 1978.
114. Ahling, B. and Lindskog, A., Thermal destruction of PCB and hexachlorobenzene, *Sci. Total Environ.,* 10, 51, 1978.
115. Wheatley, G. A. and Hardman, J. A., Indications of the presence of organochlorine insecticides in rainwater in Central England, *Nature,* 207, 486, 1965.
116. Weibel, S. R., Weidner, R. B., Cohen, J. M., and Christianson, A. G., Pesticides and other contaminants in rainfall and runoff, *J. Am. Water Works Assoc.,* 58, 1075, 1966.
117. Tarrant, K. R. and Tatton, J. O. G., Organochlorine pesticides in rainwater in the British Isles, *Nature,* 219, 725, 1968.
118. Pearce, P. A., Reynolds, L. M., and Peakall, D. B., DDT residues in rainwater in New Brunswick and estimate of aerial transport of DDT into the Gulf of St. Lawrence, 1967—68, *Pestic. Monit. J.,* 11, 199, 1978.
119. Masahiro, O. and Takahisa, H., Alpha- and gamma-BHC in Tokyo rainwater (December 1968 to November 1969), *Environ. Pollut.,* 9, 283, 1975.

120. Bevenue, A., Hylin, J. W., Kawano, Y., and Kelley, T. W., Organochlorine pesticide residues in water, sediment, algae, and fish, Hawaii — 1970—71, *Pestic. Monit. J.,* 6, 56, 1972.

121. Osterroht, C. and Smetacek, V., Vertical transport of chlorinated hydrocarbons by sedimentation of particulate matter in Kiel Bight, *Mar. Ecol. Prog. Ser.,* 2, 27, 1980.

122. Wells, D. E. and Johnstone, S. J., The occurrence of organochlorine residues in rainwater, *Water Air Soil Pollut.,* 9, 271, 1978.

123. Tanabe, S., Hidaka, H., and Tatsukawa, R., PCBs and chlorinated hydrocarbon pesticides in Antarctic atmosphere and hydrosphere, *Chemosphere,* 12, 277, 1983.

124. Schrimpff, E., Thomas, W., and Herrmann, R., Regional patterns of contaminants (PAH pesticides and trace metals) in snow of Northeast Bavaria and their relationship to human influence and orographic effects, *Water Air Soil Pollut.,* 11, 481, 1979.

125. Murty, A. S., unpublished.

126. McElroy, A. D., Chiu, S. Y., Nebgen, J. W., Aleti, A., and Vandegrift, A. E., Water pollution from nonpoint sources, *Water Res.,* 9, 675, 1975.

127. Anon., Sediment is nations' main water pollution burden, *Environ. Sci. Technol.,* 2, 993, 1968.

128. Sonzogni, W. C., Chesters, G., Coote, D. R., Jeffs, D. N., Konrad, J. C., Ostry, R. C., and Robinson, J. B., Pollution from land runoff, *Environ. Sci. Technol.,* 14, 148, 1980.

129. Bradshaw, J. S., Loveridge, E. L., Rippee, K. P., Peterson, J. L., White, D. A., Barton, J. R., and Fuhriman, D. K., Seasonal variations in residues of chlorinated hydrocarbon pesticides in the water of the Utah Lake drainage system 1970—1971, *Pestic. Monit. J.,* 6, 166, 1972.

130. Braun, H. E. and Frank, R., Organochlorine and organophosphorus insecticides: their use in eleven agricultural watersheds and their loss to stream waters in southern Ontario, Canada, 1975—77, *Sci. Total Environ.,* 15, 169, 1980.

131. Penrose, D. L. and Lenat, D. R., Effects of apple orchard runoff on the aquatic macrofauna of a mountain stream, *Arch. Environ. Contam. Toxicol.,* 11, 383, 1982.

132. The effects of pesticides on fish and wildlife, FWS Circ. 226, Fish and Wildlife Service, U.S. Department of the Interior, 1965, in Truhlar, J. F. and Reed, L. A., Occurrence of pesticide residues in four streams draining land-use areas in Pennsylvania, 1969—71, *Pestic. Monit. J.,* 10, 101, 1976.

133. Caro, J. H., Freeman, H. P., and Turner, B. C., Persistence in soil and losses in runoff of soil incorporated carbaryl in a small watershed, *J. Agric. Food Chem.,* 22, 860, 1974.

134. Hamelink, J. L. and Waybrant, R. C., DDE and lindane in a large-scale model lentic ecosystem, *Trans. Am. Fish Soc.,* 105, 124, 1976.

135. Helling, C. S., Kearney, P. C., and Alexander, M., Behavior of pesticides in soils, *Adv. Agron.,* 23, 147, 1971 in Gerakis, P. A. and Sficas, A. G., Eds., The presence and cycling of pesticides in the ecosphere, *Residue Rev.,* 52, 69, 1974.

136. Bailey, G. W. and White, J. L., Review of adsorption and desorption of organic pesticides by soil colloids, with implications concerning pesticide bioactivity, *J. Agric. Food Chem.,* 12, 324, 1964.

137. Kobylinski, G. J. and Livingston, R. J., Movement of mirex from sediment and uptake by the hogchoker, *Trinectes maculatus, Bull. Environ. Contam. Toxicol.,* 14, 692, 1975.

138. Kenaga, E. E., Predicted bioconcentration factors and soil sorption coefficients of pesticides and other chemicals, *Ecotoxicol. Environ. Saf.,* 4, 26, 1980.

139. Sharom, M. S., Miles, J. R. W., Harris, C. R., and McEwen, F. L., Behavior of 12 insecticides in soil and aqueous suspensions of soil and sediment, *Water Res.,* 14, 1095, 1980.

140. Gaynor, J. D. and Volk, V. V., Runoff losses of atrazine and terbutryn from unlimed and limed soil, *Environ. Sci. Technol.,* 15, 440, 1981.

141. Caro, J. H. and Taylor, A. W., Loss of dieldrin from soils under field conditions, *J. Agric. Food Chem.,* 19, 379, 1971.

142. Willis, G. H. and Hamilton, R. A., Agricultural chemicals in surface runoff, ground water, and soil. I. Endrin, *J. Environ. Qual.,* 2, 463, 1973.

143. Ritter, W. F., Johnson, H. P., Lovely, J. W., and Molnau, M., Atrazine, propachlor, and diazinon residues on small agricultural watersheds, *Environ. Sci. Technol.,* 8, 38, 1974.

144. White, A. W., Barnett, A. P., Wright, B. G., and Holladay, J. H., Atrazine losses from fallow land caused by runoff and erosion, *Environ. Sci. Technol.,* 1, 740, 1967.

145. Frank, P. A., Herbicidal residues in aquatic environments, in *Fate of Organic Pesticides in the Aquatic Environment,* Faust, S. D., Ed., Advances in Chemistry Series 111, American Chemical Society, Washington, D.C., 1972, chap. 6.

146. Suzuki, M., Yamato, Y., and Akiyama, T., Occurrence and determination of a herbicide benthiocarb in rivers and agricultural drainages, *Water Res.,* 11, 275, 1977.

147. Suzuki, M., Yamato, Y., and Akiyama, T., Fate of herbicide CNP in rivers and agricultural drainages, *Water Res.,* 12, 777, 1978.

148. Pionke, H. B. and Chesters, G., Pesticide-sediment-water interactions, *J. Environ. Qual.,* 2, 29, 1973.

149. Wauchope, R. D., The pesticide content of surface water draining from agricultural fields — a review, *J. Environ. Qual.,* 7, 459, 1978.

150. Martell, J. M., Rickert, D. A., and Siegel, F. R., PCB's in suburban watershed, Reston, *Va. Environ. Sci. Technol.,* 9, 872, 1975.

151. Harper, D. B., Smith, R. V., and Gotto, D. D., BHC residues of domestic origin: a significant factor in pollution of freshwater in Northern Ireland, *Environ. Pollut.,* 12, 223, 1977.

152. Buhler, D. R., Rasmusson, M. E., and Nakaue, H. S., Occurrence of hexachlorophene and pentachlorophenol in sewage and water, *Environ. Sci. Technol.,* 7, 929, 1973.

153. Fry, D. M. and Toone, C. K., DDT-induced feminization of gull embryos, *Science,* 213, 922, 1981.

154. Jukes, T. H., DDT in the sewers, *Science,* 218, 494, 1982.

155. Furr, A. K., Lawrence, A. W., Tong, S. S. C., Grandolfo, M. C., Hofstader, R. A., Bache, C. A., Gutenmann, W. H., and Lisk, D. J., Multielement and chlorinated hydrocarbon analysis of municipal sewage sludges of American cities, *Environ. Sci. Technol.,* 10, 683, 1976.

156. Kopperman, H. L., Kuehl, D. W., and Glass, G. E., Chlorinated compounds found in waste-treatment effluents and their capacity to bioaccumulate, in *Proc. Conf. Environ. Impact of Water Chlorination,* Oak Ridge, Tenn., Jolley, R. L., Ed., Oak Ridge National Laboratory, Energy Research and Development Administration, and US Environmental Protection Agency, 1976, 327.

157. Holden, A. V., Source of polychlorinated biphenyl contamination in the marine environment, *Nature,* 228, 1220, 1970.

158. Holden, A. V. and Marsden, K.,, The examination of surface waters and sewage effluents for organochlorine pesticides, *J. Proc. Inst. Sew. Purif.,* 3, 3, 1966.

159. Bopp, R. F., Simpson, H. J., Olsen, C. R., and Kostyk, N., Polychlorinated biphenyls in sediments of the tidal Hudson River, New York, *Environ. Sci. Technol.,* 15, 210, 1981.

160. Södergren, A., Djirsarai, R., Gharibzadeh, M., and Moinpour, A., Organochlorine residues in aquatic environments in Iran, 1974, *Pestic. Monit. J.,* 12, 81, 1978.

161. Hsieh, D. P. H., Archer, T. E., Munnecke, D. M., and McGowan, F. E., Decontamination of noncombustible agricultural pesticide containers by removal of emulsifiable parathion, *Environ. Sci. Technol.,* 6, 826, 1972.

162. Shuman, F. L., Jr., Stojanovic, B. J., and Kennedy, M. V., Engineering aspects of the disposal of unused pesticides, pesticide wastes, and pesticide containers, *J. Environ. Qual.,* 1, 66, 1972.

163. Archer, T. E., Removal of 2,4-dichlorophenoxyacetic acid (2,4-D) formulations from noncombustible pesticide containers, *Bull. Environ. Contam. Toxicol.,* 13, 44, 1975.

164. Lamberton, J. G., Thomson, P. A., Witt, J. M., and Deinzer, M. L., Pesticide container decontamination by aqueous wash procedures, *Bull. Environ. Contam. Toxicol.,* 16, 528, 1976.

165. Bays, L. R., Pesticide pollution and the effects on the biota of Chew Valley Lake, *Environ. Pollut.,* 1, 205, 1971.

166. Lawless, E. W., The pollution potential in pesticide manufacturing, TS-00-72-04, Environmental Protection Agency, June 1972, in Chian, E. S. K., Bruce, W. N., and Fang, H. H. P., Removal of pesticides by reverse osmosis, *Environ. Sci. Technol.,* 9, 53, 1975.

167. Kveseth, N. J., Residues of DDT in a contaminated Norwegian lake ecosystem, *Bull. Environ. Contam. Toxicol.,* 27, 397, 1981.

168. Teasley, J. I., Identification of a cholinesterase-inhibiting compound from an industrial effluent, *Environ. Sci. Technol.,* 1, 411, 1967.

169. Borsetti, A. P. and Roach, J. A. G., Identification of Kepone alteration products in soil and mullet, *Bull. Environ. Contam. Toxicol.,* 20, 241, 1978.

170. Greve, P. A. and Wit, S. L., Endosulfan in the Rhine River, *J. Water Pollut. Fed. Control,* 43, 2338, 1971.

171. Deelstra, H., Power, J. L., and Kenner, C. T., Chlorinated hydrocarbon residues in the fish of Lake Tanganyika, *Bull. Environ. Contam. Toxicol.,* 15, 689, 1976.

172. Pierce, R. H., Brent, C. R., Williams, H. P., and Reeves, S. G., Pentachlorophenol distribution in a freshwater ecosystem, *Bull. Environ. Contam. Toxicol.,* 18, 251, 1977.

173. Wells, D. E. and Cowan, A. A., Vertebral dysplasia in salmonids caused by the herbicide trifluralin, *Environ. Pollut.,* 29, 249, 1982.

174. Perry, J. A., Pesticide and PCB residues in the Upper Snake River ecosystem, southeastern Idaho, following the collapse of the Teton dam, 1976, *Arch. Environ. Contam. Toxicol.,* 8, 139, 1979.

175. Anderson, D. W., Castle, W. T., Woods, L. A., Jr., and Ayres, L. A., Residues of *o,p'*-DDT in southern California coastal sediments in 1971, *Bull. Environ. Contam. Toxicol.,* 29, 429, 1982.

176. Buckler, D. R., Witt, A., Jr., Mayer, F. L., and Huckins, J. N., Acute and chronic effects of Kepone and mirex on the fathead minnow, *Trans. Am. Fish. Soc.,* 110, 270, 1981.

177. Picer, M., Picer, N., and Ahel, M., Chlorinated insecticide and PCB residues in fish and mussels of east coastal waters of the Middle and North Adriatic sea, 1974—75, *Pestic. Monit. J.,* 12, 102, 1978.

178. Westoo, G. and Noren, K., Polychlorinated 2-amino-diphenyl ethers in fish, *Ambio,* 6, 232, 1977.

179. Menzie, C. A., Potential significance of insects in the removal of contaminants from aquatic systems, *Water Air Soil Pollut.*, 13, 473, 1980.

180. Seba, D. B. and Corcoran, E. F., Surface slicks as concentrators of pesticides in the marine environment, *Pestic. Monit. J.*, 3, 190, 1969.

181. Duce, R. A., Quinn, J. G., Olney, C. E., Piotrowicz, S. R., Ray, B. J., and Wade, T. L., Enrichment of heavy metals and organic compounds in the surface microlayer of Narragansett Bay, Rhode Island, *Science*, 176, 161, 1972.

182. Eisenreich, S. J., Elzerman, A. W., and Armstrong, D. E., Enrichment of micronutrients, heavy metals, and chlorinated hydrocarbons in wind-generated lake foam, *Environ. Sci. Technol.*, 12, 413, 1978.

183. Moody, R. P., Greenhalgh, R., Lockhart, L., and Weinberger, P., The fate of fenitrothion in an aquatic ecosystem, *Bull. Environ. Contam. Toxicol.*, 19, 8, 1978.

184. Södergren, A., Origin of ^{14}C and ^{32}P labelled lipids moving to and from freshwater surface microlayers, *Oikos*, 33, 278, 1979.

185. Platford, R. F., The environmental significance of surface films. II. Enhanced partitioning of lindane in thin films of octanol on the surface of water, *Chemosphere*, 10, 719, 1981.

186. Platford, R. F., Carey, J. H., and Hale, E. J., The environmental significance of surface films. I. Octanol-water partition coefficients for DDT and hexachlorobenzene, *Environ. Pollut.*, 83, 125, 1982.

187. Naqvi, S. M. and de la Cruz, A. A., Mirex incorporation in the environment: residues in nontarget organisms — 1972, *Pestic. Monit. J.*, 7, 104, 1973.

188. Schaefer, M. L., Peeler, J. T., Gardner, W. S., and Campbell, J. E., Pesticides in drinking water — waters from the Mississippi and Missouri Rivers, *Environ. Sci. Technol.*, 3, 1261, 1969.

189. Dupuy, A. J. and Schulze, J. A., Selected water quality records for Texas surface waters, 1970 water year, Texas Water Development Board, Rep. 149, Austin, Texas, in Coppage, D. L. and Matthews, E., Brain-acetylcholinesterase inhibition in a marine teleost during lethal and sublethal exposures to 1,2-dibromo-2,2-dichloroethyl dimethyl phosphate (naled) in sea water, *Toxicol. Appl. Pharmacol.*, 31, 128, 1975.

190. Miles, J. R. W. and Harris, C. R., Insecticide residues in water, sediment and fish of the drainage system of the Holland Marsh, Ontario, 1972—1975, *J. Econ. Entomol.*, 71, 125, 1978.

191. Coppage, D. L., Matthews, E., Cook, G. H., and Knight, J., Brain acetylcholinesterase inhibition in fish as a diagnosis of environmental poisoning by malathion, *O,O*-dimethyl *S*-(1,2-dicarbethoxyethyl) phosphorodithioate, *Pestic. Biochem. Physiol.*, 5, 536, 1975.

192. Lowden, G. F., Saunders, C. L., and Edwards, R. W., *Proc. Soc. Water Treat. Exam.*, 18, 275, 1969; quoted in Holden, A. V., The effects of pesticides on life in fresh waters, *Proc. R. Soc. London, Ser. B*, 180, 383, 1972.

193. Frank, R. and Sirons, G. J., Chlorophenoxy and chlorobenzoic acid herbicides; their use in eleven agricultural watersheds and their loss to stream waters in southern Ontario, Canada, 1975—77, *Sci. Total Environ.*, 15, 167, 1980.

194. Finlayson, B. J., Acute toxicities of the herbicides Komeen and hydrothol-191 to golden shiner *(Notemigonus crysoleucas)*, *Bull. Environ. Contam. Toxicol.*, 25, 676, 1980.

195. Greve, P. A., Potentially hazardous substances in surface waters, *Sci. Total Environ.*, 1, 173, 1972.

196. Ahnoff, M. and Josefsson, B., Polychlorinated biphenyls (PCB) in Göta river water, *Ambio*, 4, 172, 1975.

197. Kahanovitch, L. and Lahav, L., Occurrence of pesticides in selected water sources in Israel, *Environ. Sci. Toxicol.*, 8, 762, 1974.

198. Yamato, Y., Suzuki, M., and Akiyama, T., Persistence of BHC in river water in the Kitakyushu district, Japan, 1970—74, *Bull. Environ. Contam. Toxicol.*, 14, 380, 1975.

199. Herzel, F., Chlorkohlenswasserstoff-Insektizeds in Oberflachenwassern, *Bundesgesundheitsblatt*, 14, 175, 1971.

200. Laska, A. L., Bartell, K., and Laseter, J. L., Distribution of hexachlorobenzene and hexachlorobutadiene in water, soil, and selected aquatic organisms along the lower Mississippi River, Louisiana, *Bull. Environ. Contam. Toxicol.*, 15, 535, 1976.

201. Sackmauerová, M., Palušová, O., and Szokolay, A., Contribution to the study of drinking water, Danube water and biocenose contamination with chlorinated insecticides, *Water Res.*, 11, 551, 1977.

202. Frank, R., Braun, H. E., and Holdrinet, M. V. H., Residues from past uses of organochlorine insecticides and PCB in waters draining eleven agricultural watersheds in southern Ontario, Canada, 1975—77, *Sci. Total Environ.*, 20, 255, 1981.

203. Kellogg, R. L. and Bulkely, R. V., Seasonal concentrations of dieldrin in water, channel catfish, and catfish-food organisms, Des Moines River, Iowa — 1971—73, *Pestic. Monit. J.*, 9, 186, 1976.

204. Barber, R. T. and Warlen, S. M., Organochlorine insecticide residues in deep sea fish from 2,500 m in the Atlantic Ocean, *Environ. Sci. Technol.*, 13, 1146, 1979.

205. Halter, M. T. and Johnson, H. E., A model system to study the desorption and biological availability of PCB in hydrosoils, *Aquatic Toxicology and Hazard Evaluation,* ASTM STP 634, Mayer, F. L. and Hamelink, J. L., Eds., American Society for Testing and Materials, Philadelphia, 1977, 178.

206. Zitko, V., The analysis of aquatic sediments for organic compounds, in *Contaminants and Sediments,* Vol. 2, Baker, R. A. and Arbor, A., Eds., Ann Arbor Science, Ann Arbor, Mich., 1980, 89.

207. Mauck, W. L., Mayer, F. L., and Holz, D. D., Simazine residue dynamics in small ponds, *Bull. Environ. Contam. Toxicol.,* 16, 1, 1976.

208. Odum, W. E., Woodwell, G. M., and Wurster, C. F., DDT residues absorbed from organic detritus by fiddler crabs, *Science,* 164, 576, 1969.

209. Frank, R., Holdrinet, M., Braun, H. E., Thomas, R. L., Kemp, A. L. W., and Jaquet, J. M., Organochlorine insecticides and PCBs in sediments of Lake St. Clair (1970—1974) and Lake Erie (1971), *Sci. Total Environ.,* 8, 205, 1977.

210. Choi, W. W. and Chen, K. Y., Association of chlorinated hydrocarbons with fine particles and humic substances in nearshore surficial sediments, *Environ. Sci. Technol.,* 10, 782, 1976.

211. Lotse, E. G., Graetz, D. A., Chesters, G., Lee, G. B., and Newland, L. W., Lindane adsorption by lake sediments, *Environ. Sci. Technol.,* 2, 353, 1968.

212. Fay, R. R. and Newland, L. W., Organochlorine insecticide residues in water, sediment, and organisms, Aransas Bay, Texas — September 1969—June 1970, *Pestic. Monit. J.,* 6, 97, 1972.

213. Nicholson, H. P., Webs, H. J., Lauer, G. J., O'Brien, R. E., Grzenda, A. R., and Shanklin, D. W., Insecticide contamination in a farm pond. I. Origin and duration, *Trans. Am. Fish. Soc.,* 91, 213, 1962.

214. Wolfe, N. L., Zepp, R. G., Paris, D. F., Baughman, G. L., and Hollis, R. C., Methoxychlor and DDT degradation in water: rates and products, *Environ. Sci. Technol.,* 11, 1077, 1977.

215. Di Toro, D. M. and Horzempa, L. M., Reversible and resistant components PCB adsorption-desorption isotherms, *Environ. Sci. Technol.,* 16, 594, 1982.

216. Haque, R., Schmedding, D. W., and Freed, V. H., Aqueous solubility, adsorption and vapor behavior of polychlorinated biphenyl Aroclor 1254, *Environ. Sci. Technol.,* 8, 139, 1974.

217. Boucher, F. R. and Lee, G. F., Adsorption of lindane and dieldrin pesticides on unconsolidated aquifer sands, *Environ. Sci. Technol.,* 6, 538, 1972.

218. Särkka, J., Hattula, M. L., Janatuinen, J., and Paasivirata, J., Mercury and chlorinated hydrocarbons in plankton of Lake Päijänne, Finland, *Environ. Pollut.,* 16, 41, 1978.

219. Nau-Ritter, G. M., Wurster, C. F., and Rowland, R. G., Partitioning of (^{14}C) PCB between water and particulates with various organic contents, *Water Res.,* 16, 1615, 1982.

220. Simmons, M. S. and Kotz, K. T., Association studies of polybrominated biphenyls in aquatic systems, *Bull. Environ. Contam. Toxicol.,* 29, 58, 1982.

221. Steen, W. C., Paris, D. F., and Baughman, G. L., Partitioning of selected polychlorinated biphenyls to natural sediments, *Water Res.,* 12, 655, 1978.

222. Hamelink, J. L., Waybrant, R. C., and Ball, R. C., A proposal: exchange equilibria control the degree chlorinated hydrocarbons are biologically magnified in lentic environments, *Trans. Am. Fish. Soc.,* 100, 207, 1971.

223. Frank, R., Thomas, R. L., Holdrinet, M., Kemp, A. L. W., and Braun, H. E., Organochlorine insecticides and PCB in surficial sediments (1968) and sediment cores (1976) from Lake Ontario, *Int. Assoc. Great Lakes Res.,* 5, 18, 1979.

224. Hutchinson, G. E., *A Treatise on Limnology,* Vol. I, John Wiley & Sons, New York, 1957, chap. 7.

225. Miller, C. W., Zuckerman, B. M., and Charig, A. J., Water translocation of diazinon-C^{14} and parathion-S off a model cranberry bog and subsequent occurrence in fish and mussels, *Trans. Am. Fish. Soc.,* 95, 345, 1966.

226. Muir, D. C. G., Pitze, M., Blouw, A. P., and Lockhart, W. L., Fate of terbutryn in macrophyte-free and macrophyte-containing farm ponds, *Weed Res.,* 21, 1981.

227. Thingvold, D. A. and Lee, G. F., Persistence of 3-(trifluoromethyl)-4-nitrophenol in aquatic environments, *Environ. Sci. Technol.,* 15, 1335, 1981.

228. Brooker, M. P. and Edwards, R. W., Aquatic herbicides and the control of water weeds, *Water Res.,* 9, 1, 1975.

229. Metcalf, R. L., Sangha, G. K., and Kappor, I. P., Model ecosystem for the evaluation of pesticide biodegradability and ecological magnification, *Environ. Sci. Technol.,* 5, 709, 1971.

230. Sharom, M. S., Miles, J. R. W., Harris, C. R., and McEwen, F. L., Persistence of 12 insecticides in water, *Water Res.,* 14, 1089, 1980.

231. Sethunathan, N., Siddaramappa, R., Rajaram, K. P., Barik, S., and Wahid, P. A., Parathion: residues in soil and water, *Residue Rev.,* 68, 91, 1977.

232. Weber, K., Degradation of parathion in sea water, *Water Res.,* 10, 237, 1976.

233. Wolfe, N. L., Zepp, R. G., and Paris, D. F., Carbaryl, propham and chloropropham: a comparison of the rates of hydrolysis and photolysis with the rate of biolysis, *Water Res.,* 12, 565, 1978.

234. Aly, O. A. and El-Dib, M. A., Studies on the persistence of some carbamate insecticides in the aquatic environment. I, *Water Res.,* 5, 1191, 1971.
235. Ivie, G. W., Bull, D. L., and Veech, J. A., Fate of diflubenzuron in water, *J. Agric. Food Chem.,* 28, 330, 1980.
236. El-Dib, M. A. and Aly, O. A., Persistence of some phenylamide pesticides in the aquatic environment. I. Hydrolysis, *Water Res.,* 10, 1047, 1976.
237. El-Dib, M. A. and Aly, O. A., Persistence of some phenylamide pesticides in the aquatic environment. II. Adsorption on clay minerals, *Water Res.,* 10, 1051, 1976.
238. El-Dib, M. A. and Aly, O. A., Persistence of some phenylamide pesticides in the aquatic environment. III. Biological degradation, *Water Res.,* 10, 1055, 1976.
239. Eichelberger, J. W. and Lichtenberg, J. J., Persistence of pesticides in river water, *Environ. Sci. Technol.,* 5, 541, 1971.
240. Lee, G. F., Hughes, R. A., and Veith, G. D., Evidence for partial degradation of toxaphene in the aquatic environment, *Water Air Soil Pollut.,* 8, 479, 1977.
241. Merna, J. W., Bender, M. E., and Novy, J. R., The effects of methoxychlor on fishes. I. Acute toxicity and breakdown studies, *Trans. Am. Fish. Soc.,* 101, 298, 1972.
242. Royer, L. M., Bioassay method for the determination of toxaphene in lake water, *J. Fish. Res. Board Can.,* 23, 723, 1966.
243. Watson, J. R., Seasonal variation in the biodegradation of 2,4-D in river water, *Water Res.,* 11, 153, 1977.
244. Clark, J. M. and Matsumura, F., Metabolism of toxaphene by aquatic sediment and a camphor-degrading pseudomonad, *Arch. Environ. Contam. Toxicol.,* 8, 285, 1979.
245. Patil, K. C., Matsumura, F., and Boush, G. M., Metabolic transformation of DDT, dieldrin, aldrin, and endrin by marine microorganisms, *Environ. Sci. Technol.,* 6, 629, 1972.
246. Stojanovic, B. J., Kennedy, M. V., and Shuman, F. L., Jr., Edaphic aspects of the disposal of unused pesticides, pesticide wastes, and pesticide containers, *J. Environ. Qual.,* 1, 54, 1972.
247. Quirke, J. M. E., Marei, A. S. M., and Eglinton, G., The degradation of DDT and its degradative products by reduced iron (III) porphyrins and ammonia, *Chemosphere,* 8, 151, 1979.
248. Wahid, P. A. and Sethunathan, N., Involvement of hydrogen sulphide in the degradation of parathion in flooded acid sulphate soil, *Nature (London),* 282, 401, 1979.
249. Adhya, T. K., Sudhakar-Barik, and Sethunathan, N., Fate of fenitrothion, methyl parathion and parathion in anoxic sulfur-containing soil systems, *Pestic. Biochem. Physiol.,* 16, 14, 1981.

Chapter 2

PESTICIDE RESIDUES IN FISH

I. INTRODUCTION

Even as it was realized that DDT-type compounds began to spread far and wide in the ecosystem, and their residues were recorded in the abiotic and biotic samples from unexpected places like the Antarctic, attempts were afoot to determine whether such residues could be present in natural fish populations too. At about the same time, the reports that carnivorous animals, especially those at the higher trophic levels, may concentrate lipophilic compounds in their tissues at several hundred to several thousand times the ambient concentrations in the environment,[1] led to concerted efforts at monitoring the residue levels in fish in nature. The development of gas chromatographic techniques (particularly that employing an electron capture detector) for residue analysis in the early 1960s has proved to be a boon, and over the last 2 decades, much information has accrued on the different types of compounds that accumulate in fish tissues. Although much of this information concerns the species of only a few countries of the world, reflecting the high degree of awareness of environmental problems in those countries, the patterns of accumulation of pesticide residues by fish are now well documented and the processes involved are fairly well understood. In this chapter, the residue levels in fish from different parts of the world are reviewed, and the reasons for the variations and fluctuations in the residue concentration in fish are also examined. The care that should be exercised in employing ultrasensitive analytical tools and the pitfalls of mistaken identity are also emphasized.

II. ANALYTICAL METHODOLOGY

A. Transport of Samples to the Laboratory

The first step in determining the residue load of fish is the collection and transportation of the samples to the laboratory. A biopsy technique to extract small samples of muscle without harming the fish was described.[2] More commonly, fish are collected in the field and transported to the laboratory in the frozen condition. Since transportation from distant places to the laboratory can often be a problem, preservation in 4% formaldehyde or 10% phenol was studied. Two pigeons, force-fed daily with a gelatin capsule containing 5 mg of dieldrin and 10 mg of DDT, for 5 days, were sacrificed and the livers were finely minced and divided into 10 equal portions. Half of these samples were preserved in formaldehyde and the other in phenol, at room temperature ranging between 10 to 27°C. Preserved tissues were analyzed the same day, and also 5 and 10 days, 4 months, and 1 year later.[3] There was a slight loss of weight in formalin (1% between 5 and 10 days, 6% in 4 months and 10% in 1 year), whereas with phenol, the results were irregular, there being weight loss in the beginning and weight gain later. With both the preservatives, the residues were stable and extractable. Unlike phenol, formalin did not completely inhibit the post-mortem conversion of p,p'-DDT to p,p'-DDD; only 10.5% of the original DDT was present 1 year after preservation. The total DDT (Σ DDT), however, was not significantly different at 0 hr and at the end of 1 year. No residues were extracted by either of the preservatives, as revealed by the analysis of the preservatives. Formalin was chosen and phenol was rejected because of possible column (gas chromatographic) difficulties and also because of weight changes in the tissue.[3] In another study, tissues were stored in 4% formalin for at least 2 days before being transported to the laboratory, where they were held at 10°C.[4] Pick et al.[5]

transported tissues of birds and fish to the laboratory in glass jars containing formalin, and the tissues were stored at 4°C until extracted within 2 months. Deubert et al.[6] reported fixing fish muscle tissue in 4% formalin or Bouin's fixative; either method yielded residue data in the same range as those obtained from frozen samples. Miles et al.[7] observed no loss of Abate® residues in fish samples preserved for 3 weeks in 10% formalin, containing 5% sodium thiosulfate. Hence, in instances where freezing of samples and transportation in the frozen state are not possible, formalin, preextracted with a suitable solvent, may be employed to preserve the samples.

B. Analysis

Among different classes of pesticides, the poorly water soluble, lipophilic compounds (mostly organochlorine [OC] compounds) are taken up by organisms and deposited in tissues. Hence, residue analytical methods are developed with an emphasis on extraction of the lipid, using a nonpolar solvent or more commonly a combination of polar-nonpolar solvents. The extract is concentrated and cleaned of coextractives by column chromatography (usually a column of Florisil®, alumina or silicic acid, or occasionally, two different columns) or gel permeation chromatography (GPC). The eluate is concentrated or diluted, depending on the residue concentration and analyzed by gas chromatography (GC). The various steps in the extraction of residues from biological or nonbiological materials and cleanup from coextractives are described in detail in the Pesticide Analytical Manual (PAM).[8] Appropriate modifications of this general residue method, developed to yield a good recovery of a specific compound, or to suit the needs of a laboratory or to circumvent a specific problem, are too numerous to mention here. Hesselberg and Johnson[9] described a method of column extraction of residues from fish and fish-food with a recovery of the various compounds in the range of 95 to 99%. The authors reported that their cold, column extraction method was superior to the blending method (recommended in PAM) in recovering DDT metabolites and polychlorinated biphenyls (PCBs), and in many cases the standard error of the mean between replicate samples was less for the former method than for the latter. Hattula[10] compared four solvent systems, each used with cold (column) or hot (soxhlet) extraction methods, using a lean (pike), medium fatty (perch), and a fatty (bream) fish to test the extraction efficiency. With lean fish, soxhlet extraction with methanol and chloroform, 1:1 (v/v) gave the best extraction. For perch, a medium fatty fish, extraction was highest by soxhlet with 1:1 (v/v) 25% n-hexane in acetone and 10% diethyl ether in petroleum ether. For very fatty fish, soxhlet extraction with methanol and chloroform, 1:1 (v/v) or cold extraction with this solvent combination gave the best extraction and recovery. Cold extraction with any of the solvent combinations employed gave a lower recovery than soxhlet extraction with methanol:chloroform (1:1). The steam codistillation method for extracting pesticide residues from biological materials extracts very little lipid and hence requires no cleanup and gives 80% or more recovery.[11] Ernst et al.[12] employed a cold, column extraction method similar to that of Hesselberg and Johnson,[9] but instead of acetonitrile and Florisil® cleanup, they used an alumina column, followed by a Florisil® column cleanup for the analysis of marine biotic samples.

As none of the methods usually gives 100% recovery of the residues, the actual percentage of recovery is calculated after fortifying a part of the sample with a known quantity of a standard pesticide or a combination of many pesticides and all sample values are usually corrected for this recovery. Occasionally the values were reported without being corrected for recovery.[13,14] Holden[15] opined that addition of known quantities of compounds and subsequent extraction can rarely correct for the actual recovery, as the recovery of a compound added to a matrix is not equivalent to that of the substance accumulated through normal biological processes. Although Holden's point on the actual integration of the residue molecules with the living matrix is valid, in view of the wide variation in the recovery of residues from biological material, (ranging from 70 to 110%), correction for recovery seems advisable for purposes of comparability of results between different laboratories. At times recovery is estimated by exposing the fish to radioactively labeled substances and measuring the radioactivity in various tissues. It was stated that Jensen et al.[16] held the conventional recovery experiments as not being satisfactory as they are based on a post-mortem addition of a standard. According to Hattula,[10] the recovery is relevant only if labeled substances have been added to the live animal and the radioactivity remaining in the tissues is measured. However, this approach is open to criticism because the presence of radioactivity in a tissue is not equivalent to the presence of the original compound, as the parent compound may be metabolized, or conjugated with more polar substances in the process of elimination, or the radioactive moiety of the breakdown products may be incorporated in other molecules.[17-20] In a model ecosystem study on the uptake and degradation of methoprene, an insect growth regulator, by bluegills, the fish had a surprisingly large amount of radioactivity after 4 to 6 weeks of exposure. If the radioactivity were to be due to the presence of the original compound, one would have concluded that the compound was bioaccumulated several thousand times; however, less than 0.1% of the measured radioactivity was in the form of methoprene and its primary metabolites, the rest being present in such natural products like cholesterol, proteins, free fatty acids, and glycerides.[21] It has been emphasized that "radioassay is a gross, nonspecific measuring technique which cannot distinguish one carbon-14 containing compound from another . . . the carbon-14 measured might be as parent compound, various metabolites, or even as part of some natural product . . . "[22] Hence, it is not advisable to depend on radioisotope studies alone to measure the percentage of uptake or deposition.

GC and such other fine analytical methods need to be handled with care and the identification of the compounds should be confirmed by another method before its routine use in a laboratory. Gunther,[23] in an excellent paper on the interpretation of pesticide residue data, cited many instances of mistaken analytical identity. He listed such mistaken identifications as sulfur being identified as aldrin, p-dichlorobenzophenone identified as dicofol, unknown artifacts interpreted as DDT, and inorganic phosphate in human urine identified as alkyl phosphates resulting from exposure to organophosphate (OP) compounds, etc. Maini and Collina[24] reported that soil extracts, upon standing in daylight for 2 days, developed a spurious peak that would be normally identified as p,p'-DDT, owing to photochemical reactions in the solvent phase. Because of the reaction of Kepone® with acetone and methanol used for extraction and cleanup, formation of products that could have been identified as metabolic products of Kepone® was noticed.[25] Well-established methods and techniques, too, can sometimes lead to erroneous conclusions, as in the case of the use of hexane, (which is the most often used GC injection solvent) with which the appearance of "ghost peaks" was detected while Kepone® was being analyzed.[26] Formation of impurities either on the column or during cleanup or while concentrating the extract with a rotary evaporator was described in the analysis of pentachlorophenol (PCP) from biological materials.[27] Several peaks that could have been interpreted as oxychlordane, heptachlor epoxide, and nonachlor if confirmatory tests were not applied were reported while analyzing human adipose tissue.[28]

Mistaken identity and confusion of one compound with another even while using a sensitive analytical tool like GC is nowhere else better illustrated than in the case of DDT and PCBs. Soon after the electron capture detector was employed for detecting OC compounds, several researchers reported the finding of GC peaks having the same retention time as the DDT group compounds; within a few years the presence of "residues of DDT group'' [sic] was reported from the biotic and abiotic samples of even the Arctic and Antarctic. Indeed, DDT had attained ubiquity by that time, but not all the peaks really corresponded to the retention time of DDT, as was observed by a few of the researchers who reported the presence of other unidentified peaks with almost the same retention time or nearer to that of *p,p'*-DDE.[29,15] It was not until Jensen[30] correctly identified that the then unidentified peaks belong to a separate class of compounds, viz., PCBs, that this confusion was cleared. It is only from 1968 to 1970 that attempts have been made to separate DDT from PCBs and the former correctly quantified. Hence, in all the studies on DDT prior to 1968 to 1970 (when an electron capture detector was employed), the values in all probability included PCBs, too, and should not be taken as the true concentration of the reported residues. After 1970, methods have been standardized to separate DDT groups from PCBs. While analyzing environmental samples it has become customary to analyze both these groups, as the methods of extraction, cleanup, and analysis are the same for both.

The danger of PCBs being interpreted as mirex has been pointed out by Markin et al.[31] Analyzing the same composite sample of fish in the National Pesticide Monitoring Program (NPMP) in the U.S.,[32] one laboratory reported the presence of heptachlor epoxide and the other did not in the early years after the identity of PCBs was established. A reinvestigation of the sample indicated that what had been identified as heptachlor epoxide might have been a PCB peak. GC peaks, corresponding to the retention times of heptachlor, heptachlor epoxide, γ-HCH (hexachlorocyclohexane), aldrin, and dieldrin were identified in the extracts of soil samples collected in 1910, i.e., 30 years before the insecticidal properties of DDT were discovered and environmental use of DDT commenced![33]

Residues tentatively identified as *o,p'*-DDD, *p,p'*-DDT, and Strobane® from fish samples collected from Rybinsk Reservoir in the U.S.S.R. and analyzed at Borok (U.S.S.R.) could not be confirmed when the samples were reanalyzed using the same methods at the Columbia National Fisheries Research Laboratory (CNFRL), Missouri.[34]

The foregoing discussion emphasizes the care needed in interpreting the analytical data. The mere presence of a peak on a gas chromatogram should mean nothing unless the presence of the compound is confirmed by appropriate confirmatory techniques. This point cannot be overemphasized because, despite the fact that residue analytical techniques are carefully developed by chemists, they are universally employed by other specialists who may not understand the intricacies involved in the analysis. Fortunately, after the development of the tiered system of toxicity testing (see Chapter 8, Volume II) reliance on a few isolated determinations of pesticide residues for environmental hazard evaluation has ceased, but yet acceptability for human consumption is still linked with residue concentration in food items in many countries. Hence, all residue analysts should exercise utmost caution in determining and reporting the concentration of residues in fish and other such materials, especially at the lower end of the values. Gunther[23] opined that most residue data below 0.1 mg/kg are analytically not very meaningful.

As much as it is necessary to confirm the presence of pesticide residues in samples, there is also a need to evolve new methods and sensitive tools to identify compounds hitherto unidentified. As has been pointed out by Kuehl et al.,[35] improved and sophisticated analytical techniques reveal the presence of many more types of organic contaminants than hitherto suspected. The current residue analytical methodology to study the extent of xenobiotic contamination of the environment and biota are unduly biased in favor of nonionic compounds[36] and leave out all ionic compounds, some of which, like PCP, are as widespread as some of the more commonly studied nonionic compounds.[37,38]

III. PESTICIDE RESIDUES IN FISH FROM DIFFERENT REGIONS OF THE WORLD

There is extensive information on residues in fish from different parts of the globe. In the following section only some representative reports are reviewed. The residues reported in fish of different countries, in general, reflect two points: (1) the intensity of the use of pesticides and (2) the general level of awareness of the environmental problems in those countries. It is not surprising to find that much of the data on residues in fish come from two regions — North America, and the countries surrounding the Baltic. Reports from other regions are scanty or not available, perhaps because of low level of use or lack of general awareness of the problems of environmental contamination.

A. North America
1. U.S.

Museum specimens of six species of fish from Lake Michigan collected between 1929 and 1966 and stored in ethyl alcohol were analyzed to determine the years in which the various contaminants started appearing in fish. DDT and its metabolites appeared in fish samples for the first time in 1949, i.e., within 4 years after the environmental application of DDT had commenced; dieldrin appeared in 1955.[39] PCBs, which were produced in the U.S. for the first time in 1929, appeared only in 1949. In a 3-year study (1965 to 1967) on the residues in fish from the watersheds of Massachusetts, Σ DDT in individual fish varied from undetectable levels to 49.1 mg/kg (dry weight basis). Different species collected from the same locality had different concentrations of residues. During the 3-year study period, an increasing trend in pesticide concentration was noticed.[40] The total DDT content of channel catfish collected from 18 sites in the watersheds of Nebraska in 1964 was 2.2 to 92.2 mg/kg and that of dieldrin 0.1 to 6.7 mg/kg.[41] Largemouth bass kept in cages in the Lost River system draining into Tule Lake and Klamath Lake Refuges in California had 97 and 107 μg/kg endrin in 1965 and 1966.[42] In fish collected from all over the U.S., in 1967 and 1968, as part of the NPMP (see Section IX), DDT and its metabolites were found in all but 6 out of 590 composited samples of 62 species of fish. The DDT values ranged up to 45 mg/kg (wet weight, whole fish).[43] Up to 2 mg/kg dieldrin was found in about 75% of the samples. Heptachlor, heptachlor epoxide, HCH, and chlordane were the other compounds recorded. Out of seven laboratories involved in the analysis, only one laboratory reported the presence of PCBs in the samples, but attributed it to the bottle cap liners in which the cross-check samples were stored. The highest quantity of DDT found was in a perch taken from the Delaware River and was more than nine times the FDA (U.S. Food and Drug Administration) tolerance limit in operation at that time. In 1969, 28,000 lb of contaminated coho salmon from Lake Michigan were seized by the FDA, as the DDT concentration in the coho was around 19 mg/kg.[44] Pinfish and Atlantic croakers collected in the estuary near Pensacola, Fla. in 1964 and 1965 were reported to have usually less than 0.1 mg/kg DDT, and the highest quantity recorded was 1.3 mg/kg.[45] In Lake Poinsett, in South Dakota, lindane, heptachlor, heptachlor epoxide, dieldrin, DDT, DDE, DDD, and toxaphene were recorded in 1968 to 1969.[46] DDT and its metabolites were found in all of the 147 samples collected in 1969. Σ DDT ranged from 0.03 mg/kg (Kenai River, Alaska) to 57.8 mg/kg in channel catfish caught in the St. Lucie Canal, Indiantown, Fla.[32] Channel catfish, white perch, and largemouth bass had consistently higher levels, whereas bluegills and bullheads had low levels. The average total OC residue levels in different species ranged from 1937 μg/kg in bigmouth buffalo to 5700 μg/kg in the northern pike. Uptake of mirex that had leached from fire ant bait by mosquitofish and green sunfish was reported.[47] Following the treatment of a rice field-marshland ecosystem in Texas with aldrin, dieldrin was recorded in the spotted gar (275 μg/kg).[48] While aldrin persisted in the other organisms of the ecosystem for only 2 to 4 weeks, aldrin was detected in the spotted gar up to the 7th week. Uptake as well as elimination of aldrin by this species was observed to be slower than in the other species. The highest concentration of aldrin and dieldrin were, however, detected in the menhaden. DCPA (dimethyl tetrachloro tetraphthalate), a herbicide, was reported from five species of fish (all values in μg/kg): mullet (555 in skin, 159 in flesh, and 231 in viscera), Rio Grande perch (468 in liver, 420 in ovaries, and 217 in flesh), spotted sea trout (472 in liver and 55 in flesh), menhaden (0 to 8.2), and redfish (18 in liver and 132 in testes) was recorded.[49] Residues of hexachlorobenzene (HCB), originally wrongly identified as β-HCH in the NPMP of fall 1970, ranged from less than 1 μg/kg in paddlefish to 62 mg/kg in carp.[50] In 1970, DDT was found in all the catfish samples obtained from 54 commercial catfish farms sampled in Arkansas, whereas dieldrin, endrin, and toxaphene were present in 89, 76, and 96% of the samples.[51] The residue levels of one or more of the compounds were higher than the FDA tolerance limits in 15% of the samples, the levels being exceeded in 2% of the samples by DDT, 6% of the samples by aldrin-dieldrin, 4% of the samples by endrin, and 7% of the samples by toxaphene. All the fish-feed samples from 43 farms had detectable residues. High levels of HCB (71.8 to 379.8 μg/kg) were reported in mosquitofish from the lower reaches of the Mississippi.[52] Between 1970 and 1974, the mean levels of DDT in fish declined, although high concentrations were still recorded in areas of intense use of DDT; dieldrin and endrin levels remained unchanged whereas the levels of toxaphene increased.[53] Viewed in the light of the recommendations of the U.S. National Academy of Sciences Water Quality Criteria, OC residue levels in freshwater fish may have represented a hazard to piscivores at 71% of the places sampled in 1970 and at 66% of the places sampled in 1974.[55] The levels of DDT and PCBs recorded in dover sole, a flatfish collected near a municipal sewage outfall in southern California, were DDT — 0.1 to 45 mg/kg in 1971 to 1972 and 0.04 to 26 mg/kg in 1974 to 1975, and PCBs — not detectable to 6.2 mg/kg in 1971 to 1972 and 0.03 to 2.8 mg/kg in 1974 to 1975.[54] Declining levels of DDT, DDE, and PCBs in 1978 in comparison with those in 1971 were reported from 20 species of fish from the Gulf of Mexico;[55] *p,p'*-DDT values ranged from less than 0.1 μg/kg in the muscle of several species of fish to 50 μg/kg in the liver of shark; *p,p'*-DDE values ranged from 2 μg/kg in the muscle of sand trout to 83 μg/kg in the liver of shark. The mean residue levels in the fish of this region were 60 μg/kg PCBs and 50 μg/kg total DDT in 1971, and 26 μg/kg and 10 μg/kg, respectively, in 1978. In a survey of the young-of-the-year fish (which indicates the contamination in the last 12 months or less) in North Carolina, 97% of the samples in 1972, 43% in 1975, 38% in 1974, 45% in 1975, and 18% in 1976 had DDT, but the average Σ DDT values were almost constant at 0.02 to 0.04 mg/kg.[56]

In the U.S., the Environmental Protection Agency (EPA) banned the use of DDT, effective from the last day of 1972,[57] and suspended the production and use of aldrin and dieldrin in 1974.[58] On the basis of systems analysis and assuming that DDT would be carried between trophic levels by mass transfer, Harrison et al.[59] estimated that the equilibrium time of DDT in the ecosystem would lie between four times the longevity of the longest lived species and the sum of the longevity of all the species occupying all the trophic levels in an ecosystem. They concluded that even if no more DDT were to be added to the biosphere, its concentration in certain species at the higher trophic levels would continue to rise for some years and that a long time is needed before the top carnivores respond to the input of DDT. Bloom and Menzel[60] criticized the assumption of Harrison et al. that all the DDT ingested by an organism is retained. Assuming steady state condition, Bloom and Menzel suggested that the time required for 98.2% reduction of DDT (if all applications are halted) is about 27 years. Woodwell et al.[61] and Hamelink and Waybrant[62] also held that equilibrium conditions would be achieved much sooner in lentic systems than that predicted by Harrison et al. The rapid decline in DDT levels in fish in the U.S. and other regions since the imposition of the ban on DDT, suggests that its turnover is much faster and although DDT may continue to persist in the ecosystem for some time to come, peak values have occurred much earlier than had been predicted by Harrison et al.

2. Canada

Concentration of DDT group compounds was reported to be low after 20 years of DDT use for the control of blackfly larvae (1948 to 1967) in the Saskatchewan River.[63] DDT and DDD levels were 0.01 to 0.15 mg/kg and DDE was 0.01 to 0.06 mg/kg in nine species of fish. Zitko[64] reported PCBs, p,p'-DDT, p,p'-DDE, p,p'-DDD in marine and freshwater fish in New Brunswick and Nova Scotia; the levels recorded in the various species were: p,p'-DDT, 0.01 to 0.63; p,p'-DDE, 0.01 to 0.56; p,p'-DDD, not detectable to 0.37; HCB, 0.001 to 0.019; and PCBs, 0.02 to 4.93 (all values in mg/kg). The methyl mercury content of American eels caught in Nova Scotia was less than the tolerance limit prescribed for human consumption (0.5 mg/kg) in 1972.[65] PCP residues were recorded in fish in eastern Canada.[66] Frank et al.[67] reported 0.032 to 323 mg/kg of total DDT in 26 species of fish collected in the Bay of Quinte in Ontario; comparable dieldrin values were 0.001 to 0.254 mg/kg. Low levels of residues were reported from the fish of the Fraser River[68] in 1972 to 1973. Hargrave and Phillips[69] reported low levels of DDT in fish caught in relatively uncontaminated St. Margaret's Bay, Nova Scotia (all values in µg/kg, wet weight): 8 in the carcass, 9 in muscle, and 625 in liver of cod; 2 in muscle, 4 in carcass, and 9 in the gonad of winter flounder; 14 to 47.5 in whole body of American plaice; 0.8 in carcass, 6.5 in muscle, and 72.3 in liver of haddock; 5.3 in muscle and 2430 in the liver of thorny skate. The presence of higher quantities of p,p'-DDT than p,p'-DDE, contrary to the reports from elsewhere, is suggestive of direct contamination of the Bay with DDT adsorbed onto particulate matter. In a survey on the pesticide residues in 10 species of fish from Lake Simcoe in central Ontario, Frank et al.[70] recorded a downward trend in the total DDT content between 1970 and 1976; o,p'-DDT was observed in 1970, but not later; p,p'-DDE was the major component of total DDT. Dieldrin values also showed a downward trend, whereas chlordane and heptachlor epoxide were recorded for the first time in 1975 to 1976. Within 2 years after the banning of DDT in Canada, 0.2 to 1.5 mg/kg (whole body, fresh weight) levels of DDT were recorded in the northern pike.[71] The residue levels in fish from Cold Lake, Alberta, were found to be highest in pike > whitefish > cisco > white sucker.[72] Kaiser[73] recorded higher concentrations of PCB than OC residues in Great Lakes whitefish and lamprey. In lake whitefish, the following levels of residues were observed in 1978 (µg/kg, whole body weight basis), HCB, 4 to 34; α-HCH, 2 to 26; heptachlor epoxide, 17 to 86; γ-chlordane, 3 to 243; α-chlordane, 9 to 202; dieldrin, 13 to 215; endrin, 2 to 54; DDE, 80 to 4890; p,p'-DDT, 25 to 554; o,p'-DDT, 2 to 509; and PCBs, 243 to 14,700. Changing trends in contaminant levels in any population are not easy to discern because of the large variations in residue concentration among samples, which requires analysis of larger samples, more effort, and hence higher expenditure. To overcome this difficulty, Kaiser[73] used contaminant ratio (DDE/DDT; DDT/Σ DDT, etc.) both within species and between two food chain related species (in this case sea lamprey and its host — whitefish) to gain a greater degree of accuracy in determining the contaminant abundance. Such ratios, according to Kaiser, are analogous to the use of internal standards and increase the accuracy while reducing the number of samples required. Interspecies contaminant quotients between a lamprey and its host are highly useful in recognizing recent trends in contaminant levels. Using this approach, he concluded that DDT levels are declining whereas those of PCBs and DDE are not, and may perhaps continue to increase in Lake Huron, possibly through atmospheric inputs.

3. Great Lakes

The Great Lakes occupy a unique position in the world because they represent the largest total mass of freshwater draining a large catchment area. As much as raptorial birds like the peregrine falcon helped focus public attention on the environmental abuses resulting from the excessive use of DDT, the coho salmon in Lake Michigan has played an equally important role in creating a general awareness of the environmental hazards of DDT group compounds. Coho was not originally an inhabitant of the Great Lakes, but was introduced as an important sport fish in the 1960s and has attained the status of a multimillion dollar business. With the discovery that coho in Lake Michigan was highly contaminated and unfit for human consumption, sport fishing collapsed.

In 1970, fish from Lake Michigan was reported to have 2 to 7 times the residue load of fish from the other Great Lakes.[74] Even within Lake Michigan, bloaters, alewives, small lake trout, and American smelt from the southern end of the lake had higher residue burden than those of the same size group and same species from the northern end. Fish from Lake Ontario and Lake Huron contained one half, and those from Lake Erie one half to one third, the residue content of the same species from Lake Michigan in 1970. Fish from Lake Superior had the lowest concentration among the Great Lakes fish.[74] All but 1 of the 80 samples of fish collected from Lake Erie in 1970 to 1971 contained either DDT or its metabolites or both, the average values being 0.06 to 0.42, DDE; 0.07 to 0.52, DDD; 0.03 to 0.25, DDT; and 0.18 to 0.9, total DDT (all values in mg/kg, wet weight basis).[75] Species at the lower levels of the food pyramid and rough fish had the lowest values, while sport fish like coho salmon had the highest values. Σ DDT content of fish in Lake Erie was, in general, found to be low in 1972.[76] Although mirex was never registered in Canada as an insecticide and does not seem to have been used in any of the States in the U.S. having rivers and streams draining into Lake Ontario, mirex was reported as a contaminant of fish from Lake Ontario.[77] The low level contamination of Lake Superior fish was once again confirmed by the lower levels of total DDT in lake trout from Lake Superior than lake trout from Lake Michigan or Lake Cayuga, N.Y., in 1971.[78] The low levels of OC contaminants in Lake Superior fish are attributable to the relatively little agricultural runoff into the lake and also to the low population density around the lake. Increased incidence of goiter in the coho salmon of Great Lakes, that may or may not have been caused by increased body contaminant burden, was reported by Leatherland and associates.[79-81] A considerable quantity of HCB has been reported from Lake Ontario salmonids (80 in lake trout, 62 in rainbow trout, and 36 in coho salmon, all values in µg/kg, wet weight basis).[82] Variation in the OC and PCB levels in Great Lakes coho salmon, caught at different sites in a given lake, was rather small, indicating that contaminant levels to which the fish were exposed were spatially integrated. This may reflect the greater mobility of coho salmon throughout a lake. Other piscivorous species had a much greater variation than coho, suggesting a somewhat restricted movement. Hence Norstrom et al.[83] asserted that it is possible to use coho as an indicator species to understand the extent of contamination of the Great Lakes.

B. Europe

Major contributions to the environmental monitoring of pesticide residues in fish in Europe have come from countries near and around the Baltic. In Norway, the use of DDT as an insecticide (except against pine weevil) has been prohibited since October 1970.[84] Until then, heavy use of DDT on fruit orchards resulted in high DDT levels in the biota, especially from the southwestern coast. Cod caught in 1969 from Dalsfjorden had total DDT content of 0.57 to 2.15 mg/kg (wet weight) whereas those caught from Sonefjorden, near an intensive fruit growing area, had a residue level of 1.98 to 33 mg/kg (wet weight).[85] Cod sampled in 1971, had 90 to 135 mg/kg (wet weight) in livers; on a fat weight basis the highest residue concentration recorded was 576 mg/kg.[84] The residue content of fish decreased as one moved towards the mouth of the fjord. On a fat weight basis, the total DDT content of liver of fish caught in the Kristiansand fjord in 1975 was 0.1 in herring and 1 in the flounder (mg/kg); PCB levels were somewhat higher: 0.4 in herring, 6.3 in codling, and 1.7 in saithe (mg/kg); HCB levels were more fluctuating and sometimes high — 0.07 in herring and 27.1 in flounder.[86] Fish accumulated tri-, tetra-, penta-, and hexachlorobenzene, octachlorostyrene, and PCBs in an area polluted by industrial effluents.[87] Cod collected from 16 localities in Norway in 1976 had total DDT of 0.1 to 1.9 (and a single wayward value of 14.5); PCB, 0.7 to 7.5; and HCB, 0.02 to 2.3 (all values in mg/kg, wet weight basis).[88] Isolated pockets of contamination, as in the vicinity of a plant nursery school near Lake Ørsjøen in southern Norway, still showed high total DDT levels (14 mg/kg) in 1975 to 1976.[89] In Lake Mjøsa, low but steady levels of OCs in biological material were recorded from 1974 to 1979, indicating constant low level input of OCs from the catchment area and perhaps through atmospheric deposition.[90] The presence of toxaphene and other chlorinated terpene residues, many of which could not be correctly identified, was reported from the Baltic, North Sea, and Lake Vattern in southern Sweden.[91] On fat weight basis, the quantities (mg/kg) of various compounds recorded, respectively, in char and herring were chlordane, 0.5 and 0.6; Σ DDT, 8 and 6.8; Σ PCB, 11, and 7.9 and chlorinated terpenes (toxaphene) 9 and 13. Jensen et al.[92] considered that the levels of chlorinated hydrocarbons in the animals of the Baltic in 1965 to 1968 were five to ten times those of the biota from the North Sea and Atlantic.

The Baltic, like Lake Michigan, is one of the most highly polluted regions of the world. Detailed studies on the contaminant levels of the Baltic fauna showed that residue levels are higher in the Baltic than in the freshwaters surrounding the Baltic.[93] Jensen et al.[92] reported 4.1 to 53 mg/kg Σ DDT and 0.5 to 20 mg/kg PCB in various species of fish caught in the Baltic during 1965 to 1968; on the Swedish west coast, the levels of Σ DDT and PCB in various species of fish during the same period were, respectively, 0.3 to 3.9 and 0.4 to 16 mg/kg (fat weight). The contaminant levels reported in the ovary and liver of Baltic flounder in 1981 were (values μg/kg, wet weight) DDD-DDE 3.1 to 92 in ovary; PCB, 5 to 517 in ovary and 5 to 730 in liver; α-HCH, 0.7 to 6 in ovary and 2.9 to 13.9 in liver; and γ-HCH, 0.4 to 5.6 in ovary and 3.6 to 13.4 in liver.[94] In Finland, the level of use of DDT and other compounds was in general very low compared with that of the other countries — from 1953 to 1971, only 229 tons of DDT was used; use of other compounds in the same period was — lindane, 100; endrin, 6.8; dieldrin, 4; and aldrin, 1.5 ton. Since 1971 the sale of aldrin and dieldrin and that of DDT, except for purposes of treatment of forest nurseries, was prohibited in Finland.[93]

The Turku Archipelago, on the southwestern coast of Finland and Lake Päijänne, the second largest lake in Finland, have been extensively sampled and studied to determine the levels and trends of contaminant accumulation in Finland. The DDT and PCB levels in herring and pike collected in 1972 from Turku Archipelago were (all values in mg/kg): herring — DDT, 0.098 to 1.8 (fresh weight basis) and 4.6 to 27 (fat weight basis); PCBs, 0.19 to 1.4 (fresh weight basis) and 5.4 to 28 (fat weight basis); and pike — DDT, 0.016 to 0.052 (fresh weight basis) and 5.3 to 20 (fat weight basis); PCBs, 0.025 to 0.066 (fresh weight basis) and 12 to 32 (fat weight basis). In pike, when values are expressed for ovary fat alone, values approached 100 mg/kg Σ DDT and 190 mg/kg PCB.[95] The variation in the Σ DDT content of herring for different regions of the Baltic was much more marked than the variation in the concentration of PCBs, indicating the presence of regional influences in the transfer of the DDT group compounds to the Baltic, but the presence of a larger, widespread and more diffuse source (atmosphere?) for PCBs. In Lake Päijänne, biota from different trophic levels were analyzed from 1972 to 1974; both Σ DDT and PCB concentrations of the biota were declining in some parts of the lake, whereas in certain other parts, only DDT was declining.[96] The methyl mercury content of pike and Baltic herring from the Turku Archipelago in 1977 varied considerably between individuals from the same populations.[97] Särkka et al.[98] concluded that in Lake Päijänne, in 1978, the mercury and PCB content of fish was decreasing, whereas there was no indication of change in the Σ DDT content of fish. In an extensive survey of the residue concentration and trends from year to year, Hattula et al.[93] analyzed over 1750 samples (biota) from Lake Päijänne. Between 1970 and 1975, there was a clear downward trend of Σ DDT and PCB concentration in fish from this lake. For instance, the Σ DDT concentration of perch in different areas was 0.031 to 0.16 in 1970 and 0.003 to 0.007 in 1975 (mg/kg, fresh weight); in bream, Σ DDT concentration in 1970 was 0.022 to 0.064, whereas in 1975 it was 0.008. Likewise, the PCB concentration in perch in 1970 was 0.4 to 0.6 and 0.033 to 0.069 in 1974. These values, when compared with similar values from other areas or countries, whether in 1970 or in 1975, are rather low, indicating the relatively lesser dimension of the contaminant problem in Lake Päijänne.[93] Extensive monitoring of contaminant levels in Finnish wildlife, as Part of the OECD (Organization for Economic Cooperation and Development) monitoring program (see Section IX), indicated consistent decreasing trends of Σ DDT and PCB in Finland between 1973 and 1978.[99] Although chlordane was not used either in Sweden or Finland, 0.02 to 0.05 mg/kg chlordane was recorded in fish tissues in 1979.[100] In samples of fish collected in 1980 from Lake Päijänne, statistical treatment of the data by way of covariance analysis to eliminate the influence of fat showed increasing trends of PCB and DDE from 1972 to 1980, contrary to the earlier findings from the same lake.[101] In the same study, 10 to 70 μg/kg (fresh weight) PCB contamination of pike was reported. On the other hand, Moilanen et al.[102] concluded on the basis of statistical evaluation that time trends of PCB and DDT compounds in Finnish fish indicate a decrease from 1972 to 1982. Simultaneously, the levels of chlordane in the Baltic fish were on the rise; the 1975 levels of 0.22 to 0.61 μg/kg in the herring rose to 0.39 to 0.83 mg/kg in 1982. Likewise, in the muscle of pike, the 1971 values of 0.38 to 1.04 mg/kg rose to 2.39 to 6.3 mg/kg in 1982.[102] In the same study, an overall decline in PCB levels was observed between 1978 to 1982, as was also the case in an earlier study covering the period 1972 to 1978. The levels were not coming down any more rapidly between 1978 and 1982 than in the previous study period. One reason for this slow decline, despite the fact that PCBs were banned in Sweden in 1971, and their use in Finland was insignificant, is that perhaps there has been a steady atmospheric input of PCBs into the Baltic. In another study conducted in 1981, HCB levels were found to be on the increase in Finnish fish, compared with the previous years.[103]

Viewed in the light of its importance as an intensively fished area, information on the residue content of fish of the North Sea is meager. The PCB and Σ DDT levels in cod and herring collected in 1972 from the central North Sea were of the same magnitude as those recorded in the fish from the German Bight, British coast, and Dutch coast.[104] Reporting on the OC residue levels of Lake Constance and the Rhine River in 1976, Eichner[105] noted that while DDT was steadily declining, HCB and PCB levels were increasing. The average DDT concentration in the flatfish *Glyptocephalus cynoglossus* from Skagerrak was reported as 3 to 7.7; PCB, 10 to 37; and HCB, 0.12 to 0.63 (mg/kg, lipid weight basis).[106] In the German Wadden Sea and the Weser estuary, p,p'-DDD, DDE, α- and γ-HCH, and dieldrin levels in the range of 1 to 10 μg/kg, wet weight basis (47 to 370 μg/kg, lipid weight basis) were reported in 1976; the PCB levels were at one to two orders of magnitude higher.[107] The average values of DDT in the liver of cod in 1978, 1979, and 1980 were 2.5, 1.7, and 1.3 mg/kg, indicating a steadily declining trend.[108] On an average, samples originating from the Baltic were more heavily contaminated than those from the North Sea.[109]

HCB levels in fish in West Germany were highest in those caught in rivers, which according to the authors, might be due to unfiltered sewage discharged into the streams.[110]

In the North Adriatic Sea, goby fish (*Gibius* sp.) collected in 1974 to 1975 had 37 to 166 μg/kg Σ DDT and 75 to 157 μg/kg PCB.[111] From the Aegean Sea, all of the 142 fish and mollusc samples collected in 1975 to 1979 were contaminated with DDT and PCBs; Σ DDT in five species of fish was 23 to 1,200 μg/kg and PCB was 310 to 2,600 μg/kg;[112] aldrin and HCB were also recorded.

In Ireland, in 1966, lindane, aldrin, and dieldrin, all in the range of 0.01 to 0.6, and *p,p'*-DDT in the range of 0.03 to 0.7 (mg/kg) were reported from salmon and trout.[113] In 1972 an analysis of the tissues of stickleback, char, and trout in Iceland did not show the presence of PCB or DDT or its metabolites in any of the tissues of the first two species or in trout muscle. In the liver of trout less than 0.01 mg/kg Σ DDT and 0.13 mg/kg PCB were detected, reflecting the relatively uncontaminated nature of this remote island. These low-level contaminants indicate aerial transport from the continental land masses.[114] In a coordinated program on the pollution profiles of the North Atlantic, North Sea, Baltic, and Mediterranean, organized by the International Council for the Exploration of the Sea (ICES), cod was selected as the best species of fish for this type of comparison over a wide area.[115] In the survey for 1974 to 1976, the Σ DDT levels in the cod, plaice, and sole in the North Sea were often low; PCBs were always detected, but at a low level (< 0.18 mg/kg in 1976); of the DDT group, DDE was the predominant member, and often DDT and DDD were below detection limits. Only in a few instances did the total pesticide residues in cod taken from the Southern Bight exceed 1 mg/kg, the highest value recorded being 3.25 mg/kg. In the Baltic Sea, Σ DDT values were in the range of 1 to 230 μg/kg, average values being in the range of 15 to 55 μg/kg; values from Finland and German Democratic Republic were lower. The highest values of DDT reported from the Baltic in this survey was 27 mg/kg (wet weight); PCB concentration was generally in the range of 10 to 80 μg/kg; values from Finland and German Democratic Republic were lower; highest values of PCB in the Baltic were in the range of 1 to 12 mg/kg (wet weight). In the North Atlantic, the reported residue values were higher in the cod taken off the east coast of Canada than those taken off the west coast of Europe.[115]

C. Other Regions

Elsewhere, pesticide residues at comparatively lower levels than in fish from North America or the Baltic, have been reported from Iran, Jordan, Sudan, Lake Nubia, Lake Tanganyika, and South Africa. In a survey conducted in 1974 in Iran, the Σ DDT on fat weight basis, from *Barbus* sp. was 60.6 mg/kg from the Shahpour River and 196 mg/kg from the Kupor River. OC residues of fish from lakes and reservoirs were, in general, less than 25 mg/kg (fat weight). In one specimen of *Salmo gairdneri* the DDT was 88 mg/kg (fat weight) and in one specimen of *Alburnoides bipantatur*, Σ DDT was 279 mg/kg. The Σ DDT from the muscle of the sturgeon from the Caspian Sea was 21 to 471 and in the eggs 91 to 1783 μg/kg (fresh weight); lindane was also occasionally recorded.[116] In Jordan, in 1971, the Σ DDT residues in fish were 0.37 mg/kg in carp, 2.6 mg/kg in benith, and 3.34 mg/kg in sardines.[117] In the fish from Lake Nubia, Sudan, Σ DDT residue concentration was 2 to 184 μg/kg; elsewhere in Sudan, 0.3 to 2.9 mg/kg Σ DDT has been reported in different species.[4,118] Total DDT values of 0.7, 0.73, and 0.38 mg/kg were reported, respectively, from *Limnothrissa, Stoloth-rissa,* and *Luciolates* caught in Lake Tanganyika in 1971.[119] In two man-made lakes in South Africa, Harbeespoort and Vöelvlei Dams, dieldrin (0.25 mg/kg) and DDT (0.75 mg/kg, dry weight) were recorded in 1977.[120]

Very low level contamination of fish tissues has been reported from Mexico, Australia, and New Zealand. Levels of dieldrin and endrin were higher than DDT (all below 10 μg/kg, wet weight) in several species of fish collected in two lagoons in northwest Mexico.[121] In a general survey carried out in Tasmania, Australia in 1975 to 1977, Σ DDT concentrations reported were 0.01 to 3.6 in brown trout and 2.8 to 3.6 in rainbow trout (all values, mg/kg). In 1971 to 1972, 0.084 mg/kg Σ DDT, 0.042 mg/kg dieldrin, and 0.005 mg/kg heptachlor epoxide were reported from New Zealand fish.[122]

A survey of fish in Japan revealed the presence of total chlordane in 1977 to 1979; chlordane concentration in Japanese fish were in the range of 3 to 489 μg/kg.[123] Oxychlordane, trans-, and cis-chlordane, and cis-nonachlor were identified from gobyfish from Tokyo Bay.[124] The herbicide, CNP (1,3,5-trichloro-2-[4-nitrophenoxy]benzene), has also been reported from goby fish from Tokyo Bay, the concentration being 2.6 to 91,400 in liver and 0.1 to 360 in muscle (μg/kg).[125] The herbicide 2,4,6-trichlorophenyl p-nitrophenyl ether was identified from rainbow trout grown in Japan.[126] About 23 μg/kg of γ-chlordane was reported from freshwater fish.[127]

The above survey underlines the following points. (1) Although DDT and its analogs are ubiquitous, their concentration has not continued to rise to alarming proportions in the ecosystem, as had been projected by some studies. Soon after they were banned in many countries, the concentration of OC compounds in the biota started to decline. (2) The concentration of compounds hitherto not suspected to be environmentally hazardous, like toxaphene and chlordane, is on the increase.[128,129] (3) HCB, which was once used as a fungicide, is present in the biota, especially fish, at a greater level than what would have resulted from its pesticidal use alone. It is now known to be a by-product in many industrial processes involving chlorination and has proved to be recalcitrant in the environment. Over the years, the concentration of HCB in fish has been increasing and the signs are that it will continue to rise. (4) Compounds like PCP, despite their moderate water solubility, may prove hazardous to fish and other aquatic organisms because of their high concentration in water (up to 500 ng/ℓ), as has been reported in the Weser Estuary and the German Bight.[37,38] (5) There are many regions of the world like India where OC compounds have been employed extensively during the last few years, but the profiles of contamination of fish are largely unknown. (6) Sophisticated and improved methodologies are likely to bring into light the existence of hitherto unexpected environmental contaminants.

IV. TYPES AND RANGE OF RESIDUES IN FISH

A. Compounds

Usually only persistent compounds like the OCs are recorded in the tissues of fish. Although some of them are as toxic, if not more toxic than OCs, OPs are rarely concentrated in the fish tissues.

In an extensive survey of fish in the course of the NPMP in the U.S. in the fall of 1969, DDT and its metabolites were found in all 147 samples collected. Dieldrin was present in all but 10 samples; isomers of HCH (including lindane) were found in all but 15 of the 147 samples. No residues of aldrin, endrin, and toxaphene were detected in the analyses made[32] but the absence of toxaphene may be due to the limitation of the technique, rather than its actual absence, as improved and better techniques later demonstrated its presence all over the world.[130,131] Cis- and trans-nonachlor, which are minor components of technical chlordane, and cis- and trans-chlordane were recorded in herring and cod from the Atlantic.[132] Aldrin is epoxidized to dieldrin in nature, and in fish it is mostly dieldrin that is recorded. Generally the ratio of dieldrin to aldrin in fish is 10:1, but in catfish having 1440 μg dieldrin per kilogram, 910 μg/kg aldrin was detected.[133] Endrin is found very rarely in samples from nature; while DDT, dieldrin, HCH, and chlordane were recorded quite often during the NPMP survey in the U.S. in 1967, endrin was recorded only at three stations.[43] Methoxychlor, which is closely related to DDT, is much less persistent; 17 weeks after an application of methoxychlor to control black fly larvae in the Saskatchewan River, no residues could be found in fish.[134] Accumulation of Dursban® and diazinon in fish was very low and amounted to less than 1 mg/kg following the treatment of a tidal marsh with these two compounds.[135]

Within the DDT group, the relative proportion of the different components has been discussed. In the environmental samples, o,p'-DDT is very rarely recorded and only DDE and DDD are reported as metabolites. Addison and Zinck[136] stated that the rate of production of other degradation products of DDT like DDMU and DDMS is too slow to lead to appreciable accumulation of either. *Fundulus heteroclitus,* obtained from estuarine waters for studying the effect of DDT on reproduction, had a background contamination of 170 μg DDT per kilogram, of which p,p'-, and o,p'-isomers accounted for 50% of the observed quantity, while DDD (20 μg), DDE (20 μg), and DDMU (45 μg) accounted for the rest.[137] In general, in environmental samples, DDE is the predominant component of Σ DDT. In a model ecosystem, DDT degraded mostly to DDE and very little to DDD.[138] In an analysis of the fauna of New Jersey saltmarsh p,p'-DDE was found in 97% of the samples (vertebrates and invertebrates); p,p'-DDD was found in all fish samples, but in only 82% of the total samples (invertebrates and vertebrates) in 1967 and in 42% in 1975; p,p'-DDT was found in 86% of the samples in 1967, but only in 6% of the samples in 1973. In 1967, p,p'-DDD was the predominant component; in 1973 samples, p,p'-DDE was the more predominant component, with no detectable p,p'-DDT in many samples.[139] In marine organisms from the Aegean Sea, p,p'-DDE was reported to constitute 60 to 90% of the Σ DDT; p,p'-DDT was not present in all samples, but when present, its concentration was equal to or less than that of DDE; the concentration of DDD was less than that of p,p'-DDT.[112] In the livers of New England marine fish, in general, the concentration of DDE was more than that of DDT, but in the dogfish the reverse was true.[56] The higher quantity of DDT in dogfish in this instance is indicative of recent contamination and is usually not expected in a fish collected 160 km offshore 10 years after the virtual termination of the use of DDT. In other areas, dogfish had low p,p'-DDT concentration, with p,p'-DDE as the principal component of Σ DDT. Similarly, in *Xiphias gladius,* collected in the Aegean Sea, the DDT concentration was reported to be higher than that of DDE.[112] Likewise, in a majority of fish species collected from Lake Päijänne, Finland, p,p'-DDE was the dominant component of DDT, but in vendace p,p'-DDT constituted the major component.[98] In a survey of fish from the North Atlantic, the relative proportions of the different components was found to vary from group to group, as shown in Table 1. In fish, p,p'-DDE followed by p,p'-DDT were the more important components of Σ DDT.[140]

In fish samples from the Po River, in Italy, p,p'-DDE was the major component and p,p'-DDT was not detected.[141] Of the total DDT reported from trout eggs, fry, and fish feed, concentration of DDE was twice that of the other two components combined.[142] In fish from the eastern states of Canada, p,p'-DDE and p,p'-DDT together accounted for 80 to 95% of the Σ DDT, with the former being the principal component.[64] DDE was the most common and major component of Σ DDT in natural fish populations of the Smoky Hill River in western Kansas,[143] in the fish of the North Atlantic[115] (in the latter p,p'-DDT and p,p'-DDD were not detected in many cases),

Table 1

RELATIVE PROPORTIONS OF DDT
COMPONENTS IN FISH AND OTHER
ORGANISMS FROM NORTH ATLANTIC

	Components of Σ DDT (%)		
Group	p,p′-DDE	p,p′-DDD	p,p′-DDT
Bivalves	51	36	13
Crustacea	84	12	4
Groundfish	45	14	41
Pelagic fish	45	17	38

Data modified from Sims, G. G., Campbell, W. R., Zemlyak, F., and Graham, J. M., *Bull. Environ. Contam.
Toxicol.*, 18, 697, 1977.

and in the livers of larger fish. A higher percentage of *p,p′*-DDT indicates that the animal had been exposed to the compound in the recent past, i.e., contamination is of recent origin. Hargrave and Phillips[69] reported that fauna from St. Margaret's Bay, an area far removed from areas of intense application of pesticides, had a higher *p,p′*-DDT component in filter feeding animals. The authors suggested that atmospheric transport and adsorption of *p,p′*-DDT onto particulate matter might have been the main source of the undegraded component there. In remote lakes of the northeastern U.S. very low levels of DDE and neither DDT nor DDD were recorded.[144]

When cutthroat trout were exposed to different concentrations of DDT in water or through flood, the proportion of the three components of Σ DDT depended on the concentration or dosage of DDT administered. Those batches of fish that were exposed to lower concentration of DDT or those that received lower doses of DDT through food, as well as control fish, had a larger proportion of DDE, whereas those lots of fish that were exposed to higher concentration of DDT or received higher doses of DDT, had a higher proportion of *p,p′*-DDT.[145] Another interesting observation was that although the fish that received lower quantities of DDT had the same residue levels (Σ DDT) as control fish, they had a higher percent of DDT and lesser amounts of DDE than the control fish. After force feeding brook trout with 114 mg of radioactive DDT, five times at weekly intervals, eggs were collected and reared. One day after the eggs were laid, 7% of the DDT had been converted to DDE; as development progressed, the DDE content steadily rose, being 12.5% on the 40th day and 33.2% on the 80th day; DDD accounted for only 5.1% on the 80th day.[146] Suckers under 2 years had a slightly greater concentration of DDE than DDD, whereas older members had a higher concentration of DDD than DDE. It was suggested that metabolic changes associated with sexual maturation, especially, steroidogenesis might have caused this differ-ence.[147] Rarely was DDD the major component of total DDT. In general, it appears that under normal, natural conditions *p,p′*-DDD constitutes only a minor component of Σ DDT except when the fish pick up DDD directly from the sediments. DDD has been reported to have been produced as a result of post-mortem changes, even when the tissues were preserved at −14°C and also when stored in formalin.[3] Evidently, when the fish has enough time to metabolize the compound, DDD is the endproduct.

B. Range of Values

The extent to which the observed environmental contaminant levels represent the true population picture needs some special mention. In a discussion on the distribution of pesticide residues in natural populations, Moriarty[148] pointed out that the largest

source of variation in values is observed between individual samples from a population. The distribution of contaminant values is not normal around the mean, but is
skewed, with a long tail towards the upper end of the range. The range found between
the minimum and maximum concentration is often of the order of two magnitudes. As
a result, a few individuals may be carrying higher quantities and hence may be much
more affected by the residues than others. Another corollary of such a distribution is
that unless great effort is made at collecting a random sample, the sample may consist
of the most affected or the least affected representatives of the population. Even in
samples collected at the same time of the year and comprising specimens of the same
size, weight, and sex, standard deviation of the order of 30 to 40% of the mean is
reported to be very common.[149] In an interlaboratory comparison of methods, the
coefficient of variation of the results varied from 33 to 71%.[15] Holden[15] emphasized
that large variation exists in the residue levels of different members of the same population collected at the same time, and data from such samples show skewness rather
than normal distribution; hence, homogenizing equal aliquots from the individuals and
carrying out single analysis would not give a true picture.

In the second OECD interlaboratory comparison of analytical procedures, agreement in the analysis of standards and spiked samples was good, with a coefficient of
variation of 2 to 3%, but in the analysis of wildlife samples, the coefficient of variation
was 30.6%. Commenting on these results, Holden[150] concluded "the number of individual analyses required is consequently large if a reasonably accurate estimate of the
mean level of contamination is to be obtained." The size of the population sample
would have to be very high if small changes in the contamination level are to be identified; at least 50 individuals would be required to detect a 25% difference between
means. In a study on the total DDT residues in seven specimens of yearling pinfish,
the range of values was 0.5 to 13.7 mg/kg. The authors concluded that a composite
sample of at least 10 specimens was required to obtain a representative sample.[45]

V. RESIDUES IN DIFFERENT SIZE AND AGE GROUPS OF FISH

A. Size vs. Residue Concentration

Size-related effect on the uptake of residues has been noted by several authors. In
nature, the concentration of DDT and dieldrin was observed to increase with the age
of lake trout and walleye in the Great Lakes. As the fish grew, the total quantity of
body fat as well as the percent of fat increased; hence the fish were able to store more
pesticide.[74] Concentration of DDT in Great Lakes trout increased with length (hence
age); in the 50 to 150 mm length group, DDT concentration was 1.3 mg/kg, whereas
in the 558 to 684 mm length group, DDT concentration was 18.1 mg/kg from the
southern part of Lake Michigan.[151] PCB residues in Lake Cayuga trout also increased
with age, with a significant positive correlation between age and PCB concentration.[152]
Similar results have been reported in the case of lake trout. The levels of Σ DDT were
1 mg/kg in 1-year-old fish and 14 mg/kg in 12-year-old fish. In the age group studied
(5 to 8 years old), female trout had higher residue levels than males.[153] Heavier and
older specimens of tuna had higher concentration of DDT and PCB residues; tunas
weighing more than 600 lb had 5.4 and 4.2 mg/kg PCBs and DDT, respectively,
whereas those weighing less than 600 lb had 2.8 and 2.3 mg/kg, respectively. This
trend, however, does not seem to be universally valid, as another batch of tuna, weighing 500 to 600 lb had 0.9 and 0.7 mg/kg DDT and PCB residues.[140] According to
Monod and Keck,[154] the influence of age is more important in the male than in the
female of several species, as shown in Table 2.

Higher levels of OCs in larger herring (average weight 222 g, and 0.54 PCB, 0.43 Σ
DDT, and 0.006 HCB) than in smaller herring (average weight 59 g, and 0.32 PCB,

Table 2

PCB CONCENTRATION (MG/KG LIPID) IN THE MALES AND FEMALES OF
TWO SPECIES OF FISH FROM LAKE LEMAN

Fish	Gills		Muscle		Liver		Abdominal fat		Kidney	
	Male	Female	Male	Female	Male	Female	Male	Female	Male	Female
Roaches (3—6 years)	6.9—14	5.8—8	5.7—15	7—11	5.3—21	9.1—12	9.7—23	4.5—9.8	7.6—13	6—12
Chars (3—6 years)	4.8—24	11—22	22—41	13—22	15—38	9.4—17	25—40	16—22	12—29	11—15

Data modified from Monod, G. and Keck, G., *Bull. Environ. Contam. Toxicol.*, 29, 570, 1982.

0.19 Σ DDT, and 0.004 HCB, all values in mg/kg, wet weight) collected from the same area was noticed.[64] A positive relationship between weight of cod and liver DDT residue levels[85] and between size of fish and whole body residues of diazinon was reported.[155] *Salvelinus namaycush* collected from Lake Simcoe, in central Ontario, between 1970 and 1976, showed a difference in the accumulation of DDT in fish over and under 4 kg weight.[70] It was estimated that the fish under 4 kg (average weight 2.9 kg) were in the 5 to 8 year age group and those over 4 kg were 10 to 15 years old. Frank et al.[70] explained that the older group would have been exposed to DDT in water as well as in food for at least 5 years (in Canada, restrictions on aerial application of DDT for mosquito control were imposed in 1966 and legislative restrictions on all uses, in 1970) and for another 5 years only through the food chain; the younger fish would have accumulated their body burdens mostly through the food chain. The larger fish had a total DDT load of 161 and the younger ones 122 in 1970 (mg/kg, lipid weight basis). The total DDT levels in 1975 to 1976 were 149 in larger fish and 11.6 in younger fish. Similarly in the 1975 to 1976 samples, eggs taken from smaller *S. namaycush* had very low Σ DDT residues, whereas those obtained from larger fish had significantly higher residues (respectively, 11.1 and 163 mg/kg, lipid weight basis).[70]

The DDE and PCB levels in lake trout of Lake Cayuga correlated positively with the age of fish.[156] A similar relationship was observed between age and residue concentration in pike from the Richelieu River in Canada.[71] Mean concentration of DDT in channel catfish did not increase with age as uniformly as with body length, the mean Σ DDT concentration being more in larger fish than in smaller fish.[157] On the other hand, the PCB concentration in Lake Michigan trout was related more to age of fish rather than to the size.[158] The dieldrin concentration in the channel catfish correlated with age, sex, and lipid content.[13] Lieb et al.[159] reported that after equilibrium concentrations were reached, rainbow trout continued to accumulate PCBs at the same rate at which they grew, i.e., while the total quantity of PCB in the body steadily increased, there was no increase in the concentration of PCBs.

Contrary to the above reports on the positive relationship between size and residue concentration in various species, Kellogg and Bulkley[160] found that dieldrin concentrations in larger catfish were not always higher than in smaller fish. Further, Bulkley[157] questioned the assumption that older, larger, or fatty fish contain a higher residue concentration than younger, smaller, or leaner fish. Also, no difference in the OC levels of 3- to 9-year-old lagesild (*Coregonus albula*) collected in Lake Mjøsa, in Norway, could be detected.[90] Giam et al.[161] noticed no correlation between size and residue in regions of low pollution, but such a relationship existed in areas where the contaminant levels in the biota were high. In an experimental study on the levels of DDT in cutthroat trout exposed to DDT via water or food, no correlation was observed between the residue load and either sex or size of the fish.[145]

One reason for the conflicting reports on the presence or absence of a positive correlation between residue concentration and size, residue concentration and age, residue concentration, and reproductive state, etc. may lie in the way the residue concentration is expressed. Residue concentrations are usually reported on the basis of wet tissue weight (sometimes whole body weight) or extractable lipid weight. Very high and inconsistent variation in the residue concentration of landlocked salmon in Sebago Lake, Maine, was reported.[162] Hence, the 39 males collected were separated into three age groups which were further subdivided into lean and fat fish. DDD and DDE content increased with lipid and age; dieldrin showed a positive correlation with lipid only. DDT was significantly higher in fish at ages III+ and IV+, but not in fish at V+ age (for details of the age groups, the original paper may be consulted). Anderson and Fenderson[162] recommended that complete randomization of the samples should be given up and that the samples should be grouped according to the age and fat condition of the fish. Similarly, Bulkley et al.[13] considered that lipid content and metabolic rate may be more important factors than size.

B. Development Stage vs. Residue Concentration

No significant difference in the concentration of Σ DDT (on the basis of wet tissue weight) was observed between the males and females of channel catfish in the prespawning season.[157] On the contrary, the PCB concentration in the ovaries of Atlantic tomcod was lower than that in the testes of fish collected from the same locality.[163] In the dogfish a peculiar situation has been reported by Butler and Schutzmann.[56] Dogfish metabolize DDT very slowly and about 85% of the absorbed DDT is stored in the liver. This species requires 18 to 20 years to attain maturity and the first eggs that are formed receive the major part of DDT mobilized from the mother. Since DDT is poorly metabolized, the young dogfish stores the DDT it receives, again in the liver, until it passes on its load to its first brood of eggs. The phenomenon may be repeated every 20 years or so for a few generations. Likewise, the female Atlantic salmon is the primary source of PCB in the eggs, although the latter may be taking up PCB directly from water also.[164] DDT residue load in the eggs of coho salmon taken from Lake Michigan was two to five times that of eggs taken from coho of Lake Superior, which is in accordance with the known levels of contamination of these two lakes and their biota. Eggs of *S. gairdneri* had a total DDT concentration of 256 µg/kg of which 235 µg/kg was DDE.[116] The OC residue levels in the eggs of several species of fish from the Iowa and Mississippi Rivers were studied.[165] Levels of dieldrin were highest in all species and correlated well with the previously reported high levels of dieldrin in fish of Iowa streams. The residue levels recorded (µg/kg, wet weight basis) were dieldrin, 37 to 950; DDE, 64 to 360; DDT, 15 to 175; DDD, 32 to 180; aldrin, 162 to 175; chlordane, 72 to 350, and heptachlor epoxide, 5 to 76 in channel catfish eggs; dieldrin, 79 to 455; DDE, 110 to 190; DDT, 46 to 48; DDD, 76 to 107; and heptachlor epoxide, 10 to 69 in largemouth bass eggs; dieldrin, 142; DDE, 190; DDT, 69; DDD, 98; and heptachlor epoxide, 13 in walleye eggs; and dieldrin, 115; DDE, 57; DDT, 16; DDD, 30; and heptachlor epoxide, 13 in northern pike eggs. The relatively higher percentage of DDD of the Σ DDT in the eggs, in comparison with its generally reported low percentage in the adult fish, is noteworthy. When lake trout eggs, sacfry, and sacfry in which the yolk sac had been absorbed were experimentally exposed to 2,5,2′,5′-tetrachlorobiphenyl (TCB) (^{14}C-labeled), maximum portion (87%) of the TCB, taken up by the egg in 4 hr, was present in the yolk. In contrast, when the sacfry were exposed, about 70% of the absorbed TCB was in the tissues and the rest in the yolk. Sacfry in which the yolk was completely absorbed took up TCB more quickly and in higher quantities.[166] The body concentration of various contaminants in five species of fish and their eggs from Lakes Ontario and Erie, decreased by 5% in smallmouth bass, increased by about 10% in rainbow trout and white sucker and did not change in the white bass and yellow perch as a result of spawning.[167] In experimental studies, higher concentrations of residues were found in eggs of cutthroat trout exposed to higher concentration of DDT.[145]

VI. RELATIONSHIP BETWEEN LIPID CONTENT AND RESIDUE LOAD

Many authors express the residue content on the basis of extractable lipid. Discussing the variation observed in the DDT stored in the various tissues of brown trout, Holden[168] opined that a better assessment might be obtained if the DDT concentration was expressed in terms of extractable lipid rather than tissue weight. The choice of the solvent, according to Holden, will determine the amount of lipid extracted, although he employed carbon tetrachloride, because of its better extraction of DDT, rather than its lipid-extracting properties. Reinert[74] noted wide variation in the pesticide concentrations of different size groups of various species of Great Lakes fish; these differences between size groups and different species could be reduced by expressing the residue concentration on the lipid weight basis. He also suggested that a positive relationship existed between lipid content and residue concentration. In general, a positive correlation between lipid content and residue concentration of the tissues of marine organisms was observed, the residue concentration per lipid weight being highest in the muscle.[169] Sugiura et al.[170] and Monod and Keck[154] also arrived at a similar conclusion; the former stated that the accumulation factors of one compound in different species of fish were correlated with the lipid content of the fish; the latter noted a positive relationship between lipid content and PCB concentration of different organs of fish. A positive correlation was reported between DDT levels and lipid content of fish from San Francisco Bay.[171] The uptake and bioaccumulation of PCBs, when expressed on a wet weight basis in female fathead minnows, were thrice that of males; the concentration of Aroclor® 1248 and 1260, when expressed on a lipid basis, however, was essentially the same in both sexes.[172] In experimental exposure of fathead minnows to DDT, residue values correlated with lipid values.[173] Toxaphene residue concentration in bluegills correlated with the lipid content rather than the weight of fish.[174] The persistence and quantities of chlordane in the tissues of redhorse suckers (*Mixostoma macrolepidotum*) were directly related to the lipid content. The net assimilation from food was also influenced by the extent of adiposity of the fish. The results of the study by Roberts et al.[175] showed that the steady state concentration of chlordane in the fish did not exceed the steady state concentration of chlordane in the diet unless the lipid content of the fish was high. PCP residues in fatty fish like eel were reported to be higher than those in lean fish like pike.[176] PCB residue load in the female fathead minnows during spawning was twice that of the males, which was attributable to the change in the lipid content during spawning.[172,177]

Although all the above-cited works suggest a direct relationship between the lipid content and total residue concentration, other workers found no such correlation; no relationship was noted between PCB concentration and lipid content of striped bass collected from the Hudson River.[178] Keck and Raffenot[179] could establish no relation between the lipid content of different tissues of fish and the levels of PCB. Further, they noted that although salmonids had a much higher muscle lipid content, the PCB concentration of the muscle of a lean fish — chub — was much higher. In chinook and coho salmon, the lipid content was related negatively with PCB and DDE levels; DDT showed no correlation at all with the lipid.[180] The lack of correlation is perhaps due to the mobilization of fat during the period immediately preceding spawning. The authors considered that expressing the residue content on a fat basis could be misleading. Although the lipid content of 2-year-old cod caught off the Finnish coast did not vary appreciably, considerable variation in the OC content of the cod tissues was reported.[100] Zitko and Carson[181] pointed out that on the basis of the steric factors, isopropyl PCBs should be more soluble in lipids than the PCBs, and consequently should be accumulated by the aquatic organisms to a greater extent than Aroclor® 1242. In practice, accumulation of isopropyl PCBs is less than that of PCBs. The presence of the isopropyl group renders them amenable to oxidation and excretion. Although, in general, higher Σ DDT concentration was found in animals rich in lipid, the residue concentration in whole organisms or muscle tissue did not correlate well with lipid content.[69] Kleinert et al.[182] reported that the relationship between DDT levels and percentage of fat was not well defined and was insignificant in fish from Wisconsin. Bulkley[157] pointed out that fish with the highest fat content (11%) contained less DDT in muscle than those that had less than 1% fat in muscle. Henderson et al.[32] could not establish a definite correlation between lipid content and insecticide residues. The condition of the organisms is also very important, stressed organisms absorbing more contaminants. Tadpoles that were reared at a higher density per unit volume of water absorbed a higher quantity of DDT although they had a lower lipid content (420 mg of DDT, with 18 mg lipid per gram weight) than those reared at a lower density and had a higher lipid content (110 mg of DDT, with 23 mg lipid per gram weight).[183] Moreover, the lipid content of individual members of a population may vary as much as 100%. The percentage of lipid in the herring from the same school may vary between 2 and 10, and expressing residue concentration by lipid weight causes variation in the expressed values too.[10] Further, expressing residue concentration on lipid weight basis may not give a true picture. Holden,[168] who advocated the expression of residue concentration on lipid basis, reported that the amount of solvent extractable lipid in the brain was high, yet the concentration of DDT in brain was low in comparison with other tissues. Although the lipid content was the same, guppies acclimated to salt water bioconcentrated three times more α-HCH than those acclimated to freshwater.[184] PCB concentration in chinook and coho salmon was twice that of yellow perch, even though the lipid content of all three species was the same.[185] Variation in percent body fat could explain the levels of residues within a particular species, but did not explain differences in concentration in different species.[186] Grzenda et al.[187,188] did not find any correlation between dieldrin concentration and tissue lipid content and hence questioned the belief that lipid solubility is the most important factor in residue buildup. After equilibrium concentration of PCB in rainbow trout was reached, the relative concentration of PCB in lipid remained constant, although the absolute quantity increased.[159] Allison et al.[145] rightly emphasized: "The distribution of the reported components [of DDT, *sic*] is probably not a function of the lipid content of the various organs but may reflect individual rates of uptake and discharge and of metabolic formation and degradation." Pointing out that maximum concentration of DDE was found in larger individuals, Hamelink and Waybrant[62] commented that the larger individuals display a higher concentration of contaminants regardless of the lipid content because of a multicompartment, countercurrent distribution in operation in the body of fish, which would permit maximum extraction efficiency. The retention of a xenobiotic chemical is not only a function of uptake and partitioning into the body lipid, but also that of elimination, the body concentration being the result of the equilibrium achieved between uptake, deposition, metabolism, and excretion. Although rainbow trout had a higher body lipid content than that of yellow perch, the elimination of 4-chlorobiphenyl (2,5,2′,5′-TCB) was similar in both species, indicating that lipid content is not a primary determinant of the rate of retention in the body.[189]

The absorption and retention of residues by fish seem to depend not only on the lipid content within the body but on many intricate factors without. Vanderford and

Hamelink[190] demonstrated that Σ DDT and dieldrin concentration in fish negatively correlated with turbidity and the trophic state in nine natural lakes, in contrast to which the residue concentration in fish was positively correlated with turbidity and the trophic state of the lake in five man-made reservoirs in Indiana. In the former, adsorption to seston (mostly algal particles) made the pesticide molecules nonavailable to the fish, whereas in the latter, adsorption to suspended soil particles acted as a sustained source.

Yet another reason for the observed inconsistency between lipid content and residue concentration may be the method used for extracting the lipid. It is well known that not all types of lipids are extractable. For instance, of the lipids in the pyloric caeca, which often contain high residue loads, only 10% of the lipids was extractable, whereas depot fat contained 80 to 90% extractable lipids.[191] Roberts et al.[175] suggested that the lipid content of the tissues should be expressed in terms of total neutral lipid, since phospholipids do not appear to form part of the lipid pool involved in pesticide storage. Although separate methods for extraction of lipids and pesticide residues have been adopted by a few workers,[32,53] there was no significant difference in the amount of endrin extracted from the brain of *Gambusia* following extraction of the tissue by hexane or chloroform-methanol,[192] the latter being the most widely employed solvent system for maximum recovery of lipids.

Phillips[193] recommended the expression of residue concentration both on wet weight and lipid weight basis, which perhaps helps reduce the variability among samples. As was emphasized by Hamelink and Spacie[194] "residue-lipid content correlations do not necessarily prove a cause and effect relationship." The relationship between lipophilicity and uptake of xenobiotic compounds by fish is discussed in detail in the next chapter.

VII. SEASONAL CHANGES IN PESTICIDE RESIDUE LEVELS IN FISH AND OTHER CONSIDERATIONS

A. Influence of Seasons

Seasonal variation in residue concentration is related to the season of application on land, and the transport to the aquatic environment, as well as the condition of the fish, extent of feeding, stage of reproduction, and the like. Coho salmon in Lake Michigan accumulated the maximum concentration of DDT between June and August preceding the spawning migration.[151] The first year class fish in 1965 had a concentration of 2 to 4 mg/kg from September to next June, but the concentration increased to 12.3 mg/kg by August 1966. The rapid increase before spawning is attributable to the increase in the total lipid content of the fish. Such a marked increase, however, was not noticeable in coho salmon of comparable age collected from Lake Erie. The reason for the difference, in part, was that coho from Lake Erie were half the weight of coho of comparable age from Lake Michigan. Correlations of PCB concentration in carp from Saginaw Bay, Lake Huron with size and weight of fish were highest in spring and summer.[195] The levels of Σ DDT and heptachlor in fish surveyed in the U.S. during NPMP in 1967 to 1968 were higher in fall than in spring; those of dieldrin, however, were higher in spring than in fall.[43] Concentration of pesticides in water and biota of the Lost River system (California) peaked in the summer growing season.[42] The DDT and PCB levels in roach and perch taken from the discharge point of a nuclear power plant correlated with the temperature of water and were substantially higher in spring and early summer and stable in late summer and autumn.[196] In Oliver Lake, the Σ DDT levels in fish decreased from summer to fall and increased in spring, high residue values in fish coinciding with the period of maximum runoff following spring rains.[190] Vanderford and Hamelink[190] described the seasonal changes in the residue concentration of fish associated with the spring and fall turnover in Oliver Lake. Maximum PCB levels occurred in the fish of Lake Roxen, in Sweden, in the spring and early summer and decreased rapidly thereafter.[197] This increase in the spring of 1975 was not the result of spring overturn, as there was mixing of water all through the warm winter of 1974 to 1975, and yet a maximum occurred in the spring, which was perhaps related to the spawning activity in May. The rate of mirex loss from treated baits was lower during fall and winter[198] and was presumably related to environmental temperatures. Cod from Norwegian fjords had the highest DDT residues in May.[84] No significant difference existed in dieldrin concentration between the various length groups of catfish in June, but a significant difference did develop later.[13] Seasonal trends in the mixed function oxidase activity, leading to differences in rates of metabolism of xenobiotic chemicals was reported in roaches from a polluted environment.[199]

Significant seasonal changes in residue concentration, observed when the concentration was expressed on tissue weight basis, disappeared when the concentration was expressed on lipid weight basis.[71] Zabik et al.[200] and Henderson et al.[32] reported minimal seasonal variation in residue loads. Nonmigrating juveniles of winter flounders were supposed to indicate seasonal patterns of accumulation much better than migrating adults.[201]

B. Influence of Trophic Level

Trophic level seems to have little influence on body residue levels. Biological magnification was not evident in small species occupying higher trophic levels.[143] Although the cyprinid *Varichorhinus* sp. belonged to a lower trophic level than *Salmo* sp. both had the same amount of Σ DDT.[116] No significant difference in the residues of trifluralin in fish belonging to different trophic levels was detected. Thus the residue burden in fish seems to be influenced more by other factors like lipid content, size and condition of the body, reproductive stage, etc., rather than by its mere position in the food pyramid.

C. Pesticide Residues in Fish and Spatial Considerations

The physical characters and other environmental conditions of the water body are also important factors that determine the levels of residue contamination in the fish. The work of Vanderford and Hamelink[190] on the relationship between the degree of eutrophication and the residue concentration in largemouth bass has already been discussed. The residue concentrations of animals of various types of water bodies are enclosed ponds > free flowing creeks > larger bodies like lakes > contiguous bay estuaries.[47] Fish species living in similar environments and depending on the same food had similar concentration of pollutants.[111] In general, in the freshwater environment, Σ DDT is accumulated to the same extent as, or more than, PCBs. In the marine environment, distinctly more PCBs are accumulated by the same species as is shown by salmon from the Miramichi River in Canada after they migrated to the sea. Residues in fish of lakes in recreational areas were higher than those in fish from larger lakes like Lake Ontario and Lake Erie.[202] When rivers drain dryland farming areas, the transport of residues to the aquatic ecosystem and hence consequent uptake by fish were less.[143]

Freshwater fish, in general, have higher residue burdens than marine fish.[90,141] Estuarine fish and fish from coastal areas have higher residue levels than those from open ocean waters.[203] Bottom dwelling coastal fish have higher levels than the pelagic forms from open oceans.[204] Deep sea dwelling fish had higher residue loads than pelagic fish like cod from the same locality.[205] It was suggested that higher levels in the bottom dwellers were due to higher levels of residues adsorbed to the bottom and suspended sediments.[186] Bottom feeders are known to aggregate very high quantities of dieldrin.[133]

The high levels of DDD observed in the bottom feeding carps correlated well with the DDD content of the top 12 cm of the sediment.[206]

VIII. DISTRIBUTION OF RESIDUES IN DIFFERENT BODY TISSUES

The distribution of residues in different parts of the fish body is of some interest for the humans. Usually, only the fillet or edible portion used for human consumption is analyzed. On the other hand, a carnivorous fish or bird would not discriminate between the so-called "edible and nonedible" parts and hence from the environmental point of view the residues of the whole body are of interest. Residues in the whole body are usually greater than the concentration in the edible part.[147] Head slices of fish, which usually have more lipid are also reported to have higher concentration of pesticides, but when the residue concentration is expressed on fat weight basis, the difference in the concentration in head slices or body muscle was not marked.[200] The fatty, median muscle and belly flap contained the highest amount of residues.[200] It is suggested that the residue concentration could be reduced by trimming. Reinert and Bergman,[151] who also reported higher residue content from belly flap, however, felt that trimming would be of little benefit.

Among the different organs, liver and muscle are often analyzed for residues. The relative proportion of metabolites of DDT was the same in muscle and liver.[207] The residue concentration in muscle was more than that of the liver,[4,159,169] whereas the reverse was also reported.[56,115,208] Relatively high concentrations of residues were found in testes, ovaries, and eggs in fish.[48,116,143] Finally, enrichment of the residue concentration in fish oils was observed.[50,209-213]

IX. MONITORING THE PESTICIDE RESIDUES IN THE ENVIRONMENT

Monitoring is the repetitive observation of one or more segments of the environment to ascertain the levels and temporal trends of contaminants in the environment on a region-, state-, nation-, or multination-wide basis.[214] The best known among the monitoring programs to ascertain pesticide residues and other contaminants in the environment is the NPMP in the U.S., which was organized in pursuance of the recommendation of the President's Science Advisory Committee Report.[215] The monitoring of contaminants in fish commenced in 1967, with fish being collected from 50 stations in the U.S. In 1967 and 1968, fish were collected in spring and again in fall. Since 1969, collections have been made only in the fall (collections were suspended in 1976) and by 1980, the number of stations was increased to 117. The number of contaminants analyzed was 8 in the beginning and increased to 20 by 1980. Details of the NPMP have been described by Henderson et al.,[43] Schmitt et al.,[53] Schmitt et al.,[216] and Ludke and Schmitt.[214]

In the U.S., the NPMP has served the following useful purposes: (1) It has helped in discerning the trends in the levels of some important problem compounds like DDT. The steady decline in DDT concentration in U.S. fish samples is now clearly established (Figure 1). (2) Areas of prolonged and persistent contamination are identified and efforts are made to identify the source and magnitude of the regional problem. (3) Appearance of any new contaminants in the environmental samples is immediately identified and the program suitably altered to keep track of the trends of the newly identified contaminants. Thus, PCBs were added to the list in 1969 and HCB in 1971. (4) Based on the results of analyses, new analytical approaches are devised.[214]

A multination attempt to monitor OC residues in the wildlife was organized in 1967 to 1968 involving 17 laboratories in 11 countries by the OECD. The precision with

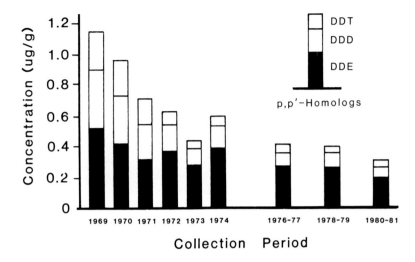

FIGURE 1.   Geometric mean concentrations of *p,p'*-DDT homologs in freshwater fish, 1969 to 1981. U.S. Fish and Wildlife Service, NPMP. (From Schmitt, C. J., Zajicek, J. L., and Ribick, M. A., *Arch. Environ. Contam. Toxicol.,* in press. With permission.)

which the different laboratories analyzed and reported the values, in the standards provided, was evaluated.[150] As a second part of the program, the background contamination in four species was sought to be identified. In 1969 to 1971 the program was slightly enlarged to include species of wildlife from both terrestrial and aquatic environments. Subsequently, this program has been extended, with part of the emphasis being on the evaluation of the comparability of methods of analysis between different laboratories. The objectives of such a monitoring, similar to that organized by the NPMP have been outlined by Holden.[15] The ICES carried out a coordinated monitoring program for the Baltic, North Sea, and North Atlantic. Beginning in 1972, baseline studies on pollution levels were made.[115] The ICES considered that cod was best suited to monitor the contaminant levels in various parts of the marine environment covered by this survey.

Residue methods, like the short term toxicity tests, may be used to monitor the environmental stress to which the organism is subjected. Since the death of channel catfish exposed to endrin occurred only after a threshold value of endrin in blood was reached, Mount et al.[217] proposed that endrin concentration of blood in fish could be used as a diagnostic tool to confirm the suspicion that endrin had caused death. Likewise, Mount and Boyle[218] proposed that the blood concentration of parathion could be used as a confirmation of the cause of death in the event of suspicion of fishkills in nature because of environmental contamination by parathion. On the other hand, based on the experience of uptake by caged fish, which contained less residues than wildfish in the same stretch of river following application of methoxychlor to control black fly larvae, Lockhart et al.[219] considered that residue methods could not be relied upon as environmental tools.

While residue methods have helped in discerning the trends of accumulation of environmental contaminants and in identifying hazardous compounds, Niimi[220] utilized the information on the PCB residue burden of lake trout and coho salmon from Great Lakes in a novel way to estimate the annual gross growth efficiency. The food intake was estimated from annual increases in body residue loads of PCBs, assuming 100 or 80% assimilation and little or poor metabolism and elimination. The annual growth was estimated from age vs. weight relationship.

X. CONCLUSIONS

Residues of persistent pesticides have been reported from different parts of the globe. Much of this information is based on studies conducted in two regions: North America and the Scandinavian countries. In these regions, declining trends in the residue burdens of fish have been evident since the banning of many OC insecticides in the western countries. Even as the DDT group compounds are on the decline, the concentrations of other problematic compounds like HCB and toxaphene are on the increase. Elsewhere, the available information, though meager, indicates lower buildup of residues than in North America or certain parts of Europe. The recent increase in the application of OC compounds in developing countries is an immediate cause for concern in those countries. Since DDT-type compounds are known to spread far and wide, the escalated use of these compounds in developing countries may eventually contribute to the continued presence of these compounds in the fish of other regions.

In general, the residue burden seems well correlated with the lipid content, size, and age, though certain exceptions are known. Among the DDT group, DDE constitutes the major component. Trophic level has little influence on the residue burden of fish. Residue levels are higher in detrivores than in others; in freshwater fish than in marine fish and in lipid-rich organs like gonads than in other tissues.

Ever since it was realized that persistent pesticides are environmentally hazardous, attempts have been afoot in a few countries to monitor the trends of residue concentrations in fish and other biota. The NPMP is the best known and the most well organized among all such attempts. Since the ban imposed on such chemicals, the levels of DDT and other OC insecticides in the environment as well as the biota have been decreasing in the U.S. and other countries. In Europe, such a monitoring is organized by the OECD and the ICES.

REFERENCES

1. Hunt, E. G. and Bischoff, A. L., Inimical effects on wildlife of periodic DDD applications to Clear Lake, *Calif. Fish Game,* 46, 91, 1960.
2. Moy, D. C. and Dredge, M. C. L., A novel biopsy technique for monitoring environmental contaminants in fish, *Bull. Environ. Contam. Toxicol.,* 22, 35, 1979.
3. French, M. C. and Jefferies, D. J., The preservation of biological tissue for organochlorine insecticide analysis, *Bull. Environ. Contam. Toxicol.,* 6, 460, 1971.
4. Elzorgani, G. A., Abdulla, A. M., and Ali, M. E. T., Residues of organochlorine insecticides in fishes in Lake Nubia, *Bull. Environ. Contam. Toxicol.,* 22, 44, 1979.
5. Pick, F. E., de Beer, P. R., and van Dyk, L. P., Organochlorine insecticide residues in birds and fish from the Transvaal, South Africa, *Chemosphere,* 10, 1243, 1981.
6. Deubert, K. H., Timmerman, J. S., and McCloskey, L. R., Effects of fixation on the extraction of dieldrin and p,p′-DDT from muscle tissue, *Bull. Environ. Contam. Toxicol.,* 9, 54, 1973.
7. Miles, J. W., Dale, W. E., and Churchill, F. C., Storage and analysis of samples of water, fish, and mud from environments contaminated with Abate, *Arch. Environ. Contam. Toxicol.,* 5, 29, 1976.
8. Pesticide Analytical Manual, Food and Drug Administration, Washington, D.C., 1977, 1.
9. Hesselberg, R. J. and Johnson, J. L., Column extraction of pesticides from fish, fish food and mud, *Bull. Environ. Contam. Toxicol.,* 7, 116, 1972.
10. Hattula, M. L., Some aspects of the recovery of chlorinated residues (DDT-type compounds and PCB) from fish tissue by using different extraction methods, *Bull. Environ. Contam. Toxicol.,* 12, 301, 1974.
11. Veith, G. D. and Kiwus, L. M., An exhaustive steam-distillation and solvent-extraction unit for pesticides and industrial chemicals, *Bull. Environ. Contam. Toxicol.,* 17, 631, 1977.
12. Ernst, W., Schaefer, R. G., Goerke, M., and Eder, G., Auf Arbeitung von Meerestierer fur die Bestimmung von PCB, DDT, DDE, DDD, γ-HCH and HCB, *Z. Anal. Chem.,* 272, 358, 1974.

13. Bulkley, R. V., Kellogg, R. L., and Shannon, L. R., Size-related factors associated with dieldrin concentrations in muscle tissue of channel catfish *Ictalurus punctatus, Trans. Am. Fish. Soc.,* 105, 301, 1976.
14. Dimond, J. B., Getchell, A. S., and Blease, J. A., Accumulation and persistence of DDT in a lotic ecosystem, *J. Fish. Res. Board Can.,* 28, 1877, 1971.
15. Holden, A. V., Organochlorines — an overview, *Mar. Pollut. Bull.,* 12, 110, 1981.
16. Jensen, S., Renberg, L., and Verz, R., Rep. PCB Conf. II, Stockholm, December 1972, National Swedish Environment Protection Board, Publications 1973: 4E; as cited in Hattula, M. L., Some aspects of the recovery of chlorinated residues (DDT-type compounds and PCB) from fish tissue by using different extraction methods, *Bull. Environ. Contam. Toxicol.,* 12, 301, 1974.
17. Eberhardt, L. L., Meeks, R. L., and Peterle, T. J., Food chain model for DDT kinetics in a fresh-water marsh, *Nature,* 390, 60, 1971.
18. Addison, R. F., Zinck, M. E., Leahy, J. R., Metabolism of single and combined doses of ^{14}C-aldrin and ^{3}H-p,p′-DDT by Atlantic salmon (*Salmo salar*) fry, *J. Fish. Res. Board Can.,* 33, 2073, 1976.
19. Stalling, D. L. and Huckins, J. N., Metabolism of 2,4-dichlorophenoxyacetic acid (2,4-D) in bluegills and water, *J. Agric. Food Chem.,* 26, 447, 1978.
20. Huckins, J. N. and Petty, J. D., Dynamics of isopropylphenyl diphenyl phosphate in fathead minnows, *Chemosphere,* 12, 799, 1983.
21. Quistad, G. B., Schooley, D. A., Staiger, L. E., Bergot, B. J., Sleight, B. H., and Macek, K. J., Environmental degradation of the insect growth regulator methoprene. IX. Metabolism by bluegill fish, *Pestic. Biochem. Physiol.,* 6, 523, 1976.
22. Krzeminski, S. F., Gilbert, J. T., and Ritts, J. A., A pharmacokinetic model for predicting pesticide residues in fish, *Arch. Environ. Contam. Toxicol.,* 5, 157, 1977.
23. Gunther, F. A., Interpreting pesticide residue data at the analytical level, *Residue Rev.,* 76, 155, 1980.
24. Maini, P. and Collina, A., Photochemically induced artifact in the analysis of soil for residues of organochlorine pesticides, *Bull. Environ. Contam. Toxicol.,* 14, 593, 1975.
25. Skaar, D. R., Johnson, B. T., Jones, J. R., and Huckins, J. N., Fate of Kepone and mirex in a model aquatic environment: sediment, fish and diet, *Can. J. Fish. Aquat. Sci.,* 38, 931, 1981.
26. Hodgson, D. W., Kantor, E. J., and Mann, J. B., Analytical methodology for the determination of Kepone residues in fish, shellfish, and hi-vol air filters, *Arch. Environ. Contam. Toxicol.,* 7, 99, 1978.
27. Huckins, J. N. and Petty, J. D., Problems associated with the purification of pentachlorophenol for biological studies, *Bull. Environ. Contam. Toxicol.,* 27, 836, 1981.
28. Atallah, Y. H., Whitacre, D. M., and Polen, P. B., Artifacts in monitoring-related analysis of human adipose tissue for some organochlorine pesticides, *Chemosphere,* 1, 17, 1977.
29. Holmes, D. C., Simmons, J. H., and Tatton, J. O'G., Chlorinated hydrocarbons in British wildlife, *Nature,* 216, 227, 1967.
30. Jensen, S., Report of a new chemical hazard, *New Sci.,* 32, 612, 1966.
31. Markin, G. P., Hawthorne, J. C., Collins, H., L., and Ford, J. H., Levels of mirex and some other organochlorine residues in seafood from Atlantic and Gulf coastal states, *Pestic. Monit. J.,* 7, 139, 1974.
32. Henderson, C., Inglis, A., and Johnson, W. L., Organochlorine insecticide residues in fish — Fall 1969 National Pesticide Monitoring Program, *Pestic. Monit. J.,* 5, 1, 1971.
33. Frazier, B. E., Chesters, G., and Lee, G. B., Apparent organochlorine insecticide contents of soils sampled in 1910, *Pestic. Monit. J.,* 4, 67, 1970.
34. Mayer, F. L., Petty, J. D., Kozlovskaya, V. I., and Flerov, B. A., The determination of residual amounts of organochlorine pesticides in the Rybinsk Reservoir fish, *Hydrobiol. J.,* 17, 63, 1982.
35. Kuehl, D. W., Leonard, E. N., Welch, K. J., and Veith, G. D., Identification of hazardous organic chemicals in fish from the Ashtabul River, Ohio, Wabash River, Indiana, *J. Assoc. Off. Anal. Chem.,* 63, 1238, 1980.
36. Glass, G. E., Strachan, W. M. I., Willford, W. A., Armstrong, F. A. I., Kaiser, K. L. E., and Lutz, A., Organic contaminants, in *The Waters of Lake Huron and Lake Superior, Vol. 2* (Part B), *Lake Huron, Georgian Bay, and the North Channel.* Rep. Int. Jt. Comm. Upper Great Lakes Ref. Group., Windsor, Ontario, 577—590, 667—670, 1977.
37. Ernst, W. and Weber, K., The fate of pentachlorophenol in the Weser Estuary and the German Bight, *Veroeff. Inst. Meeresforsch. Bremerhaven,* 17, 45, 1978.
38. Weber, K. and Ernst, W., Levels and pattern of chlorophenols in water of the Weser Estuary and the German Bight, *Chemosphere,* 11, 873, 1978.
39. Neidermyer, W. J. and Hickey, J. J., Chronology of organochlorine compounds in Lake Michigan fish, 1929—66, *Pestic. Monit. J.,* 10, 92, 1976.
40. Lyman, L. D., Tompkins, W. A., McCann, J. A., Residues in fish, wildlife, and estuaries, *Pestic. Monit. J.,* 2, 109, 1968.

41. Stucky, N. P., Pesticide residues in channel catfish from Nebraska, *Pestic. Monit. J.*, 4, 62, 1970.
42. Godsil, P. J. and Johnson, W. C., Pesticide monitoring of the aquatic biota at the Tule Lake National Wildlife Refuge, *Pestic. Monit. J.*, 1, 21, 1968.
43. Henderson, C., Johnson, W. L., and Inglis, A., Organochlorine insecticide residues in fish (National Pesticide Monitoring Program), *Pestic. Monit. J.*, 3, 145, 1969.
44. Anon., DDT: U.S. legislators propose nationwide ban . . . , *Environ. Sci. Technol.*, 3, 419, 1969.
45. Hansen, D. J. and Wilson, A. J., Jr., Significance of DDT residues from the estuary near Pensacola, Fla., *Pestic. Monit. J.*, 4, 51, 1970.
46. Hannon, M. R., Greichus, Y. A., Applegate, R. L., and Fox, A. C., Ecological distribution of pesticides in Lake Poinsett, South Dakota, *Trans. Am. Fish. Soc.*, 99, 496, 1970.
47. Naqvi, S. M. and de la Cruz, A. A., Mirex incorporation in the environment: residues in nontarget organisms — 1972, *Pestic. Monit. J.*, 7, 104, 1973.
48. Ginn, T. M. and Fisher, F. M., Jr., Studies on the distribution of flux of pesticides in waterways associated with a ricefield-marshland ecosystem, *Pestic. Monit. J.*, 8, 23, 1974.
49. Miller, F. M. and Gomes, E. D., Detection of DCPA residues in environmental samples, *Pestic. Monit. J.*, 8, 53, 1974.
50. Johnson, J. L., Stalling, D. L., and Hogan, J. W., Hexachlorobenzene (HCB) residues in fish, *Bull. Environ. Contam. Toxicol.*, 11, 393, 1974.
51. Crockett, A. B., Wiersma, G. B., Tai, H., and Mitchell, W., Pesticide and mercury residues in commercially grown catfish, *Pestic. Monit. J.*, 8, 235, 1975.
52. Laska, A. L., Bartell, C. K., and Laseter, J. L., Distribution of hexachlorobenzene and hexachlorobutadien in water, soil and selected aquatic organisms along the lower Mississippi River, Louisiana, *Bull. Environ. Contam. Toxicol.*, 15, 535, 1976.
53. Schmitt, C. J., Ludke, J. L., and Walsh, D. F., Organochlorine residues in fish: National Pesticide Monitoring Program, 1970—74, *Pestic. Monit. J.*, 14, 136, 1981.
54. McDermott-Ehrlich, D., Young, D. R., and Heesen, T. C., DDT and PCB in flatfish around southern California municipal outfalls, *Chemosphere*, 7, 453, 1978.
55. Giam, C. S., Chan, H. S., and Neff, G. S., Phthalate ester plasticizers, DDT, DDE and polychlorinated biphenyls in biota from the Gulf of Mexico, *Mar. Pollut. Bull.*, 9, 249, 1978.
56. Butler, P. A. and Schutzmann, R. L., Bioaccumulation of DDT and PCB in tissues of marine fishes, *Aquatic Toxicology*, ASTM STP 667, Marking, L. L. and Kimerle, R. A., Eds., American Society for Testing and Materials, Philadelphia, 1979, 212.
57. Anon., EPA bans most DDT uses, readies lead action, *Environ. Sci. Technol.*, 6, 675, 1972.
58. Glass, G. E., Strachan, W. M. I., Willford, W. A., Armstrong, F. A. I., Kaiser, K. L. E., and Lutz, A., Organic contaminants, in *The Waters of Lake Huron and Lake Superior, Vol. 3 (Part B), Lake Superior Rep. Int. Jt. Comm., Upper Great Lakes Ref. Group,* Windsor, Ontario, 417—429, 499—502, 1977.
59. Harrison, H. L., Loucks, O. L., Mitchell, J. W., Parkhurst, D. F., Tracy, C. R., Watts, D. G., and Yannacone, V. J., Jr., A systems analysis provides new insights for predicting long-term impacts of DDT in ecosystems, *Science*, 170, 503, 1970.
60. Bloom, S. G. and Menzel, D. B., Decay time of DDT, *Science*, 172, 213, 1971.
61. Woodwell, G. M., Craig, P. P., and Johnson, H. A., DDT in the biosphere — where does it go?, *Science*, 174, 1101, 1971.
62. Hamelink, J. L. and Waybrant, R. C., DDE and lindane in a large-scale model lentic ecosystem, *Trans. Am. Fish. Soc.*, 105, 124, 1976.
63. Fredeen, F. J. H., Saha, J. G., and Royer, L. M., Residues of DDT, DDE, and DDD in fish in the Saskatchewan River after using DDT as a blackfly larvicide for twenty years, *J. Fish. Res. Board Can.*, 28, 105, 1971.
64. Zitko, V., Organochlorine pesticides in some freshwater and marine fishes, *Bull. Environ. Contam. Toxicol.*, 6, 464, 1971.
65. Freeman, H. C. and Horne, D. A., Total mercury and methylmercury content of the American eel (*Anguilla rostrata*), *J. Fish. Res. Board Can.*, 30, 454, 1971.
66. Zitko, V., Hutzinger, O., and Choi, P. M. K., Determination of pentachlorophenol and chlorobiphenylols in biological samples, *Bull. Environ. Contam. Toxicol.*, 12, 649, 1974.
67. Frank, R., Armstrong, A. E., Boelens, R. G., Braun, H. E., and Douglas, C. W., Organochlorine insecticide residues in sediment and fish tissues, Ontario, Canada, *Pestic. Monit. J.*, 7, 165, 1974.
68. Albright, L. J., Northcote, T. G., Oloffs, P. C., and Szeto, S. Y., Chlorinated hydrocarbon residues in fish, and shellfish of the lower Fraser River, its estuary, and selected locations in Georgia Strait, British Columbia — 1972—73, *Pestic. Monit. J.*, 9, 134, 1975.
69. Hargrave, B. T. and Phillips, G. A., DDT residues in benthic invertebrates and demersal fish in St. Margaret's Bay, Nova Scotia, *J. Fish. Res. Board Can.*, 33, 1692, 1976.
70. Frank, R., Holdrinet, M. V. H., Desjardine, R. L., and Dodge, D. P., Organochlorine and mercury residues in fish from Lake Simcoe, Ontario 1970—76, *Environ. Biol. Fish.*, 3, 275, 1978.

71. Boileau, S., Baril, M., and Alary, J. G., DDT in northern pike *(Esox lucius)* from the Richelieu River, Quebec, Canada, 1974—75, *Pestic. Monit. J.,* 13, 109, 1979.
72. Tsui, P. R. P. and McCart, P. J., Chlorinated hydrocarbon residues and heavy metals in several fish species from the Cold Lake area in Alberta, Canada, *Int. J. Environ. Anal. Chem.,* 10, 277, 1981.
73. Kaiser, K. L. E., Early trend determination of organochlorine contamination from residue ratios in the sea lamprey (*Petromyzon marinus*) and its lake whitefish (*Coregonus clupeaformis*) host, *Can. J. Fish. Aquat. Sci.,* 39, 571, 1982.
74. Reinert, R. E., Pesticide concentrations in Great Lakes fish, *Pestic. Monit. J.,* 3, 233, 1970.
75. Carr, R. L., Finsterwalder, C. E., and Schibi, M. J., Chemical residues in Lake Erie fish — 1970—71, *Pestic. Monit. J.,* 6, 23, 1972.
76. Kelso, J. R. M. and Frank, R., Organochlorine residues, mercury, copper and cadmium in yellow perch, white bass and smallmouth bass, Long Point Bay, Lake Erie, *Trans. Am. Fish. Soc.,* 103, 577, 1974.
77. Kaiser, K. L. E., Mirex: an unrecognized contaminant of fishes from Lake Ontario, *Science,* 185, 523, 1974.
78. Parejko, R., Johnson, R., and Keller, R., Chlorohydrocarbons in Lake Superior lake trout *(Salvelinus namaycush), Bull. Environ. Contam. Toxicol.,* 14, 480, 1975.
79. Leatherland, J. F. and Sonstegard, R. A., Lowering of serum thyroxine and triiodothyronine levels in yearling coho salmon, *Oncorhynchus kisutch,* by dietary mirex and PCBs, *J. Fish. Res. Board Can.,* 35, 1285, 1978.
80. Moccia, R. D., Leatherland, J. F., and Sonstegard, R. A., Increasing frequency of thyroid goiters in coho salmon (*Oncorhynchus kisutch*) in the Great Lakes, *Science,* 198, 425, 1977.
81. Moccia, R. D., Leatherland, J. F., Sonstegard, R. A., and Holdrinet, M. V. H., Are goiter frequencies in Great Lakes salmon correlated with organochlorine residues?, *Chemosphere,* 7, 649, 1978.
82. Niimi, A. J., Hexachlorobenzene (HCB) levels in Lake Ontario salmonids, *Bull. Environ. Contam. Toxicol.,* 23, 20, 1979.
83. Norstrom, R. J., Hallet, D. J., and Sonstegard, R. A., Coho salmon (*Oncorhynchus kisutch*) and herring-gulls (*Larus argentatus*) as indicators of organochlorine contamination in Lake Ontario, *J. Fish. Res. Board Can.,* 35, 1401, 1978.
84. Bjerk, J. E., Residues of DDT in cod from Norwegian fjords, *Bull. Environ. Contam. Toxicol.,* 9, 89, 1973.
85. Stenersen, J. and Kvalvag, J., Residues of DDT and its degradation products in cod liver from two Norwegian fjords, *Bull. Environ. Contam. Toxicol.,* 8, 120, 1972.
86. Brevik, E. M., Organochlorines in fish and crabs from the Kristiansand fjord in Norway, *Nord. Veterinaermed.,* 30, 375, 1978.
87. Rygg, B., Chlorinated aromatic hydrocarbons in fish from an area polluted by industrial effluents, *Sci. Total Environ.,* 10, 219, 1978.
88. Brevik, E. M., Bjerk, J. E., and Kveseth, N. J., Organochlorines in codfish from harbours along the Norwegian coast, *Bull. Environ. Contam. Toxicol.,* 20, 715, 1978.
89. Kveseth, N. J., Residues of DDT in a contaminated Norwegian lake ecosystem, *Bull. Environ. Contam. Toxicol.,* 27, 397, 1981.
90. Brevik, E. M., Organochlorine residues in fish from Lake Mjøsa in Norway, *Bull. Environ. Contam. Toxicol.,* 26, 679, 1981.
91. Jansson, B., Vaz, R., Blomkvist, G., Jensen, S., and Olsson, M., Chlorinated terpenes and chlordane components found in fish, guillemot and seal from Swedish waters, *Chemosphere,* 8, 181, 1979.
92. Jensen, S., Johnels, A. G., Olsson, M., and Otterlind, G., DDT and PCB in marine animals from Swedish waters, *Nature,* 224, 247, 1969.
93. Hattula, M. L., Janatuinen, J., Särkka, J., and Paasivirta, J., A five-year monitoring study of the chlorinated hydrocarbons in the fish of a Finnish lake ecosystem, *Environ. Pollut.,* 15, 121, 1978.
94. Westernhagen, H. V., Rosenthal, H., Dethlefsen, V., Ernst, W., Harms, U., and Hansen, P.-D., Bioaccumulating substances and reproductive success in Baltic Flounder *Platichthys flesus, Aquat. Toxicol.,* 1, 85, 1981.
95. Linko, R. R., Kaitaranta, J., Rantamaki, P., and Eronen, L., Occurrence of DDT and PCB compounds in Baltic herring and pike from the Turku Archipelago, *Environ. Pollut.,* 7, 193, 1974.
96. Paasivirta, J., Hattula, M. L., Särkka, J., Janatuinen, J., Pitkanen, M., and Kurkirinne, T., On the analysis and appearance of the organic chlorine compounds in the Lake Päijänne ecosystem, Organiska Mijogifteri Vatten, *NORDFORSK Miljoevardssekr. Publ.,* 2, 439, 1976.
97. Linko, R. R. and Terho, K., Occurrence of methyl mercury in pike and Baltic herring from the Turku Archipelago, *Environ. Pollut.,* 14, 227, 1977.
98. Särkka, J., Hattula, M. L., Paasivirta, J., and Janatuinen, J., Mercury and chlorinated hydrocarbons in the food chain of Lake Päijänne, Finland, *Holarctic Ecol.,* 1, 326, 1978.
99. Paasivirta, J. and Linko, R., Environmental toxins in Finnish wildlife. A study on time trends of residue contents in fish during 1973—1978, *Chemosphere,* 9, 643, 1980.

100. Wickstrom, K., Pyysalo, H., and Perttila, M., Organochlorine compounds in the liver of cod *(Gadus morhua)* in the Northern Baltic, *Chemosphere*, 10, 999, 1981.
101. Paasivirta, J., Särkka, J., Aho, M., Aho, K. S., Tarhanen, J., and Roos, A., Recent trends of biocides in pikes of the Lake Päijänne, *Chemosphere*, 10, 405, 1981.
102. Moilanen, R., Pyysalo, H., Wickstrom, K., and Linko, R., Time trends of chlordane, DDT, and PCB concentrations in pike *(Esox lucius)* and Baltic herring *(Culpea harengus)* in the Turku Archipelago, Northern Baltic Sea for the period 1971—1982, *Bull. Environ. Contam. Toxicol.*, 29, 334, 1982.
103. Paasivirta, J., Särkka, J., Aho, K. S., Humppi, T., Kuokkanen, T., and Marttinen, M., Food chain enrichment of organochlorine compounds and mercury in clean and polluted lakes of Finland, *Chemosphere*, 12, 239, 1983.
104. Schaefer, R. G., Ernst, W., Goerke, H., and Eder, G., Residues of chlorinated hydrocarbons in North Sea animals in relation to biological parameters, *Ber. Dtsch. Wiss. Komm. Meeresforsch.*, 24, 225, 1976.
105. Eichner, M., Über Ruckstandsbestimmungen von chlorierten Insektiziden und polychlorierten Biphenylen in Fischen des Bodensees, des Oberrhenins und dessen Zuflussen sowie in diesen Gewassern, *Z. Lebensm. Unters. Forsch.*, 161, 327, 1976.
106. Eder, G., Schaefer, R. G., Ernst, W., and Goerke, H., Chlorinated hydrocarbons in animals of the Skagerrak, *Veroeff. Inst. Meeresforsch. Bremerhaven*, 16, 1, 1976.
107. Goerke, H., Eder, G., Weber, K., and Ernst, W., Patterns of organochlorine residues in animals of different trophic levels from the Weser Estuary, *Mar. Pollut. Bull.*, 10, 127, 1979.
108. Kruse, V. R. and Kruger, K. E., Organochlorpestizide in der Leber des Ostseedorsches-eine aktuale Bestandsaufnahme, *Arch. Lebensmittelhyg.*, 32, 1, 1981.
109. Luckas, B. and Lorenzen, W., Zum vorkommen von chlororganischen Pestiziden and polychlorierten Biphenylen in Meersestieren der Kusten Schleswig-Holsteins, *Dtsch. Lebensm.-Rundsch.*, 77, 437, 1981.
110. Brunn, H. and Manz, D., Contamination of native fish stock by hexachlorobenzene and polychlorinated biphenyl residues, *Bull. Environ. Contam. Toxicol.*, 28, 599, 1982.
111. Picer, M., Picer, N., and Ahel, M., Chlorinated insecticide and PCB residues in fish and mussels of east coastal waters of the middle and North Adriatic Sea, 1974—75, *Pestic. Monit. J.*, 12, 102, 1978.
112. Killkidis, S. D., Psomas, J. E., Kamarianos, A. P., and Panetsos, A. G., Monitoring of DDT, PCBs, and other organochlorine compounds in marine organisms from the North Aegean Sea, *Bull. Environ. Contam. Toxicol.*, 26, 496, 1981.
113. Eades, J. F., Pesticide residues in the Irish environment, *Nature*, 210, 650, 1966.
114. Bengtson, S. A., DDT and PCB residues in airborne fallout and animals in Iceland, *Ambio*, 3, 84, 1974.
115. Anon., Selected pollution profiles: North Atlantic, North Sea, Baltic Sea, and Mediterranean Sea, *Ambio*, 7, 75, 1978.
116. Södergren, A., Djirsarai, R., Gharibzadeh, M., and Moinpour, A., Organochlorine residues in aquatic environments in Iran, 1974, *Pestic. Monit. J.*, 12, 81, 1978.
117. Paz, J. D., Preliminary study of the occurrence and distribution of DDT residues in the Jordan watershed, 1971, *Pestic. Monit. J.*, 10, 96, 1976.
118. Zorgani, G. A. El., Residues of organochlorine pesticides in fishes in Sudan, *J. Environ. Sci. Health*, 15, 1091, 1980.
119. Deelstra, H., Power, J. L., and Kenner, C. T., Chlorinated hydrocarbon residues in the fish of lake Tanganyika, *Bull. Environ. Contam. Toxicol.*, 15, 689, 1976.
120. Greichus, Y. A., Greichus, A., Amman, B. D., Call, D. J., Hamman, D. C. D., and Pott, R. M., Insecticides, polychlorinated biphenyls and metals in African lake ecosystems. I. Harbeespoort dam, Transvaal and Vöelvlei dam, Cape Province, Republic of South Africa, *Arch. Environ. Contam. Toxicol.*, 6, 371, 1977.
121. Rosales, M. T. L. and Escalona, R. L., Organochlorine residues in organisms of two different lagoons of Northwest Mexico, *Bull. Environ. Contam. Toxicol.*, 30, 456, 1983.
122. Neuhaus, J. W. G., Brady, M. N., Siyali, D. S., and Wallis, E., Mercury and organochlorine pesticides in fish, *Med. J. Aust.*, 1, 107, 1973.
123. Yamagishi, T., Miyazaki, T., Akiyama, K., Kaneko, S., and Horii, S., Residues of chlordanes in fish and shellfish from Kanto area and its vicinity, *J. Food Hyg. Soc. Jpn.*, 22, 270, 1981.
124. Miyazaki, T., Akiyama, K., Kaneko, S., Horii, S., and Yamagishi, T., Identification of chlordanes and related compounds in Goby fish from Tokyo Bay, *Bull. Environ. Contam. Toxicol.*, 24, 1, 1980.
125. Yamagishi, T. and Akiyama, K., 1,3,5-trichloro-2-(4-nitrophenoxy) benzene in fish, shellfish, and seawater in Tokyo Bay, 1977—1979, *Arch. Environ. Contam. Toxicol.*, 10, 627, 1981.
126. Gretch, F. M., Barry, T. L., Petzinger, G., and Geltman, J., Identification of the herbicide 2,4,6-trichlorophenyl p-nitrophenyl ether in imported rainbow trout, *Bull. Environ. Contam. Toxicol.*, 23, 165, 1979.

127. Horii, S., Miyazaki, T., Kaneko, S., Akiyama, K., and Yamagishi, T., Identification of γ-chlordene in freshwater fish from the Tama River (Japan), *Bull. Environ. Contam. Toxicol.*, 26, 254, 1981.

128. White, D. H., Mitchell, C. A., Kennedy, H. D., Krynitsky, A. J., and Ribick, M. A., Elevated DDE and toxaphene residues in fishes and birds reflect local contamination in the Lower Rio Grande Valley, Texas, *Southwest. Nat.*, 28, 325, 1983.

129. Musial, C. J. and Uthe, J. F., Widespread occurrence of the pesticide toxaphene in Canadian east coast marine fish, *Int. J. Environ. Anal. Chem.*, 14, 117, 1983.

130. Bidleman, T. F. and Olney, C. E., Long range transport of toxaphene insecticide in the atmosphere of the Western North Atlantic, *Nature,* 257, 475, 1975.

131. Ribick, M. A., Dubay, G. R., Petty, J. D., Stalling, D. L., and Schmitt, C. J., Toxaphene residues in fish: identification, quantification, and confirmation at part per billion levels, *Environ. Sci. Technol.*, 16, 310, 1982.

132. Zitko, V., Nonachlor and chlordane in aquatic fauna, *Chemosphere,* 7, 3, 1978.

133. Morris, R. and Johnson, L. G., Dieldrin levels in fish from Iowa streams, *Pestic. Monit. J.,* 5, 12, 1971.

134. Fredeen, F. J. H., Saha, J. G., and Balba, M. H., Residues of methoxychlor and other chlorinated hydrocarbons in water, sand, and selected fauna following injections of methoxychlor black fly larvicide into the Saskatchewan River, 1972, *Pestic. Monit. J.,* 8, 241, 1975.

135. Marganian, V. M. and Wall, W. J., Jr., Dursban and diazinon residues in biota following treatment of intertidal plots on Cape Cod — 1967—69, *Pestic. Monit. J.,* 6, 160, 1972.

136. Addison, R. F. and Zinck, M. E., The metabolism of some DDE-type compounds by brook trout (*Salvelinus fontinalis*), in *Environmental Quality and Safety,* Suppl. Vol. 3, Coulston, F. and Korte, F., Eds., Georg Thieme Verlag, Stuttgart, 1975, 880.

137. Crawford, R. B., Effects of DDT in Fundulus: studies on toxicity, fate, and reproduction, *Arch. Environ. Contam. Toxicol.*, 4, 334, 1976.

138. Virtanen, M. T., Roos, A., Arstila, A. U., and Hattula, M. L., An evaluation of a model ecosystem with DDT, *Arch. Environ. Contam. Toxicol.*, 9, 491, 1980.

139. Klaas, E. E. and Belisle, A. A., Organochlorine pesticide and polychlorinated biphenyl residues in selected fauna from a New Jersey salt marsh — 1967 vs. 1973, *Pestic. Monit. J.,* 10, 149, 1977.

140. Sims, G. G., Campbell, J. R., Zemlyak, F., and Graham, J. M., Organochlorine residues in fish and fishery products from the Northwest Atlantic, *Bull. Environ. Contam. Toxicol.*, 18, 697, 1977.

141. Galassi, S., Gandolfi, G., and Pacchetti, G., Chlorinated hydrocarbons in fish from the River Po (Italy), *Sci. Total Environ.,* 20, 231, 1981.

142. Cuerrier, J. P., Keith, J. A., and Stone, E., Problems with DDT in fish culture operations, *Nat. Can.*, 94, 315, 1967.

143. Klaassen, H. E. and Kadoum, A. M., Pesticide residues in natural fish populations of the Smoky Hill River of Western Kansas — 1967—69, *Pestic. Monit. J.,* 7, 53, 1973.

144. Haines, T. A., Organochlorine residues in brook trout from remote lakes in the Northeastern United States, *Water Air Soil Pollut.*, 20, 47, 1983.

145. Allison, D., Kallman, B. J., Cope, O. B., and Valin, C. C. V., Insecticides: effects on cutthroat trout of repeated exposure to DDT, *Science,* 142, 958, 1963.

146. Atchison, G. J. and Johnson, H. E., The degradation of DDT in brook trout eggs and fry, *Trans. Am. Fish. Soc.,* 104, 782, 1975.

147. Kent, J. C. and Johnson, D. W., Organochlorine residues in fish, water, and sediment of American Falls Reservoir, Idaho, 1974, *Pestic. Monit. J.,* 13, 28, 1979.

148. Moriarty, F., The effects of pesticides on wildlife: exposure and residues, *Sci. Total Environ.,* 1, 267, 1972.

149. Ketchum, B. H., Zitko, V., and Saward, D., Aspects of heavy metal and organohalogen pollution in aquatic ecosystems, in *Ecological Toxicology Research,* McIntyre, A. D. and Mills, C. F., Eds., Plenum Press, New York, 1976, 75.

150. Holden, A. V., International cooperative study of organochlorine pesticide residues in terrestrial and aquatic wildlife, 1967/1968, *Pestic. Monit. J.,* 4, 117, 1970.

151. Reinert, R. E. and Bergman, H. L., Residues of DDT in lake trout *(Salvelinus namaycush)* and coho salmon *(Oncorhynchus kisutch)* from the Great Lakes, *J. Fish. Res. Board Can.,* 31, 191, 1974.

152. Bache, C. A., Serum, J. W., Youngs, W. D., and Lisk, D. J., Polychlorinated biphenyl residues: accumulation in Cayuga lake trout with age, *Science,* 177, 1191, 1972.

153. Youngs, W. D., Gutenmann, W. H., and Lisk, D. J., Residues of DDT in lake trout as a function of age, *Environ. Sci. Technol.,* 6, 451, 1972.

154. Monod, G. and Keck, G., PCBs in Lake Geneva (Lake Leman) fish, *Bull. Environ. Contam. Toxicol.,* 29, 570, 1982.

155. Kanazawa, J., Bioconcentration ratio of diazinon by freshwater fish and snail, *Bull. Environ. Contam. Toxicol.,* 20, 613, 1978.

156. Wszolek, P. C., Lisk, D. J., Wachs, T., and Youngs, W. D., Persistence of polychlorinated biphenyls and 1,1-dichloro-2,2-bis(p-chlorophenyl) ethylene (p,p'-DDE) with age in lake trout after 8 years, *Am. Chem. Soc.*, 13, 1269, 1979.

157. Bulkley, R. V., Variations in DDT concentration in muscle tissue of channel catfish, *Ictalurus punctatus,* from the Des Moines River, 1971, *Pestic. Monit. J.,* 11, 165, 1978.

158. Delfino, J. J., Toxic substances in the Great Lakes, *Environ. Sci. Technol.,* 13, 1462, 1979.

159. Lieb, A. J., Bills, D. D., and Sinnhuber, R. O., Accumulation of dietary polychlorinated biphenyls (Aroclor 1254) by rainbow trout *(Salmo gairdneri), J. Agric. Food Chem.,* 22, 638, 1974.

160. Kellogg, R. L. and Bulkley, R. V., Seasonal concentrations of dieldrin in water, channel catfish, and catfish-food organisms, Des Moines River, Iowa — 1971—73, *Pestic. Monit. J.,* 9, 186, 1976.

161. Giam, C. S., Richardson, R. L., Taylor, D., and Wong, M. K., DDT, DDE and PCBs in the tissues of reef dwelling groupers (Serranidae) in the Gulf of Mexico and the Grand Bahamas, *Bull. Environ. Contam. Toxicol.,* 11, 189, 1974.

162. Anderson, R. B. and Fenderson, O. C., An analysis of variation of insecticide residues in landlocked Atlantic salmon *(Salmo salar), J. Fish. Res. Board Can.,* 27, 1, 1970.

163. Klauda, R. J., Peck, T. H., and Rice, G. K., Accumulation of polychlorinated biphenyls in Atlantic tomcod *(Microgadus tomcod)* collected from the Hudson River Estuary, New York, *Bull. Environ. Contam. Toxicol.,* 27, 829, 1981.

164. Elson, P. F., Meister, A. L., Saunders, J. W., Saunders, R. L., Sprague, J. B., and Zitko, V., Impact of chemical pollution on Atlantic salmon in North America, *Int. Atlantic Salmon Symp. 1973,* International Atlantic Salmon Foundation, St. Andrews, New Brunswick, Canada, 1973, 83.

165. Johnson, L. G. and Morris, R. L., Chlorinated insecticide residues in the eggs of some freshwater fish, *Bull. Environ. Contam. Toxicol.,* 11, 503, 1974.

166. Broyles, R. H. and Noveck, M. I., Uptake and distribution of 2,5,2',5'-tetrachlorobiphenyl in developing lake trout, *Toxicol. Appl. Pharmocol.,* 50, 291, 1979.

167. Niimi, A. J., Biological and toxicological effects of environmental contaminants in fish and their eggs, *Can. J. Fish. Aquat. Sci.,* 40, 306, 1983.

168. Holden, A. V., A study of the absorption of ^{14}C-labelled DDT from water by fish, *Ann. Appl. Biol.,* 50, 467, 1962.

169. Ernst, W., Goerke, H., Eder, G., and Schaefer, R. G., Residues of chlorinated hydrocarbons in marine organisms in relation to size and ecological parameters. I. PCB, DDT, DDE and DDD in fishes and molluscs from the English Channel, *Bull. Environ. Contam. Toxicol.,* 15, 55, 1976.

170. Sugiura, K., Washino, T., Hattori, M., Sato, E., and Goto, M., Accumulation of organochlorine compounds in fishes. Difference of accumulation factors by fishes, *Chemosphere,* 7, 359, 1979.

171. Earnest, R. D. and Benville, P. E., Jr., Correlation of DDT and lipid levels for certain San Francisco Bay fish, *Pestic. Monit. J.,* 5, 235, 1971.

172. DeFoe, D. L., Veith, G. D., and Carlson, R. W., Effects of Aroclor 1248 and 1260 on the fathead minnow *(Pimephales promelas), J. Fish. Res. Board Can.,* 35, 997, 1978.

173. Jarvinen, A. W., Hoffman, M. J., and Thorslund, T. W., Long-term toxic effects of DDT food and water exposure on fathead minnows *(Pimephales promelas), J. Fish. Res. Board Can.,* 34, 2089, 1977.

174. Hughes, R. A. and Lee, G. F., Toxaphene accumulation in fish in lakes treated for rough fish control, *Environ. Sci. Technol.,* 7, 934, 1973.

175. Roberts, J. R., DeFrietas, A. S. W., and Gidney, M. A. J., Influence of lipid pool size on bioaccumulation of the insecticide chlordane by northern redhorse suckers *(Mixostoma macrolepidotum), J. Fish. Res. Board Can.,* 34, 89, 1977.

176. Rudling, L., Determination of pentachlorophenol in organic tissues and water, *Water Res.,* 4, 533, 1970.

177. Nebeker, A. V., Puglisi, F. A., and DeFoe, D. L., Effect of polychlorinated biphenyl compounds on survival and reproduction of the fathead minnow and flagfish, *Trans. Am. Fish. Soc.,* 103, 562, 1974.

178. Mehrle, P. M., Haines, T. A., Hamilton, S., Ludke, J. L., Mayer, F. L., and Ribick, M. A., Relationship between body contaminants and bone development in east-coast striped bass, *Trans. Am. Fish. Soc.,* 111, 231, 1982.

179. Keck, G. and Raffenot, J., Chemical contamination by PCBs in the fishes of a French River: the Furan's (Jura), *Bull. Environ. Contam. Toxicol.,* 21, 689, 1979.

180. Smith, W. E., Funk, K., and Zabik, M. E., Effects of cooking on concentration of PCB and DDT compounds in chinook *(Oncorhynchus tshawytsha)* and coho *(O. kisutch)* salmon from Lake Michigan, *J. Fish. Res. Board Can.,* 30, 702, 1975.

181. Zitko, Z. and Carson, W. G., A comparison of the uptake of PCB's and isopropyl-PCB's (chloralkylene 12) by fish, *Chemosphere,* 2/3, 133, 1977.

182. Kleinert, S. J., Degurse, P. E., and Wieth, T. L., Occurrence and significance of DDT and dieldrin residues in Wisconsin fish, *Wis. Dep. Nat. Resour. Bull.,* 41, 43, 1968.

183. Cooke, A. S., The influence of rearing density on the subsequent response to DDT dosing for tadpoles of the frog *Rana temporaria, Bull. Environ. Contam. Toxicol.,* 7, 837, 1979.

184. Canton, J. H., Wegman, R. C. C., Vulto, T. J. A., Verhoef, C. H., and Esch, G. J. V., Toxicity-, accumulation- and elimination studies of α-hexachlorocyclohexane (α-HCH) with saltwater organisms of different trophic levels, *Water Res.*, 12, 687, 1978.

185. Veith, G. D., Baseline concentrations of polychlorinated biphenyls and DDT in Lake Michigan fish, *Pestic. Monit. J.*, 9, 21, 1975.

186. Bulkley, R. V., Leung, S. Y. T., and Richard, J. J., Organochlorine insecticide concentrations in fish of the Des Moines River, Iowa, 1977—78, *Pestic. Monit. J.*, 15, 86, 1981.

187. Grzenda, A. R., Taylor, W. J., and Paris, D. F., The uptake and distribution of chlorinated residues by goldfish *(Carassius auratus)* fed a ¹⁴C-dieldrin contaminated diet, *Trans. Am. Fish. Soc.*, 100, 215, 1971.

188. Grzenda, A. R., Taylor, W. J., and Paris, D. F., The elimination and turnover of ¹⁴C-dieldrin by different goldfish tissues, *Trans. Am. Fish. Soc.*, 101, 686, 1972.

189. Guiney, P. D. and Peterson, R. E., Distribution and elimination of a polychlorinated biphenyl after acute dietary exposure in yellow perch and rainbow trout, *Arch. Environ. Contam. Toxicol.*, 9, 667, 1980.

190. Vanderford, M. J. and Hamelink, J. L., Influence of environmental factors on pesticide levels in sport fish, *Pestic. Monit. J.*, 11, 138, 1977.

191. Holden, A. V., The effects of pesticides on life in freshwaters, *Proc. R. Soc. London, Ser. B.*, 180, 383, 1972.

192. Fabacher, D. L. and Chambers, H., Uptake and storage of ¹⁴C-labeled endrin by the livers and brains of pesticide susceptible and resistant mosquitofish, *Bull. Environ. Contam. Toxicol.*, 16, 203, 1976.

193. Phillips, D. J. H., Use of biological indicator organisms to quantitate organochlorine pollutants in aquatic environments — a review, *Environ. Pollut.*, 16, 167, 1978.

194. Hamelink, J. L. and Spacie, A., Fish and chemicals: the process of accumulation, *Annu. Rev. Pharmacol. Toxicol.*, 17, 167, 1977.

195. Zabik, M. E., Merrill, G., and Zabik, M. J., Predictability of PCBs in carp harvested in Saginaw Bay, Lake Huron, *Bull. Environ. Contam. Toxicol.*, 28, 592, 1982.

196. Edgren, M., Olsson, M., and Reutergard, L., A one year study of the seasonal variations of DDT and PCB levels in fish from heated and unheated areas near a nuclear power plant, *Chemosphere*, 10, 447, 1981.

197. Olsson, M., Jensen, S., and Reutergard, L., Seasonal variation of PCB levels in fish — an important factor in planning aquatic monitoring programs, *Ambio*, 7, 66, 1978.

198. de la Cruz, A. A. and Lue, K. Y., Mirex incorporation in the environment: *in situ* decomposition of fire ant bait and its effects on two soil macroarthropods, *Arch. Environ. Contam. Toxicol.*, 7, 47, 1978.

199. Chambers, J. E. and Yarbrough, J. D., Xenobiotic biotransformation systems in fishes, *Comp. Biochem. Physiol.*, 55, 77, 1976.

200. Zabik, M. E., Olson, B., and Johnson, T. M., Dieldrin, DDT, PCBs, and mercury levels in freshwater mullet from the Upper Great Lakes, *Pestic. Monit. J.*, 12, 36, 1978.

201. Smith, R. M. and Cole, C. F., Chlorinated hydrocarbon insecticide residues in winter flounder, *Pseudopleuronectes americanus*, from the Weweantic River Estuary, Massachusetts, *J. Fish. Res. Board Can.*, 27, 2374, 1970.

202. Harris, C. R. and Mile, J. R. W., Pesticide residues in the Great Lakes region of Canada, *Residue Rev.*, 57, 27, 1975.

203. Ernst, W., Effects of pesticides and related organic compounds in the sea, *Helgol. Meeresunters.*, 33, 301, 1980.

204. Duke, T. W. and Wilson, A. J., Jr., Chlorinated hydrocarbons in livers of fishes from the Northeastern Pacific Ocean, *Pestic. Monit. J.*, 5, 228, 1971.

205. Barber, R. T. and Warlen, S. M., Organochlorine insecticide residues in deep sea fish from 2,500 m in the Atlantic Ocean, *Environ. Sci. Technol.*, 13, 1146, 1979.

206. Cairns, T. and Parfitt, C. H., Persistence and metabolism of TDE in California Clear Lake fish, *Bull. Environ. Contam. Toxicol.*, 7, 504, 1980.

207. Sims, G. G., Cosham, C. E., Campbell, J. R., and Murray, M. C., DDT residues in cod livers from the maritime provinces of Canada, *Bull. Environ. Contam. Toxicol.*, 14, 505, 1975.

208. Ernst, W. and Goerke, H., Anreicherung, Verteilung, Umwandlung und Ausscheidung von DDT-¹⁴C bei *Solea solea* (Pisces:Soleidae), *Mar. Biol.*, 24, 287, 1974.

209. Holden, A. V., The OECD, international co-operative studies of organochlorine residues in wildlife, *Environ. Qual. Saf.*, 3, 40, 1975.

210. Addison, R. F., Zinck, M. E., and Ackman, R. G., Residues of organochlorine pesticides and polychlorinated biphenyls in some commercially produced Canadian marine oils, *J. Fish. Res. Board Can.*, 29, 349, 1972.

211. Dugal, L. C., Pesticide residue in freshwater fish oils and meals, *J. Fish. Res. Board Can.*, 25, 169, 1968.

212. Musial, C. J. and Uthe, J. F., A study of the stability of polychlorinated biphenyl in fish oil, International Council for the Exploration of the Sea, ICES C. M. 1983/E: 37, Marine Environmental Quality Committee, Copenhagen, 1983.

213. Falandysz, J., Organochlorine pesticides and PCBs in codliver oil of Baltic origin, 1971—80, *Pestic. Monit. J.,* 15, 51, 1981.

214. Ludke, J. L. and Schmitt, C. J., Monitoring contaminant residues in freshwater fishes in the United States: The National Pesticide Monitoring Program, in *Proc. 3rd USA-USSR Symp. on the Effects of Pollutants upon Aquatic Ecosystems,* Swain, W. R. and Shannon, V. R., Eds., Duluth, Minn., U.S. Environmental Protection Agency, 1980, 97.

215. The President's Science Advisory Committee, Use of pesticides: a report, *Residue Rev.,* 6, 1, 1964.

216. Schmitt, C. J., Ribick, M. A., Ludke, J. L., and May, T. W., National Pesticide Monitoring Program: organochlorine residues in freshwater fish, 1976—79, Fish and Wildlife Service, U.S. Department of Interior, Washington, D.C., 1983.

217. Mount, D. I., Vigor, L. W., and Schafer, M. L., Endrin: use of concentration in blood to diagnose acute toxicity to fish, *Science,* 152, 1388.

218. Mount, D. I. and Boyle, M. W., Parathion — use of blood concentration to diagnose mortality of fish, *Environ. Sci. Technol.,* 3, 1183, 1969.

219. Lockhart, W. L., Metner, D. A., and Solomon, J., Methoxychlor residue studies in caged and wild fish from the Athabasca River, Alberta, following a single application of blackfly larvicide, *J. Fish. Res. Board Can.,* 34, 626, 1977.

220. Niimi, A. J., Gross growth efficiency of fish (K_1) based on field observations of annual growth and kinetics of persistent environmental contaminants, *Can. J. Fish. Aquat. Sci.,* 38, 250, 1981.

Chapter 3

UPTAKE AND DEPURATION OF PESTICIDE RESIDUES BY FISH

I. INTRODUCTION

Fish accumulate xenobiotic chemicals, especially those with poor water solubility, from water or food. The uptake from water occurs because of the very intimate contact with the medium that carries the chemicals in solution or suspension and also because fish have to extract oxygen from the medium by passing enormous volumes of water over their gills. Water that is transported actively (marine fish) or passively (freshwater fish) into the body (because of the difference in the osmotic concentration between the external and the internal environment), may also contribute to the uptake from water during the lifetime of a fish. The process of uptake, either through food or from water, is influenced by several factors such as the chemistry of the molecule, physical conditions of the medium, and the fish itself — its lipid content, size, stage of development, physiological activity, etc. In this chapter, the uptake of pesticide residues, their deposition in the tissues, and the processes of depuration of the residues are considered.

Before discussing the various aspects of uptake and depuration, it is necessary to define without ambiguity the different terms employed to describe the uptake of residues from water or through food. Ware,[1] in his review on the effects of pesticides on nontarget organisms, Kanazawa,[2] and Anderson and DeFoe[3] used the two terms — bioconcentration and biomagnification — interchangeably. Dobbs and Williams[4] defined bioconcentration as the process by which an organism achieves a higher concentration of a chemical than that present in its food or its medium. Könemann and Leeuwen[5] used the term bioaccumulation for the process of uptake from water. Khan and Khan[6] employed the term "biological magnification" to describe this process, but occasionally also used the term "bioconcentration" to describe the same process. The terms that have gained wide usage have been clearly defined by Brungs and Mount[7] as follows: bioconcentration is the process by which a compound is absorbed from water through gills or epithelial tissues and is concentrated in the body; bioaccumulation is the process by which a compound is taken up by an aquatic organism, both from water and through food; and biomagnification denotes the process by which the concentration of a compound increases in different organisms, occupying successive trophic levels. Whether biomagnification is a universally occurring phenomenon has been much discussed and this concept has been questioned in the recent past.

When the chemical is concentrated from water, the ratio of its concentration in the organism and water should be called "bioconcentration factor (BCF)". In the following discussion, the terms bioconcentration and bioaccumulation are used with the same significance as given by Brungs and Mount.[7]

II. BIOCONCENTRATION AND BIOACCUMULATION

A. Bioconcentration

A few representative BCFs of various compounds are shown in Table 1. Since by definition bioconcentration is the result of the uptake of the toxicant by the organism from water alone, results of studies involving bioaccumulation are not included in this table. In "Water Quality Criteria" (for various pesticides) published by the United States Environmental Protection Agency (USEPA), the BCFs are sometimes calculated on the basis of the residue concentration in water and the organism, both monitored in the field (see Table 5, in the Criteria for DDT).[8] In such cases, the reported BCF is

Table 1

REPRESENTATIVE BIOCONCENTRATION FACTORS OF SOME PESTICIDES

Compound	Species	Conc in water		Duration of exposure	BCF	Ref.
DDT	Fathead minnow	0.5—2	μg/ℓ	56—112 days	100,000	77
	Golden shiner	0.3	μg/ℓ	15 days	100,000	248
	Green fish	0.11—0.33	μg/ℓ	15 days	17,500	249
	Pinfish and Atlantic croaker	0.1—1	μg/ℓ	15 days	10,000 to 38,000	250
	Daphnia magna	8—50	μg/ℓ	24 hr	16,000 to 23,000	251
	Salmo gairdneri	133—176	μg/ℓ	84 days	21,300 to 51,300	22
Dieldrin	Sculpin	0.017—8.6	μg/ℓ	32 days	300 to 11,000	67
	Guppy	0.8—4.3	μg/ℓ	18 days	49,307	45
	Bluegill (static test)	1	μg/ℓ	48 hr	2,441	252
	Bluegill (flow-through test)	1.5	μg/ℓ	48 hr	1,727	252
Heptachlor	Sheepshead minnow	6.5—21	μg/ℓ	96 hr	7,400 to 21,300	253
	Pinfish	0.32—32	μg/ℓ	96 hr	3,800 to 7,700	253
	Spot	1.2—3.7	μg/ℓ	96 hr	3,000 to 13,800	253
Mirex	Juvenile pinfish	25—46	μg/ℓ	3 days	3,800	254
Kepone®	Sheepshead minnow juveniles	41—780	μg/ℓ	21 days	2,600	25
	Adult male	41—780	μg/ℓ	21 days	7,600	25
	Adult female	41—780	μg/ℓ	21 days	5,700	25
HCH	Pinfish	18.4—31.3	μg/ℓ	4 days	218	20
	Sheepshead minnow	41.9—108.3	μg/ℓ	4 days	490	20
	Guppy	10—1400	μg/ℓ	24 hr	500	83
Technical HCH	Pinfish edible part	1.4—36	μg/ℓ	24 hr	500	83
	Pinfish offal	1.4—36	μg/ℓ	28 days	175	20
Chlordane	Goldfish	3.4	μg/ℓ	4 days	67 to 162	168
	Sheepshead minnow	15—51	μg/ℓ	4 days	12,600 to 18,700	225
	Pinfish	5.4—15.2	μg/ℓ	4 days	3,000 to 7,500	225
HCB	Killifish	160—380	μg/ℓ	6.68 hr	65 to 710	256
	Fathead minnow	—	—	—	16,200	14
	Green sunfish	—	—	—	21,900	14
	Rainbow trout	—	—	—	5,500	14
Permethrin	Juvenile Atlantic salmon	1.4—12	μg/ℓ	89 hr	73	257
Cypermethrin	Juvenile Atlantic salmon	1.4—12	μg/ℓ	96 hr	3 to 7	257
Fenvalerate	Juvenile Atlantic salmon	1	μg/ℓ	96 hr	200	257
PCP	Trout	2	mg/ℓ	24 hr	100	258
	Killifish	57—120	μg/ℓ	168 hr	10 to 64	259
	Killifish	100—610	μg/ℓ	240 hr	8 to 50	259
Trichlorophenol	*Poecilia* female	610	μg/ℓ	36 hr	12,180	136
	Poecilia male	350	μg/ℓ	36 hr	7,000	136
Leptophos	Bluegill sunfish	240	mg/ℓ	10 days	750	10
Fenitrothion	Killifish	800	μg/ℓ	10 days	53	15
	Coho salmon underyearling	560	μg/ℓ	24 hr	16	260
Diazinon	Topmouth gudgeon	10	μg/ℓ	7 days	152	261
	Silver crucian carp	10	μg/ℓ	7 days	37	261
	Carp	10	μg/ℓ	7 days	65	261
	Guppy	10	μg/ℓ	7 days	18	261
Fluridone	Fathead minnow	140	mg/ℓ	10 weeks	64	262
2,4-D	Bluegill sunfish	3	mg/ℓ	8 days	1	263
2,4,5-T	Bluegill sunfish	3	mg/ℓ	8 days	1	263
MCPA	Trout	10—100	mg/ℓ	10—28 days	1	19

Table 1 (continued)
REPRESENTATIVE BIOCONCENTRATION FACTORS OF SOME PESTICIDES

Compound	Species	Conc in water		Duration of exposure	BCF	Ref.
Fosamine ammonium	Channel catfish	1.1	mg/ℓ	4 weeks	1	264
Hexamethyl phosphoramide	Sheepshead minnow	0.5	mg/ℓ	28 days	1	265
Benthiocarb	Fathead minnow	28	µg/ℓ	2.5 days	446 to 471	266
	Channel catfish	29	µg/ℓ	3 days	120	266
	Bluegill	28	µg/ℓ	5 days	91	266
	Longear sunfish	99	µg/ℓ	1—5 days	280 to 300	266

the result of bioconcentration as well as bioaccumulation. Hence it is not surprising to note that "Freshwater fish species bioconcentration in the field was much greater than in laboratory tests . . . "[8] While discussing the provisions of the Japanese Law on New Chemicals and the various types of tests that are to be conducted to evaluate the environmental hazards of chemical substances, Fujiwara[9] described the various steps to be adopted to calculate the extent of concentration of the test chemical by the test fish (carp) from water. As has been stressed by Macek et al.[10] much of the confusion regarding the various processes involved and their relative importance stems partly from the inconsistent use of the various terms by different authors.

1. Factors that Influence Bioconcentration

Bioconcentration is influenced by the structure of the compound, the concentration of the chemical in water, its water solubility, physiological activity of the animal (which in turn is influenced by seasonal changes), and environmental factors such as temperature, organic matter content of sediment and water, and also by population density, age, etc.

No relationship between the type of organism and the extent of bioconcentration of PCBs (polychlorinated biphenyls) was noticed.[11] On the other hand, Ernst[12] reported that the polychaete *Lanice* took up 10 times more α-HCH, γ-HCH, and PCP (pentachlorophenol) from water than did *Mytilus*. Simultaneous exposure to more than one compound did not influence the uptake of any compound; when whitesuckers were simultaneously exposed to dieldrin and Aroclor® 1232, neither compound had any influence on the uptake of the other.[13] Similarly, the uptake of p,p'-DDT or heptachlor[14] by fathead minnows or the uptake of several phosphoric acid triesters[15] was compound-specific and independent of the other compounds present simultaneously. The greater extent of bioconcentration of the more highly chlorinated PCB mixtures[11,16] is likewise related to the chemical structure of the molecule. In general, it appears that the bioconcentration of a compound is inversely related to the exposure concentration, i.e., at higher concentrations of the toxicant in water, it is bioconcentrated less and vice versa. Rainbow trout bioconcentrated 2-ethylhexyl diphenyl phosphate, 1481 ± 704 and 1147 ± 651 times when the aqueous concentration of the compound was, respectively, 5 and 50 µg/ℓ.[17] The bioconcentration of MCPA (4-chloro-2-methylphenoxy acetic acid) by trout[18] and phosphoric acid triesters by killifish[15] was independent of the exposure concentration. When pinfish were exposed to 32, 38, 64, 81.5, and 91.3 µg/ℓ of technical grade HCH (hexachlorocyclohexane), the resulting BCFs in 96 hr were, respectively, 540, 308, 554, 474, and 532.[19] Exposure of spot to 1.5, 3.4, 4.4, 7.8, and 15.9 µg Kepone® per liter, resulted in BCFs of 1133, 941, 1591,

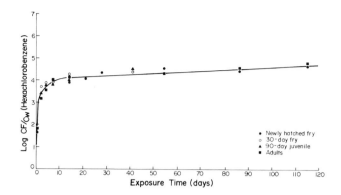

FIGURE 1.   Uptake of hexachlorobenzene in four age-classes of fat-
head minnows (*Pimephales promelas*). (From Veith, G. D., DeFoe,
D. L., and Bergstedt, B. V., *J. Fish. Res. Board Can.,* 36, 1040, 1979.
With permission.)

1385, and 1057,[20] respectively, in 96 hr. The inverse relationship between exposure
concentration and extent of bioconcentration appears valid with low polarity compounds, but not with high polarity ones. The inconsistent results in the case of Ke-
pone® and HCH are perhaps the result of nonattainment of steady state conditions.

Seasonal differences in the bioconcentration of α-HCH, γ-HCH, and PCP by the
polychaete *Lanice conchilega* were observed, although in most experiments, a constant
temperature of 10°C was chosen.[12] In general, temperature accelerates the uptake of
xenobiotic chemicals. Veith et al.[14] reported that the 32-day BCF of Aroclor® 1254
steadily increased with temperature in the case of three species of fish (Figure 1). The
temperature-dependence of the uptake was very prominent in the case of fathead minnows and green sunfish, between 5 and 15°C, whereas in the case of rainbow trout,
tested between 5 and 20°C, the temperature-dependence of bioconcentration, though
apparent, was not marked. Similarly, yearling rainbow trout, exposed to 133 to 176
ng/ℓ took up 3.76, 5.93, and 6.82 mg/kg *p,p'*-DDT at 5, 10, and 15°C, respectively.
Rainbow trout exposed to 234 to 263 ng/ℓ methyl mercury, at 5, 10, and 15°C took
up, respectively, 1.19, 1.71, and 1.96 mg/kg.[21] Bioconcentration of PCBs by brown
trout at three temperature regimes: (1) temperature selected by brown trout in thermal
effluents, (2) a constant temperature of 13°C, and (3) natural fluctuations in temperature that occur in the inshore waters, was studied. Bioconcentration was maximum in
the first and third regimes. PCB accumulation, according to Spigarelli et al.,[22] is affected by temperature because of its influence on food consumption, growth, and lipid
content.

The effect of age on the bioconcentration of chemicals was studied by Veith et al.[14]
Employing newly hatched larvae, 30- or 90-day-old juveniles, or adult fathead minnows, they found little difference in the bioconcentration of HCH by the four age
groups (Figure 2). They also concluded that the small size of the younger fish (30-day-
old), however, was a disadvantage while working with chemicals with small BCF. On
the contrary, Schimmel et al.[23] reported that the fry and juveniles of longnose killifish
bioconcentrated toxaphene, respectively, from 19,300 to 33,300 and 23,700 to 60,000
in 28 days, whereas adults bioconcentrated toxaphene 4200 to 5300 times in 14 days.
Goodman et al.[24] reported an increase in the BCF with increase in age; when sheepshead minnows were exposed to Kepone®, average BCFs were 2600 with 21-day juveniles, 2800 with 42-day juveniles, 7600 with adult males, and 5700 with adult females.

Physical surroundings and the presence of other fish also influence the extent of
uptake. It was reported recently that bluegills took up less anthracene when more fish

were present in the same tank, although the loading (biomass per unit volume) was comparable between the crowded and noncrowded conditions.[25]

Fish bioconcentrate chemicals not only when the compounds are in solution but also when they are adsorbed to the sediments. When mirex was incorporated in the sediment and fish were introduced into the overlying water, the fish had mirex residues in the liver and muscle after 4 weeks; the uptake was dose-dependent.[26] Although experimental studies such as this and other similar works[27,28] suggest that residues may leach from sediments into the overlying water column, under natural conditions, water solubility of the compound and the organic matter content of the sediment and water seem to be the factors that influence the availability of pollutants to the biota in water. The concentration of pollutants in sediments does not seem to be the best indicator of pollutant levels in the biota. While phthalic acid esters, benzo(a)pyrene, PCBs, HCB (hexachlorobenzene), and PCP were the compounds present, in that order of abundance in the sediments collected in San Luis Pass (West Galveston Bay, Tex.), no benzo(a)pyrene was detected in the biota; the concentration of HCB was the highest in crabs, whereas concentration of PCP was highest in fish.[29] Kent and Johnson[30] also noted the lack of correlation between the concentration of DDD in the sediment and that occurring in fish. Likewise, the insecticides detected in water samples were different from those detected in sediments[31] — heptachlor, endrin, and *p,p′*-DDT were detected in water whereas only dieldrin and *p,p′*-DDD were found in sediments.

BCF, to a large extent, depends on the water solubility of the compound and the partitioning into lipids (see Section VIII). In Lake Poinsett, S.D., DDT and its metabolites constituted 45%, lindane 15%, heptachlor and heptachlor epoxide 29%, aldrin 6%, and dieldrin 6% of the total insecticide load in water. In fish, the relative proportions were Σ DDT, 79%; lindane, 2%; dieldrin, 12%; and heptachlor and heptachlor epoxide, 7%; indicating that uptake by the organism is inversely related to the water solubility of a compound.[32]

B. Bioaccumulation
1. In Nature
Bioaccumulation includes uptake from both water and food. Species living in the same region may end up with different body burdens of pesticide residues because of their different feeding habits. Dieldrin residues were detected in the perch but not in the black crappies in the American Fall Reservoir, Idaho.[30] Although both species have similar food habits, mature yellow perch feed at the bottom, too, and hence the perch is more readily exposed to the contaminant than the guppy. Even within the same species, physical conditions of the water body may influence the residue load of different populations. Though catfish of comparable age and size were inhabiting two different sections of Iowa streams, those from the lower reaches had higher dieldrin concentration than those living in the upper reaches, presumably because of the greater availability of dieldrin as a result of accumulated siltation in the former locations.

2. Bioaccumulation Studies in Model Ecosystems and Outdoor Experimental Ponds
One of the first attempts at experimentally incorporating a pesticide in the aquatic systems and following the levels of the compound in different organisms is that of Smith et al.[33] who added Dursban® to glass jars and tanks containing different levels of the trophic chain. Terriere et al.[34] followed the fate of toxaphene applied to two natural lakes in Oregon and estimated the concentration factor in the different organisms. A model ecosystem — a miniature replica of natural conditions — consisting of a 25 × 30 × 45 cm glass aquarium with 15 kg of washed quartz sand and 12 ℓ of water, containing a terrestrial plant, a larval pest (salt marsh caterpillar), *Daphnia,* snail, and mosquitofish, was used by Kapoor et al.[35] to study the extent of persistence, uptake,

and degradation of methoxychlor, and other DDT analogs. Metcalf et al.[36] proposed the use of a terrestrial-aquatic model ecosystem and ^{14}C-labeled compounds as a realistic laboratory method for screening the proposed new pesticides and evaluating their environmental fate. Instead of waiting through 1 to 2 decades of wide-scale use of a pesticide in the environment, model ecosystems furnish meaningful data in a shorter time. Using such a model ecosystem, Metcalf et al. studied the environmental behavior of DDT, DDE, and DDD, the study requiring about a month and yielding, in general, the same type of insight into the environmental behavior of DDT-type compounds that could be accrued only after 20 years of study in nature. Subsequently, such model ecosystems have been widely employed and they have helped in a rapid evaluation of many different types of chemicals.

While the model ecosystem of Metcalf et al. incorporated a terrestrial part, others have attempted studying the fate of an anthropogenic chemical only in the aquatic ecosystem by employing different trophic levels, i.e., an alga or diatom, *Daphnia*, and fish. Such model ecosystems have also helped in gaining an insight into the extent of uptake and sequestering of organic chemicals by the aquatic organisms. A third approach to the experimental evaluation of the extent of uptake was to spray small natural ponds or outdoor pools containing various types of organisms.

In a model ecosystem similar to that of Metcalf et al., *Gambusia* were reported to bioaccumulate dieldrin 6100 times,[37] dianisyl neopentane 1630 times,[38] and parathion, about 335 times,[39] in 34 days. MCPA was not persistent and did not bioaccumulate.[40] While noting a good reproducibility of the results in the model ecosystems proposed by Metcalf et al. and stating that such models give reliable information on the bioaccumulation potential of a chemical and its metabolites, Virtanen et al.[41] at the same time, emphasized that the determination of accumulation factors by this kind of experiments is questionable, as the ratio of the area of terrestrial part to the water volume is too high.

Metcalf et al.[42] employed the term ecological magnification (EM) to denote the extent of uptake of a chemical from food and water and expressed it as the ratio between the concentration in the organism and water. Since the organisms in a model ecosystem (except the primary producer, i.e., alga or diatom) take up residues both from water and food, the "EM" proposed by Metcalf et al. is equivalent to the more universally used term, bioaccumulation, and the term EM should be dropped in favor of the latter.

In a purely aquatic model, Södergren[43] employed the alga, *Chlorella pyrenoidosa,* the cyprinid, *Leucaspius delineatus,* the perch, *Perca fluviatilis,* and the pike, *Esox lucius,* to study the uptake from water and also the food chain transfer of p,p'-DDT, p,p'-DDE, and Clophen A 50 (PCB). In an alga-*Daphnia*-guppy ecosystem, more dieldrin was taken up from water than from food and guppies concentrated dieldrin 49,300 times that present in water.[44] Similarly, more lindane was taken up from water in a laboratory food chain of *Chlorella-Daphnia-Gasterosteus.*[45] Johnson[46] described in detail the procedure for estimating the residue dynamics of contaminants in a freshwater food chain and proposed that Accumulation Factor (AF) (concentration in organism/concentration in water), or Water Accumulation Index (WAI), or a Food Transfer Index (FTI) may be used to describe the uptake at different levels and through different routes. In this approach, the bioconcentration or bioaccumulation of DDT is used as a benchmark for comparison of the level of uptake of other compounds. Using such a system, Skaar et al.[47] reported that Kepone® and mirex were concentrated to about 10,600 and 12,200 times by bluegill. Other works which used this type of model food chains are also reviewed in the next section.

The third approach, spraying outdoor ponds and natural aquatic systems with chosen pesticides, has also yielded useful information on the extent of uptake and accumulation by different aquatic organisms. Following the spraying of a marshland with

DDT, Eberhardt et al.[48] recorded the DDT levels in the aquatic plants, invertebrates, and fish. They proposed that DDT was distributed in two compartments, i.e., a "fast compartment", where the uptake was fast and represents the transient conditions when the concentration in water was relatively high, and a "slow compartment", which represented the long-term retention. Maximum DDT concentration was observed in both carp and green sunfish, but the authors considered that the few data they had precluded any opinion about the dominant mode of uptake of DDT by fish. Bluegills took up 1590 times more Dursban® than what was present in water within 3 days after outdoor ponds were sprayed.[49] Following the spraying of Abate® on six earthen ponds, bluegills had concentrated the compound 500 to 600 times in the case of ponds sprayed at higher levels (180 g a.i./ha) (a.i. = active ingredient) and 900 to 2300 times in those ponds sprayed at a lower level (18 g a.i./ha).

III. BIOMAGNIFICATION

It is often proposed and held as though unequivocally proved that there is a stepwise increase in the residue concentration of persistent chemicals from one trophic level to the next. This postulation, supported by studies on terrestrial animals, is supposed to be true for the aquatic world also. In a pre-PCB era publication, Woodwell et al.[50] described the distribution of DDT residues in an east coast estuary. By extensive sampling of the soil and biota at various trophic levels, the authors concluded that the concentration of DDT and its metabolites increased through successive trophic levels by more than 1000 times, with 0.04 mg/kg DDT in plankton, and 75 mg/kg in a ringbilled gull. In general, among fish, the carnivores had the highest concentration of DDT, and carnivorous birds had 10 to 100 times the levels found in fish. The concentration of DDT in birds was nearly a million times that estimated to be present in water. In a similar paper, at about the same time, Butler[51] claimed that from an estimated 1 μg/ℓ in water, DDT was concentrated to 70 μg/kg in plankton, 15 mg/kg in fish, and 800 mg/kg in the blubber of porpoise. The absence of top piscivores like largemouth bass in heavily contaminated environments that support resistant fish populations was attributed to the elimination of top carnivores through biological magnification of residues.[52] Bulkley et al.[53] reported, respectively, 0.7, 0.68, and 0.09 mg/kg of dieldrin, Σ DDT, and heptachlor epoxide in forage fish, and 1.52, 2.51, and 0.81 mg/kg dieldrin, Σ DDT, and heptachlor epoxide in piscivorous fish from the Des Moines River, Iowa, in 1977 to 1978, and concluded that these differences in the level of contamination of forage and piscivorous fish would suggest biological magnification. Of these observed differences, however, only dieldrin concentration between the two groups of fish was significantly different. While evaluating the efficiency of XAD-2 Amberlite® resin to extract pesticides and other such chemicals from water, Rees and Au[54] reported finding the following levels of PCB (μg/kg): water, 0.05; plankton, 20; invertebrates, 40; suspended solids, 400; and fish, 1400. They concluded that biomagnification was in operation.[54] Since they did not mention how the samples were collected and analyzed (the methods section described the details of extraction of xenobiotic compounds only from water), or the place of sampling, the sampling frequency, etc., it is difficult to understand how they arrived at that conclusion.

In order to verify whether pollutants are biomagnified, DDT was sprayed on ponds in three separate studies.[55] The results indicated no significant difference in the extent of uptake of DDT by fish in ponds with or without representative members of all trophic levels. Hence, Hamelink et al.[55] postulated that the well-known principle of partitioning of a solute into two immiscible solvents explains the deposition of DDT residues in fish and the uptake of DDT occurs through two stages, viz., water-blood and blood-tissue lipids. Further, the fact that exchange equilibrium is controlled solely by aqueous solubility and the partitioning of a compound into different phases is evident when the bioconcentration of two compounds differing in water-solubility is compared. Lindane, with a water-solubility of 10 mg/kg, was bioconcentrated about 1×10^2 times, whereas DDT, with a water-solubility of 1.2 μg/ℓ, was bioconcentrated to an extent of 1×10^5 to 1×10^6. Hence the bioconcentration/bioaccumulation of these compounds is the inverse of their water-solubility. Hamelink et al.[55] concluded that the concentration in the lower trophic level would not determine the concentration in the succeeding trophic levels, and that the residue concentration in each organism depends not so much on the trophic level, but on the absorption and storage phenomena which in turn depend on the solubility of a compound in the body lipids. Thus, for the first time, a plausible explanation for the accumulation process was offered and a proposal made that the uptake of chemicals depends solely on the partitioning into lipids and water. This proposal has subsequently stimulated numerous Structure-Activity Relationship studies on the uptake of xenobiotic compounds by fish (see Section VIII).

When about 2.76 g of DDE and lindane were introduced into a lime stone quarry to yield a theoretical concentration of 50 ng/ℓ in the entire water column, the concentration factors of DDE and lindane were, respectively, 2.86×10^4 to 6.35×10^4, and 170 to 448 in the zooplankton and 1.1×10^5 and 768 in the bluegill.[56] Rainbow trout introduced into the quarry 134 days after the treatment concentrated DDE 1.8×10^5 times in 108 days, as against a water concentration of less than 1 ng/ℓ. The average concentration factor for lindane was approximately 0.0007 times the average concentration factor for DDE, which was approximately the same in bluegills and invertebrates. It is very clear that the extent of bioconcentration is dependent on water-solubility rather than trophic position (lindane is about 1000 times more water-soluble than DDE). Based on water-solubility of DDE, approximately 1 mg/kg of DDE should have been concentrated in the bodies of fish. The actual concentration observed, which was less than the theoretical figure, was explained by Hamelink and Waybrant[56] as the result of the effect of size and age of fish in the quarry. According to them, larger individuals display a higher concentration factor (as was evident in their study) and smaller ones display a lower concentration factor, which may be attributable partly to the lipid reserves but more to the multicompartment, countercurrent distribution, regardless of the fat content. Even though the concentration of DDE in water was one tenth that of lindane, DDE was bioconcentrated 100 or more times than lindane. Hence, for an equivalent load of these two compounds, DDE presents a greater problem than lindane.

In nature, no relation in the levels of mirex sampled from the Mississippi Gulf coast was evident, the levels being (μg/kg) — seston, 200 to 3000; molluscs, 36 to 500; and fish, 0 to 259.[57] Similarly, in the biota sampled in the Jordan River watershed, the mean Σ DDT levels (mg/kg) recorded were water, 0.00002 to 0.0005; phytoplankton, 0.9; zooplankton, 6.5; and various species of fish, 0.37 to 3.34, showing no evidence of biomagnification.[58] In a report on the distribution of residues (especially dieldrin) in a ricefield-marshland ecosystem, it was concluded that biomagnification occurred in a stepwise process and a chronological sequence could be seen with the residues appearing first in the lower trophic levels and after a certain amount of delay, becoming available for assimilation by organisms at a higher trophic level.[59] Such arguments were put forward earlier by Harrison et al.[60] and strongly criticized by many workers.[61] An examination of the figures (Figures 2 to 5) in the paper of Ginn and Fisher,[59] however, fails to reveal any such time-lag, the levels of dieldrin reaching a peak at all trophic levels within 2 to 5 weeks after application, and continuing to decline in a similar manner up to the 15th week. It is also difficult to understand why such a biomagnification was not evident in the case of toxaphene and DDT and its metabolites, recorded

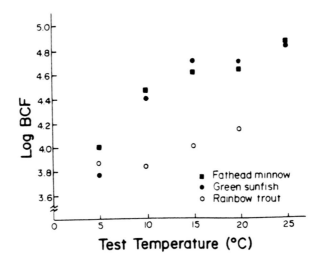

FIGURE 2.   Variation in BCF of Aroclor® 1254 with exposure temperatures for fathead minnows, green sunfish *(Lepomis cyanellus),* and rainbow trout *(Salmo gairdneri).* (From
Veith, G. D., DeFoe, D. L., and Bergstedt, B. V., *J. Fish. Res.
Board Can.*, 36, 1040, 1979. With permission.)

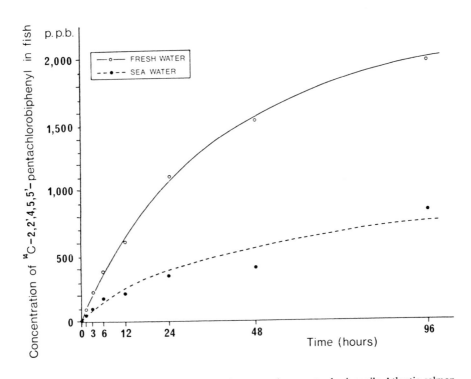

FIGURE 3.   Uptake of ^{14}C-PCB from freshwater and sea water by juvenile Atlantic salmon.
(From Tulp, M. Th. M., Haya, K., Carson, W. G., Zitko, V., and Hutzinger, O., *Chemosphere*,
8, 243, 1979. With permission. Copyright 1979, Pergamon Press.)

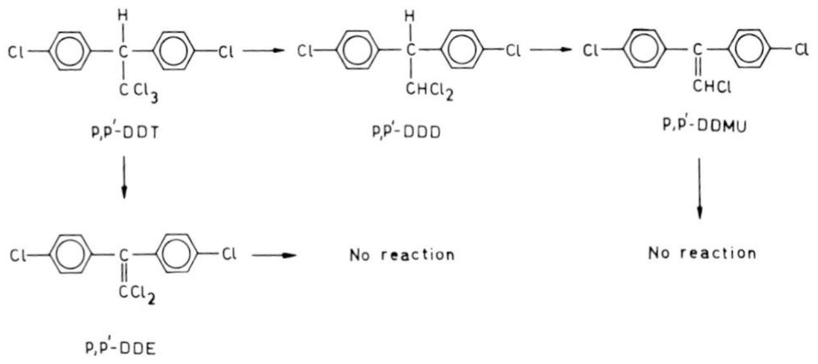

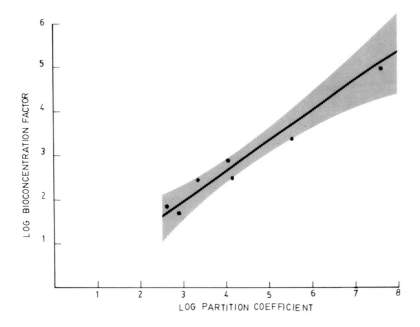

FIGURE 4.   Proposed pathway of metabolism of DDT in fish.[160]

FIGURE 5.   Linear regression between logarithms of partition coefficients and bio-concentration of various chemicals in trout muscle. (Reprinted with permission from Neely, W. B., Branson, D. R., and Blau, G. E., *Environ. Sci. Technol.,* 8, 1113, 1974.)

in the same population. In an Oklahoma stream, where high concentration of PCBs (0.23 to 7.2 mg/kg) was recorded in the sediments, but not in water, significantly higher PCB concentration was observed in filter feeders and detritus feeders than in omnivores and carnivores; the relative concentrations (mg/kg) being detritus feeder (carp and river carpsucker), 5.92; omnivore (channel catfish), 1.81; and carnivore (white bass and white crappie), 1.11; no food chain magnification was evident.

Ellgehausen et al.[62] showed that transfer of residues within the food-chain organisms amounted to 23 to 44, 3.9 to 9.1, and 9.1 to 11.9%, in the case of DDT, atrazine, and terbutryn, respectively, which means that no magnification had occurred. They found a direct relationship, with a high correlation coefficient, between transfer from one organism to another (T), and the log K_{ow} (also called log P, i.e., log octanol/water partition coefficient) as follows:

$$T = 5.35 \log K_{ow} - 9.69 \quad (r = 0.98 \text{ transfer from algae to}$$

daphnid)

$$T = 10.59 \log K_{ow} - 22.95 \ (r = 0.91 \text{ transfer from daphnid}$$

to catfish)

Using the above relation, Ellgehausen et al. calculated that a compound must have a log K_{ow} of 21.05 or a water solubility of 3.6×10^{-19} μmol/ℓ, to explain the observed levels of residue concentration in the consumer organism solely on the basis of bio-magnification. Pointing out the absurdity of such a situation, Ellgehausen et al. emphasized that the term biomagnification, denoting the buildup of residues via food chains, is indeed misleading.

The above discussion reveals that biomagnification is not of universal occurrence, at least in the aquatic ecosystem. Though it may be of local importance in a few instances, yet, in nature, other factors such as direct and intimate exposure to the toxicant (as in the case of detritus feeders), water solubility, and lipophilicity of the compound, may influence the uptake of a compound by aquatic organisms much more than transfer up the food chain. Hence, it seems advisable to refrain from using the term biomagnification except in instances of its proven occurrence, if any.

IV. UPTAKE FROM WATER OR THROUGH FOOD

Few questions in the realm of aquatic toxicology have generated as much discussion as the one on the route of uptake of pesticide residues by fish, viz., water or food. An ojective review of the various viewpoints expressed by different workers is in order before the recent trends of thinking on this question are summarized.

Macek and Korn[63] exposed brook trout to ^{14}C-DDT, through water (3 ng/ℓ, under continuous flow conditions), or through food (3 mg/kg, fed at a rate of 1.5% of the total body weight per day). After 120 days, the fish that were given DDT orally had 1.92 mg/kg; i.e., 33.5% of the total DDT administered was accumulated. The fish exposed to 3 ng/ℓ DDT, had a burden of 25.6 μg/kg, i.e., at the flow rate employed, 3.6% of the total DDT made available was retained. It was concluded that since the fish accumulated a higher percent of DDT from food than from water, accumulation through the food chain was much more important than uptake through water.

Holden[64] reported that brown trout exposed to ^{14}C-labeled DDT rapidly removed the toxicant from water, absorption was principally through gills, and much of the DDT that was taken up was stored in the body lipid. In a similar study, appreciable quantities of DDT were found in the tissues of Atlantic salmon soon after exposing it to ^{14}C-labeled DDT; it was concluded that entry through gills was the main route of uptake of DDT, and the compound was transported and distributed to all parts of the body by blood.[65] In order to determine whether death of fish was caused by the toxicant that was absorbed via gills or from swallowed water, black bullheads were operated upon and the digestive tract was tied off near the esophagus. When such fish and controls were exposed to endrin (50 μg/ℓ), death was equally rapid in both groups. Hence it was concluded that entry via gills was more important than entry through the digestive tract.[66] Chadwick and Brocksen[67] exposed reticulate sculpins to dieldrin through water or through diet (tubificid worms exposed to dieldrin until they contained a predetermined quantity of dieldrin), or through both food and water. The amount of accumulated residue depended on its concentration in water and was nearly linear and similar for different exposures. Further, when fish were given dieldrin through both food and water, accumulation was not additive, but the fish contained the same amount as those exposed to the same concentration of the compound in water alone. Murphy[68] studied the relation between body size and uptake of ^{14}C-DDT and observed that smaller fish absorbed DDT more efficiently from the medium than the larger fish. Criticizing the earlier report of Macek and Korn[63] who suggested that food chain accumulation of residues is more important, Murphy opined that had Macek and Korn used fingerling trout, they would have concluded otherwise.

In an elaborate discussion on the routes of entry of pesticides into the body, Moriarty[69] questioned the validity of the assumption of food chain magnification reported to have taken place in the biota of Clear Lake, Calif., where the death of the diving bird, western grebe *(Aechmophorus occidentalis),* was attributed to biomagnification of DDD following the spraying of the lake for controlling gnats *(Chaoborus asticto-pus).* DDD values as high as 1600 mg/kg were reported in the fatty tissues of grebes by Hunt and Bischoff.[70] Moriarty refuted the claim of Hunt and Bischoff that the level of DDD accumulation depended on the trophic position of a species, i.e., carnivorous fish have a higher content than plankton feeders. Underlining the fact that no DDD residues were detected in the plankton samples, he explained that although on a wet weight basis the residue concentration of plankton feeding and carnivorous fish appeared different, there was no significant difference when the concentration was expressed on a lipid weight basis. Moriarty concluded that aquatic organisms obtain their residue burden directly from water. He further drew support for his conclusion from the experiment of Meeks[71] who reported that in a marshland ecosystem, DDT accumulation was similar between herbivorous carp and carnivorous greenfish. Moriarty suggested that yet another reason for the higher levels of residues recorded in carnivorous species is that they pick up the prey animals that are dying, moribund, or overactive because of pesticide intoxication. Thus, according to Moriarty, selective feeding and not biomagnification would be the cause of higher residue levels in species occupying the higher levels of the food pyramid.

Reinert[44] examined the uptake of dieldrin by organisms at different levels of a simple trophic chain by exposing an alga *(Scendesmus), Daphnia,* and guppy directly to dieldrin in water and also by offering the last two species food organisms that had been previously exposed to dieldrin in water. What was interesting in these experiments was the accumulation of more dieldrin by *Daphnia* and guppy from water than from their food organisms in which residue concentration had reached equilibrium after being exposed to the same concentration of dieldrin in water. For instance, guppies exposed to 0.8 to 2.3 μg/ℓ in water accumulated 10 times more dieldrin than those guppies which were fed daphnids that had reached an equilibrium concentration of approximately 35 mg/kg, after exposure to 2.1 μg/ℓ dieldrin in water. Another very striking point was that whether the guppies were fed 10 or 20 daphnids, each containing an average of 32 mg/kg dieldrin, the resultant residue concentration was the same. Hence, Reinert concluded that both *Daphnia* and guppies accumulated more dieldrin from water than from food.

Marine polychaetes were reported to accumulate substantial quantities of DDT from very low concentrations in water; bottom feeding fish, when they fed on such polychaetes, accumulated considerable quantities of DDT in their tissues.[72] Fingerling channel catfish were exposed to endrin through food (fish were fed daily at a rate of 1% of their body weight, the feed containing 4, 0.4, 0.04, and 0.004 μg/g dry feed), or through water (0.5 and 0.25 μg/ℓ, in a continuous flow system), for 198 days and the uptake was calculated at regular intervals.[73] In the first 20 days, the fish that were given an oral dose of 4 μg/g food accumulated about 40% of the endrin provided, the percentage of uptake increasing with decreasing endrin content of the feed. In the first 4 days, fish exposed through water took up 1.6% of the endrin provided (in the higher exposure concentration), and the percent uptake decreased to less than 1 by the 20th day.

In general, in all studies on the uptake through food or water, a decreasing percentage of retention with increasing concentration of exposure has been noted by many workers. Lock[74] suggested that as a result of exposure to higher concentrations a mechanism such as increased mucus production at the respiratory surfaces and by the gut epithelium might decrease accumulation. Upon exposure to methylmercury through food and water, *Daphnia pulex* and *Salmo gairdneri* took up more methylmercury from water than from food; however, when the uptake was expressed as a percentage of the total mercury provided, a higher percentage of mercury was taken up from food than from water. It was concluded that the uptake of methylmercury was mostly from food, as practically all the methylmercury was complexed to the organic matter. In Coho salmon, the extent of retention of PCB residues given through food varied between 30 and 6% from 24 to 108 days, the percentage decreasing with time.[75]

Contrary to the report of Murphy,[68] Shannon[76] found that larger catfish initially took up more dieldrin from food and water than did smaller catfish. Fish that were exposed to 2 mg dieldrin per kilogram diet took up more residue than those exposed to 75 $\mu g/\ell$ dieldrin. Jarvinen et al.[77] exposed fathead minnows to DDT either in water (0.5 or 2 $\mu g/\ell$) or in food, or both, and analyzed the fish over a period of 266 days. The fish exposed to DDT through food were given a diet of dried, chopped clam meat, the clams having been previously exposed to 2 μg DDT per liter in a continuous flow system until equilibrium conditions were achieved (in about 8 weeks). The fish concentrated DDT from water to about one million times, whereas the mean concentration factor from food was only 1.2. Although the amount of DDT accumulated from food was not high, the presence of DDT in the food enhanced the mortality of fish significantly. The residue burden obtained from food was more-than-additive to that from water. Embryo residue levels and larval mortality of progeny derived from parents exposed via food and water were twice those of progeny derived from parents exposed to DDT only in water or food.

In a similar experiment, Jarvinen and Tyo[78] exposed fathead minnows to endrin, through water alone (0.17 and 0.28 $\mu g/\ell$), through food alone (clams, previously exposed to 0.28 μg endrin per liter, under flow-through conditions for 3 weeks, i.e., time sufficient for attaining steady state condition), or through both food and water (0.17 μg or 0.28 $\mu g/\ell$ in water and 0.17 μg or 0.28 $\mu g/kg$ in contaminated food). Results showed that higher amounts of residues were accumulated from water than food. When exposed through food alone, equilibrium concentration was achieved in 14 days. The mean concentration factor of all observations was 0.3 ± 0.01 SEM for food and 7000 ± 436 for water exposure. The highest concentration factor observed was 0.8 from food and 13,000 from water which was achieved on the 56th day of exposure to the highest concentration. Residues contributed by food were additive to those from water. Over a period of 300 days, 15% of the total body residues were accumulated from food and the remaining from water when the fish were exposed to 0.17 $\mu g/\ell$ in water and ¹⁴C-labeled endrin in food simultaneously. When exposed to 0.28 $\mu g/\ell$ in water and 0.28 $\mu g/kg$ food simultaneously, the latter accounted for only 10% of the total body burden accumulated in 300 days. Endrin, when present in food, however, significantly affected the survival of the test fish. Fish exposed to endrin through both sources had a lower survival rate than those exposed to endrin through one source only. So was the case with the embryos and larvae bred by exposed parents. This study, as well as the other study of Jarvinen et al. on DDT, indicated that uptake from water is more important than uptake through food, but the latter can prove disastrous in the long run.

Lockhart et al.[79] reported that the uptake of toxicants through gills was very substantial and rapid. For instance, as against a pretreatment level of 0.02 $\mu g/g$ (wet tissue weight) in the different tissues, the residue levels in the lower digestive tract, fat, muscle, and kidney 15 min after exposure to 300 μg methoxychlor/ℓ were 9.1 ± 3.84; 2.62 ± 1.33; 1 ± 0.17; and 4.6 ± 1.43 (μg/g wet tissue weight), respectively; 30 min after treatment, the levels were 16.9 ± 5.99; 5.12 ± 3.45; 1.29 ± 0.42; and 10.4 ± 5.24 μg/g, respectively. Such a rapid uptake suggests that gills are the primary route of uptake of residues.

In order to determine whether food is the main source of lipophilic substances, and as a consequence there is food chain magnification of substances like DDT and PCB, micro- and macroplankton and fish were sampled at the same time from the same water.[80] DDT was absent in the microplankton and it was concluded that there was no food chain magnification of lipophilic substances. On the contrary, there was a 100-fold decrease in the PCB concentration between microplankton and myctophied fish. Absence of accumulation via food is further illustrated in experiments on the accumulation of ^{14}C-toluene by bluegills. The toxicant was taken only when it was offered through the medium and not through contaminated food, that had in turn accumulated the toxicant from the medium.[81]

Evaluating the reasons for the earlier controversy regarding the relative importance of the uptake of residues by fish through food or water, Macek et al.[10] considered that one of the reasons for the controversy was the choice of environmentally unrealistic concentrations in food and water while comparing both routes of uptake. He suggested that the only way to evaluate both routes of uptake is to expose the food organisms to a particular concentration in water until steady-state was achieved and then feeding them to the consumer organisms and comparing the resulting bioaccumulation with bioconcentration in the consumer organisms exposed directly to the chemical in water at the same concentration to which the food organisms had been exposed. Such a methodology was employed by Reinert,[44] Jarvinen et al.,[77] and Jarvinen and Tyo.[78] Macek et al. also stated that the rate of feeding utilized in the experimental design is important and the feeding rates available under natural conditions should be utilized. The observation of Reinert[44] that there was no difference in the dieldrin concentration of guppies that were fed 10 or 20 *Daphnia* that had previously achieved steady-state concentration with dieldrin may be recalled in this context. To evaluate the relative importance of dietary or gill intake of residues, Macek et al.[10] exposed daphnids to ^{14}C-labeled DEHP (di-[2-ethylhexyl] phthalate), 1,2,4-trichlorobenzene (TCB), and leptophos, until steady-state was achieved (4 to 24 hr). Bluegills were exposed to one of these chemicals in water alone or through food alone, or through food and water together. Under steady-state conditions, bluegills concentrated DEHP, TCB, and leptophos 112, 183, and 146 times, respectively. The uptake through food was statistically insignificant, and the contribution of dietary uptake to the body burden when the fish were exposed both through food and water was insignificant when compared with body loads resulting from the uptake from water alone. After reexamining the earlier reports on the dietary accumulation of chemicals, Macek et al. concluded that DDT appears to be the only chemical with a potential for significant dietary accumulation (25 to 60% of the total body residues). Usually, dietary accumulation of other chemicals seems to contribute only 1 to 10% of the total body burdens, which is less than the coefficient of variation associated with the ability to measure body burdens through bioconcentration. Macek et al. also suggested that a study of depuration rates will be helpful in identifying DDT type substances, if indeed there are any, that may contribute significantly to the body burden through food organisms.

While discussing the relative importance of dietary absorption or bioconcentration of lipophilic compounds, the contribution of the water that enters the body for purposes of osmoregulation — passively (freshwater fish) or actively (marine fish) — to residue uptake has rarely been evaluated. Tulp et al.[82] attempted to evaluate the relative importance of the two routes of uptake by comparing the extent of accumulation of a compound by the same species under freshwater and marine conditions. Marine fish drink water, equivalent to approximately 5 to 12% of their body weight, daily. In freshwater fish, gills are the major entry points of water, but it is not known exactly how much water is taken in; it is known that freshwater fish excrete water equal to about 10% of their body weight per day. When the same species of migratory fish is exposed to a toxicant under otherwise identical conditions, in fresh- and sea water, the relative body burdens would show whether the uptake is primarily through gills or through food. Atlantic salmon were exposed to ^{14}C-2,2′ 4,5,5′-pentachlorobiphenyl in fresh- and sea water; the fish exposed in freshwater had higher wholebody concentration as well as higher concentration in different tissues and organs than those exposed in sea water, although the apparent concentration of ^{14}C-PCB was higher initially in the saltwater than in freshwater (Figure 3). High concentrations were found in areas of high blood flow, and tissues of low blood flow such as visceral adipose tissue reached equilibrium much more slowly. If absorption through food were to be much more important than absorption via gills, the residue loads in marine fish should be higher than those in freshwater fish, but the reverse was true in their study. Hence, the authors concluded that the primary uptake of lipophilic compounds occurs via the gills and skin. They also refuted the earlier claim of Canton et al.[83] that guppies took up three times more α-HCH in saltwater than in freshwater. Canton et al. sought to explain the increased uptake of the toxicant by guppies acclimated to saltwater as the result of drinking contaminated water for ionic balance. On the basis of the ambient concentrations, the amount of water taken in orally, and the observed body residue burden, Tulp et al. showed that guppies would have taken up (by drinking water equivalent to 10% of their body weight daily) only 1% of the observed body contaminant burden.

The contaminant burden in the marine and freshwater environment of a migratory fish like the American shad that enters the freshwater only for spawning (and does not feed during its sojourn through freshwater) would show the relative uptake through food or gills. Fish caught about 120 km upstream of the Hudson River mouth had a significantly higher level of PCB concentration than fish caught about 40 km upstream from the river mouth. Since a higher contaminant level was found in nonfeeding fish while migrating in freshwater, it was concluded that the uptake from water was evident.[84]

A marine food chain — consisting of a flagellate alga *(Duneliella* sp.), a rotifer *(Brachionus plicatilis)*, and the larva of the northern anchovy *(Engraulis modax)* — was exposed to concentrations of PCB in water representative of the near-shore conditions of southern California. The rotifer and fish were also exposed separately to food organisms that had attained steady-state upon being exposed to near-shore concentrations of PCBs. Unfed anchovy larvae accumulated the chemical to the same extent as those that were fed contaminated food.[85] The final body concentration depended on the concentration in sea water and the chlorinated hydrocarbon accumulation was evidently not a food chain phenomenon but a result of direct absorption of the chemical from sea water by the test organisms. Besides, the apparent food chain amplification of PCBs at the lower trophic levels disappeared when the concentration was calculated on a dry-weight basis. Similarly benzo(a)pyrene was taken up by clams mostly from sea water rather than from food.[86] On the other hand, Monod and Keck[87] recorded the lowest PCB levels in plankton-feeding fish (coregonines) in Lake Geneva, Switzerland, and stated that PCB levels increased in the order of increasing carnivorous feeding habits, viz., char > perch > roach. They concluded that food chain magnification was evident. A careful examination of the value reported by them, however, fails to reveal any consistent trend of increase in three out of six tissues in males and five out of six tissues in the females analyzed by them; often the residue levels in perch were lower than or comparable to those in the roach.

Another convincing piece of evidence on the relative importance of uptake via gills is contained in a report on the residue loads in Lake Simcoe, Ontario, fish between 1970 and 1976.[88] *Salvelinus namaycush* that were more than 4 kg in weight in 1976 were estimated to be 10 to 15 years old and would have been exposed to DDT in water for at least 5 years (with a simultaneous exposure to DDT in the food chain also), and for another 5 years to DDT, mainly through the food chain. Those fish that were under 4 kg in 1975 to 1976 were estimated to be 5 to 8 years old and would have been mostly exposed to DDT through the food chain only. The respective body burdens of DDT were (all values mg/kg tissue weight basis) 17.7 in 1970 and 13.3 in 1975 to 1976 in fish that were more than 4 kg in weight. The body burdens of fish below 4 kg in weight were 9.66 in 1970 and 0.97 in 1975 to 1976. These figures show that those fish that were exposed to DDT in both water and food continued to have relatively high body loads even in 1975 to 1976, while those that were born after the ban on the use of DDT in Canada in 1970, and hence were exposed to DDT mostly through the food chain, showed a dramatic decline in the total DDT residues in the body. This study clearly shows that in nature, concentration from water plays a much more significant role than accumulation through food, although the authors themselves seemed to have missed this point and stated, in a different part of their paper that, in general, the major pathway of accumulation of contaminants in fish is the food chain.

Reinert et al.[89] exposed lake trout in the laboratory to DDT or dieldrin-contaminated food or water and calculated tentatively that the uptake of DDT and dieldrin from water was 20 to 102% and 12 to 59%, respectively. The assimilation from food likewise was 20 and 17%, respectively. They tried to extrapolate the laboratory findings to the field and explain the extent to which coho salmon in Lake Michigan would sequester DDT from food and water. In a period of 104 days, between May 9, 1968 and August 22, 1968, the amount of *p,p'*-DDT in coho from Lake Michigan increased from 1.4 mg/kg in May to 14.1 mg/kg in August. Based on the average ventilation volume of 2 ℓ/min, Reinert et al. concluded that it is unlikely that such a high concentration of DDT would have been taken up through gills and hence a large part of the 12.7 mg of *p,p'*-DDT accumulated by the coho would have come from food.

In fish, rapid conversion of DDT to DDD by intestinal microflora has been reported.[90] Hence, any uptake of DDT through the digestive tract should result in elevated levels of body DDD concentration. In nature, DDE and not DDD constitutes the major component of Σ DDT (see Chapter 2), and Reinert and Bergman[91] also reported DDE as the principal constituent of Σ DDT in Great Lakes fish; therefore, uptake through food alone cannot explain the increase in the Σ DDT levels of Great Lakes fish.

If the uptake of residues is through water, then given an environment with a stable contaminant situation, the fat in all species should accumulate a given pesticide or chemical approximately to the same level, depending on the water solubility and partitioning of that chemical into the lipid phase. Such a situation, if observed in nature, would support the conclusion that accumulation is mainly through water. In order to compare the degree of accumulation of residues in different animal species from different locations, Bjerk and Brevik[92] analyzed the levels of five pollutants in the samples of aquatic biota from two locations in the Oslo Fjord area — one from the Frierfjord and another from Ora, located at the estuary of the Glomma River. In the Ora area, the sediments had a PCB content about 20 times that of DDE; but in the organisms, the PCB/DDE ratio was constant and was about 10 in all the invertebrate species studied and was close to 15 in all the fish species examined. In the Frierfjord area, PCBs, DDE, and DDT were present in minute quantities. HCB, pentachlorobenzene

(5CB), and octachlorostyrene (OCS) were present more often. The levels of 5CB in the fat of different species was about 10 times as high as in sediments. The concentrations of DDE, PCB, and 5CB lend support to the idea that direct uptake from water via respiratory organs or the general body surface is the most important route of entry. Feeding habits also are of importance; detritus-feeding brittle star had higher residue levels than the rock dwelling sea star and snail.

An attempt has been made to examine the relative importance of uptake via gills by calculating the amount of water that passes over the gills. Assuming that pesticides are extracted from water as efficiently as oxygen across the gills, Holden[93] calculated that to meet the oxygen demand of a trout with an active metabolism of 300 mg/kg/hr, about 700 ℓ of water should pass over the gills in a day. At the maximum rate of extraction, exposure to 100 ng of a toxicant would result in a theoretical concentration of 0.5 mg/kg in the fish in a week. In practice, fish exposed to 2.3 μg/ℓ dieldrin concentrated the compound about 3000 times in the muscle in 3 weeks. The actual extraction is lower than that of oxygen, presumably because of the mucus covering of the gill membrane. Neely[94] reviewed the standard and active metabolic rate coefficients for various species of fish at various temperatures. Using the ventilation volume rate, Neely proposed a method for making reasonable estimates of uptake and clearance of chemicals in fish. Rodgers and Beamish[95] measured the oxygen consumption and uptake of methylmercury by rainbow trout at 10 and 20°C. The rate of methylmercury uptake correlated positively with both oxygen consumption and methylmercury concentration. At an oxygen utilization of 33%, the percent extraction of methylmercury from water was about 8.

Addison[96] calculated the amount of DDT that may be taken up by trout ventilating about 175 mℓ water per minute per kilogram body weight, at 8°C. With a typical DDT content of 10 ng/ℓ, and at 100% assimilation efficiency, trout may concentrate approximately 900 μg DDT per kilogram body weight in a year. While stating that such levels are within the range of concentrations observed in nature, he emphasized that such a calculation assumes 100% extraction of DDT, which is unlikely, and that trout being "moderately active fish" may ventilate larger volumes of water than other sluggish fish. Hence he concluded that water is unlikely to be the main source of p,p'-DDT for fish.

Recently McKim et al.[97] measured the total flux of some selected organic chemicals across trout gills. The gill extraction efficiency varied from 7 to 60% in a single pass of the chemical across the gill. The extraction efficiency was clearly related to the octanol-water partition coefficient (K_{ow}, see Section VIII). For chemicals with a log K_{ow} value of 1 to 3 the uptake was controlled by membrane permeability and was directly related to log K_{ow}; for those with a log K_{ow} value of >3, the extraction efficiency varied between 55 and 60% and was independent of K_{ow}.

Besides examining the extent of uptake via gills, a few attempts were made to fit a model based on energy dynamics to describe the observed levels of the various pollutants in natural populations. On the basis of such a model, Norstrom et al.[98] predicted that 50 to 70% of the pollutant burden was taken up from food; although the uptake from water was 10^5 times that of the uptake from food when the concentration was the same in water and food, they postulated that faster-growing fish accumulated proportionately more from food than slow-growing fish.

Harding et al.,[99] on the basis of model simulations, concluded that it is not necessary to invoke direct uptake of DDT from sea water to explain the known levels of DDT in marine copepods. On the basis of about 60% retention of the ingested DDT under normal conditions, and 10% retention under bloom conditions, they concluded that rapidly developing *Calanus* could accumulate DDT from generation to generation and will reach equilibrium concentration after 4 to 12 generations. To what extent such models, that describe the pollutant uptake in one group of invertebrates, are suitable to describe the conditions in fish is not known. Zitko and Hutzinger[100] observed no accumulation and certainly no magnification of the PCBs in hatchery-reared Atlantic salmon that were fed contaminated food.

The above review would clearly emphasize the magnitude of the controversy regarding the relative importance of food or water as the principal means of pesticide residues by fish. Those who hold that gill ventilation affords the major opportunity for the uptake of residues base their arguments on the relative uptake from water and food that had attained equilibrium concentrations upon exposure to the contaminants in water. The main criticism against such experiments is that the fish were exposed to unrealistically high concentrations of the compound in water and also that the experiments were conducted for only a short duration.[96,101] As has already been pointed out, employing the same concentration of Aroclor® as that recorded in natural waters, Scura and Theilacker[85] showed that organisms at different trophic levels took up a higher quantity of residues from water than from food. Further, the results of the works that compared the relative uptake (1) when the fish were feeding and not feeding,[84] (2) when the fish were exposed in nature to DDT both in water and food or mainly through food,[88] (3) when water was entering through gut or through gills and general body surface,[82] and (4) the results of the study on the rapidity of uptake of a compound from water,[79] point out that given a situation where a lipophilic compound is available for absorption, both in water and food, uptake from the former is higher. It must also be pointed out that uptake from food may contribute a significant part of the total body burden in the case of rapidly growing fish. Further, in nature, the situation may be much more complicated than what has been envisaged as trophic biomagnification based on simple laboratory food chain models. In nature, each organism is intricately associated with other species in a complex food web, rather than in a simple species-to-species relationship of a food chain. While all the available evidence tilts the balance of the argument in favor of uptake from water, any conclusion that the dietary route is unimportant may be unwarranted in the light of the work of Jarvinen and associates (on the uptake of endrin and DDT) who showed that the contribution of a compound taken up through food, to the overall toxic effect, is very significant.

V. UPTAKE AND DEPURATION

A. Uptake
1. Uptake of DDT
DDT, because of its great affinity to lipid material, is taken up quickly from food and water, metabolized slowly, and stored for an extended period. ^{14}C-DDT added to rainbow trout serum was rapidly distributed among all serum lipoproteins;[102] association of residues with serum[103] or red blood cells was observed.[104] Bluegills and goldfish took up DDT rapidly after a single exposure of a few hours.[105] Percentage of uptake was inversely related to exposure concentration.[106] A major part of the deposited residue was in the form of p,p'-DDT, (>50%), followed by DDE and DDD, in that order. Likewise, the percentage retention decreased with increasing quantity administered.[107] The decreasing accumulation was attributed to elimination.[107] The uptake of DDT was higher at higher temperatures.[108,109]

The distribution pattern of accumulated DDT was independent of dosage; brain, liver, and gastrointestinal tract ranked highest, and the skeletal muscle lowest. Even during the period of elimination, this pattern was unchanged. In all the organs, more than 80% of the accumulated DDT remained unchanged. Of the ^{14}C-DDT accumulated after feeding 17 μg of DDT over a period of 4 weeks, 62% was eliminated[107] during a period of 2 months in pesticide-free water. Following the exposure of *Fundulus* to ^{14}C-DDT in water, the compound was taken up rapidly and deposited in muscle, testes, and ovaries. More DDT was incorporated in the testes than in the ovaries.[110]

Although the absolute values of DDT (lipid weight basis) in the same organ in different species of fish varied, when the values were expressed as relative concentrations (i.e., concentration in tissue ÷ concentration in the liver of the same fish × 100), the values were similar for any one type of tissue in different fish, indicating a rapid achievement of steady-state conditions.[111]

Fish are usually exposed to the toxicant via food or water, but at times the toxicant is also administered intraperitoneally. Bathe et al.[112] found that fish were less susceptible when the compound was administered i.p. For instance, the 7-day-LD 50 of DDT (given i.p.) to trout and crucian carp was, respectively, 7 and 6.5 mg/kg, whereas when the fish were exposed in water, the 96-h LC 50 was 0.06 and 0.08 mg/ℓ, i.e., nearly a 100-fold difference.

DDT, following an i.v. injection of the thorny skate, was rapidly cleared from the plasma into tissues of high blood flow and subsequently from the latter into tissues of higher lipid content.[113] Over a period of 2 to 23 days following the injection, no significant amount of metabolites could be detected in any of the tissues, indicating that the compound was metabolized and excreted to a negligible extent. During this period, about 82 to 93% of the injected dose could be accounted for in the various tissues. After a single i.m. injection of a massive dose of DDT to the catfish, *Heteropneustes fossilis* (800 mg/kg), most of the compound was retained as DDT.[114] DDE at less than 10% of the DDT content was recovered from liver, kidney, and fat bodies, and none from brain and spinal cord 24 hr after injection. The residue concentration of the brain, but not that of the body, was indicative of the signs of poisoning; the fat bodies of dead fish contained 1473 mg/kg whereas those of the surviving fish had a concentration of 2091 mg/kg.[114]

2. Uptake of Other Organochlorines (OCS)

The uptake of dieldrin from water was less than that of DDT and that of HCH less than that of the former. Exposure of bluegills and goldfish to 0.03 mg/ℓ ^{14}C-dieldrin for 5 to 9 hr resulted in an uptake of 3.8 mg/ℓ. During a 32-day depuration period in clean water, 90% of the accumulated dieldrin was lost.[105] In goldfish exposed to aldrin (0.05 mg/ℓ) for 8 hr and transferred to clean water, aldrin was rapidly converted to dieldrin. In all the tissues except visceral fat, the concentration of dieldrin increased with time. In goldfish, the conversion of aldrin to dieldrin was slower.[115] Goldfish that were fed higher doses of dieldrin accumulated higher amounts at greater rates than those given lower doses; however, the percentage of dieldrin taken up by the fish was higher in the group exposed to lower concentrations.[116] Absorption through the intestine was a slow process. Radioactivity in the tissues was attributable only to the parent compound and not to the metabolites; the highest amount of radioactivity was in the mesenteric adipose tissue and testes. Residue concentration in the ovaries increased with the stage of maturity. When goldfish were exposed to 20 μg/ℓ photodieldrin for 6 days, equilibrium was reached within 24 hr. Elimination of residue after the fish were transferred to clean water was biphasic, very rapid for the first 24 hr and slower thereafter.[117] The time required to attain equilibrium concentration of dieldrin by channel catfish depended on the initial exposure concentration. At lower exposure concentration, steady-state was reached earlier.[118]

The acute toxicity of γ-HCH is higher than that of α- and β-HCH, yet it is eliminated faster than the latter two.[119] As in the experiments with dieldrin,[118] the time taken for attaining equilibrium conditions depended on the exposure concentration. Experiments with guppies yielded similar results.[83] Uptake of endrin by channel catfish was low and elimination complete upon transfer to an endrin-free diet.[120] Heptachlor-exposed spot reached equilibrium levels within 72 hr, but eliminated the compound slowly in uncontaminated water.[121] On the other hand, equilibrium conditions were not attained by brook trout, even after 15 weeks of feeding mirex at 0.7 mg of mirex per kilogram body weight three times a week.[122] Elimination was also equally slow. The apparent decline in body residue burden was due to the growth of the fish, resulting in dilution of body residue concentration, rather than to true elimination. Other studies also confirmed that mirex was retained by fish to a high degree and eliminated little.[123] Kepone®, structurally closely related to mirex, was not taken up as much as mirex, the BCF being 1100 to 2200 for Kepone® and 12,000 to 28,000 for mirex, with fathead minnows exposed to 0.3 to 5.1 μg of Kepone® per liter and 34 μg of mirex per liter for 120 days. Upon transfer to uncontaminated water, Kepone® was eliminated in less than 7 days, whereas 46% of the mirex remained even after 56 days.

The accumulation of HCB by fish was proportional to the treatment levels but retention was highest in those that were fed lower doses.[124,125] Highest residue concentration was present in the alimentary tract and the least in the skeletal muscle. During depuration, clearance from the latter was faster and thus the edible part was rid of the contaminant first. Retention of HCB residues was longest in the liver, where HCB was metabolized to PCP.[125]

PCBs are readily taken up by fish and stored in tissues. After attaining equilibrium levels, total quantity of PCBs stored in the body continued to increase, whereas the relative concentration appeared to be constant as a result of growth. Among the PCBs, those containing fewer chlorine atoms were accumulated to a lesser extent and eliminated faster.[75] In coho salmon parr that were fed 10 μg of 3,4,3',4'-tetrachlorobiphenyl or 2,4,5,2',4',5'-hexachlorobiphenyl or 2,4,6,2',4',6'-hexachlorobiphenyl, the retention of hexachlorobiphenyls was twice that of tetrachlorobiphenyl (1.4 and 0.65 mg/kg, respectively). Upon starvation for 48 days, the ratio of hexa- to tetrachlorobiphenyls was 3 or 4 to 1.[126] Time taken for the attainment of steady-state depended on the concentration of PCBs in the feed. At the time of active uptake, residues were deposited in the muscle; starvation led to a redistribution of the residues to the non-edible parts (offal).[127] In fatty fish, 4-chlorobiphenyl was mostly stored in the skeletal muscle or carcass with the viscera and skin being of minor importance; in a lean fish, the viscera and carcass were the main areas of storage. While the residues were being cleared from the tissues of trout, even when the residue concentration in the liver was reduced to half, the residues from the muscle were not mobilized.[128]

3. Uptake of Other Pesticides

The organophosphate (OP) and carbamate compounds, because of their relatively higher water solubility, are in general taken up to lesser extent than organochlorines (OCs) and eliminated faster.[129-132] The time for achieving the highest levels of uptake and the extent of retention of OP residues by fish was directly related to the extent of persistence of a compound in water. Motsugo fish exposed to 0.6 to 1.2 mg/ℓ of diazinon, fenitrothion, malathion, carbaryl, BPMC, or XMC, attained the highest body concentrations (mg/kg) of the various compounds as follows: diazinon, 211, after 3 days; fenitrothion, 162, after 3 days; malathion, 2.4, after 1 day; carbaryl, 7.5, after 1 day; and BPMC, 4.8, after 3 days.[133] Only diazinon (17 mg/kg), fenitrothion (4.9 mg/kg), BPMC (1.2 mg/kg), and XMC (0.55 mg/kg) persisted longer than 4 weeks in the fish.

Chlorophenols, especially PCP, are now known to be ubiquitous[134] and the uptake of these compounds by fish has been little studied. Rainbow trout exposed to 25 μg/ℓ PCP for 24 hr had 16, 6.5, 6, and 1 μg/g PCP, respectively, in the liver, blood, fat, and muscle.[135] Uptake of trichlorophenol(TCP) by female guppies was more than that by the males; however, males eliminated TCP more effectively than the females.[136] Deposition of PCP upon exposure of bluegills under static conditions was highest in liver and least in muscle. As in the other studies, peak values were reached in 7 to 8 days; continued exposure thereafter, however, led to declining values in the different tissues, indicating the activation of detoxifying mechanisms.[137]

Among the herbicides, very few are taken up to a considerable extent and retained in the tissues.[138-144] Simazine was not absorbed by green sunfish through the gut, but a small quantity was taken up through water.[139] Similarly, 90% of the 2,4-D given i.p. was excreted by bluegills within 6 hr and when exposed to the toxicant in water, bluegills attained equilibrium within 24 hr.[140] Similar observations were reported with endothall.[141] Thidiazuron was rapidly excreted when given i.p. to the bluegills, whereas exposure through water resulted in a limited uptake; depuration in clean water continued for 14 days.[142] The little dinitramine that was absorbed was taken up fairly rapidly (in muscle, six times the ambient concentration in water). Depuration in clean water was also rapid. Elimination from muscle was slower than elimination from plasma and bile.[143] CNP, a herbicide, was taken up rapidly but excreted very slowly.[144]

The insect growth regulator, diflubenzuron, was taken up from water about 80 times that of the ambient concentration by white crappies and bluegills. Clearance in uncontaminated water was very fast and took less than 24 hr.[145] Methoprene, another insect growth regulator, was bioconcentrated by bluegills to a moderate extent. In clean water, bluegills were rid of 93 to 95% of the accumulated body burden in less than 2 weeks.

4. Models of Uptake

The balance of uptake and elimination of any substance by the organisms may be analyzed by compartmental models. Moriarty[69] defined a compartment as a quantity of any substance which has uniform and distinguishable kinetics of transport and metabolism. Such a compartment need not necessarily correspond to a specific tissue or an organ, but in practice it often does. One such model offered to describe uptake and deposition of xenobiotic chemicals is the mamillary model explained by Moriarty[69] and consists of a number of peripheral compartments, not communicating with one another, but with a central compartment (blood). Material transport occurs between the central and the peripheral compartments and is maintained by the intake of a chemical, exchange between different compartments, and excretion from the body. If all the variables remain constant, a steady-state will be reached and the body residue load will be maintained at a constant level (plateau level).[69]

Dvorchik and Maren[103] identified three compartments in the clearance of ^{14}C-DDT from the plasma of fish: (1) clearance from plasma, (2) distribution in the tissues of high blood flow, and (3) redistribution into lipid-rich tissues. A similar picture emerged for the uptake of HCH by rainbow trout yearlings. Following exposure of rainbow trout to lindane, initially, muscle had maximum residue concentration in 48 hr, but this was followed by a decrease in residue concentration in the muscle, and later a gradual increase with time.[146] Evidently, lindane entered the muscle tissue rapidly, reaching a peak in 48 hr. Following a redistribution of residues into other tissues, a decrease in muscle residue level was noticed.

Neely et al.[147] estimated the rate of uptake (K_1) and rate of clearance (K_2) to calculate the steady state relationship (K_1/K_2). Branson et al.[148] described an accelerated kinetic model for the calculation of BCF. Likewise, Krzeminski et al.[149] proposed a pharmacokinetic model to calculate the steady-state concentration. They proposed a two-compartment model, viz., a rapid exchange compartment (viscera) and a slow exchange compartment (tissue). The predictions based on the mathematical model were compared with experimentally derived values of a number of compounds. A good agreement was observed between the predicted and observed values.

Eberhardt[150] attempted to fit kinetic models for the uptake and retention of DDT and dieldrin, using the data published by several authors. He found that log-linear relationships were best suited to describe the relation between uptake, retention, and body size and concluded that uptake and retention experiments performed with small fish give very different results from those size groups that are to be expected in species of commercially important fish. Deviation of the residue concentration in larger species from predicted values has also been noted by Spacie and Hamelink.[151]

Norstrom et al.[152] proposed a model for pollutant uptake on the basis of fish bioenergetics and pollutant biokinetics. In this model the contribution of seasonal and annual growth to metabolism was taken into account. The uptake of pollutant from food was based on the caloric requirements for respiration and growth, coupled with concentration of the pollutant in food and the efficiency of assimilation. Similarly, uptake from water was based on the gill ventilation rate coupled with the concentration of the pollutant in water and the efficiency of assimilation via gills. Griesbach et al.[153] proposed an allometric model for pesticide bioaccumulation, taking into consideration the frequency distribution of body sizes and the appropriate allometric relationships.

5. Factors that Influence Uptake

Apart from the hydrophobicity (lipophilicity) and water solubility of a compound (which in turn depend on the molecular structure), the lipid content, age, size, sex, and physiological activity of the fish, and environmental factors such as temperature influence the rate of uptake of a xenobiotic chemical. The net assimilation of residues from food and tissue retention are dependent on the size of the lipid pool.[154] The biological half-life is also dependent on the adiposity of the fish. The rate of methylmercury uptake by rainbow trout was positively correlated with oxygen consumption and the concentration of methylmercury.[95] An increase in the temperature from 5 to 15°C resulted in the doubling of the uptake of DDT and PCBs.[109] Since a rise of 10°C results in a doubling of the metabolic rate, the observed increase in the rate of accumulation indicates a direct relationship between metabolic rate and accumulation. Female *Gasterosteus* took up more lindane than the male and the latter took up about 5.8 times more lindane at the time of spawning than at other times.[45]

B. Metabolism and Elimination of Pesticide Residues by Fish

Generally, larger fish take a longer time to eliminate the body burdens. The biodegradability and elimination of organic chemicals is mainly dependent on the atomic groups of the substituents.[155] While the uptake of residues of OC pesticides by fish is rapid, their elimination is rather slow, showing that elimination is not the reverse of uptake. Although at one time fish were supposed to be devoid of the different biochemical detoxifying mechanisms possessed by mammals, subsequent studies have proved the existence of such mechanisms in fish as well. Polar compounds that have low bioconcentration/bioaccumulation potential are poorly absorbed, quickly metabolized, and eliminated through the bile. Of nine compounds to which rainbow trout were exposed, the highest ratio of bile-to-water concentration was that of rapidly metabolized polar compounds, and the lowest ratio of bile-to-water concentration was of those compounds with poor water solubility; the latter were poorly metabolized.[156]

1. Metabolism

Among all the pesticides, degradation of DDT and mirex by fish is very slow. Little excretion of DDT through urine or gill effluate or conversion to metabolites was evident 48 hr after administering DDT to dogfish via the caudal vein, artery, or stomach tube.[103] The report of Greer and Paim,[157] that the absorbed DDT was converted to DDE and DDD within 9 hr after the exposure of salmon parr to aqueous solutions of

DDT, is contrary to other reports. DDT-exposed fathead minnows had very low concentration of DDE and no DDD in the whole body 2 weeks after exposure, but after 266 days of exposure, the DDE concentration was nearly nine times that of DDT; DDD concentration was about one third that of DDT. The concentrations of DDT, DDE, and DDD in embryos obtained from exposed fish were similar to that of the adults.[77] DDT and DDE were poorly metabolized after their i.m. injection.[158] Previous exposure of brook trout to DDT or its metabolites did not influence the subsequent rate of dechlorination of ^{14}C-DDT. The conversion of DDT to DDE is, in general, very slow but some species seem capable of metabolizing DDT faster. Salmon fry converted DDT or DDE much faster than did brook trout. Assuming first order kinetics for the process, Addison et al.[159] estimated the half-life of DDT in *Salmo salar* fry and brook trout as 60 days, and 255 to 408 days, respectively. This difference may be the result of the difference in size (Atlantic salmon fry employed were much smaller than the brook trout employed) or may reflect the differences in the ability of the two species to metabolize DDT. Following an i.v. injection of radioactive DDT and its possible degradation products — DDE, DDD, DDMS, DDNU, DDMU, DDOH, DBP, DBH, and DDA — most of the lesser polar compounds were retained by trout even 3 weeks later.[160] p,p'-DDT was converted to DDE and to a lesser extent to DDD; the latter was slowly metabolized to a limited extent to DDMU which was not excreted. DDMS was converted rapidly (in less than 24 hr) to DDNU and excreted; however, DDMS itself was not the metabolic end product of any other compound in the tissues. In fish, it seems that DDT is converted to DDE, or to DDD, and then to DDMU. Both DDE and DDMU (or even DDD) seem to be dead ends of metabolic process with no further degradation and elimination, unlike in mammals. On the basis of their extensive studies, Addison and Willis[160] summarized the metabolism of DDT in fish as shown in Figure 4.

The presence of small quantities of DDMS in Clear Lake, Calif. fish was confirmed by GC-MS studies.[161] Trace quantities of DDNU and DDNS were also recorded. All these studies indicate that DDT, DDE, or DDD, absorbed from water by fish, are poorly metabolized and that DDT is mostly converted to DDE. This would explain the higher concentrations of DDE reported in the natural fish population, especially in aged fish. The ability of intestinal microflora of fish to degrade DDT mostly to DDD rather than DDE was reported.[90,162]

Of the other OCs studied, endosulfan is poorly metabolized and is mostly converted to endosulfan sulfate.[163,164] Following the exposure of redhorse suckers to trans- and cis-chlordane, the relative quantity of trans-isomer in relation to cis-isomer decreased progressively over a 56-day period.[154] When goldfish were injected with ^{14}C-heptachlor, more than 80% of the parent compound remained at the end of 10 days.[165] Likewise, mirex was poorly metabolized by fish tissues.[123]

Pyrethroids are metabolized by both hydrolytic and oxidative processes.[166] It appears that, in general, esterases are more important in metabolizing the trans-chrysanthemates of primary alcohols, whereas oxidases are more important with the cis-chrysanthemates of primary alcohols. Pyrethroids are rapidly metabolized, as has also been reported in the case of OP compounds. No malathion residues were found 24 hr after the exposure of pinfish to 75 μg/ℓ; only malathion monoacid was recorded in the gut.[167]

2. Elimination of Pesticide Residues by Fish

Mention has already been made of the biliary path of excretion of xenobiotic chemicals. Elimination of toxicants through gills and the renal pathway also plays an important role.[168] The higher the polarity, the faster the elimination, e.g., the elimination of lindane > dieldrin > DDT.[105]

Upon transfer to clean water, complete elimination of HCH from steady-state conditions took about 30 to 50 days in rainbow trout[146] and 1 week in the spot.[20]

The uptake of endrin was rapid, but elimination in the form of conjugated metabolites was somewhat slow. The calculated half-life was 4 weeks.[169] The principal method of biotransformation of endrin was by hydroxylation followed by conjugation in the bile. Likewise, in the elimination of 1,2,4-TCB bile had the highest quantity of biotransformation products, which were in the form of highly polar compounds suggestive of conjugates.[170] Involvement of kidneys in the excretion of DDA (a metabolite of DDT) by marine fish exposed to DDA was reported;[171] however, in nature, fish are not endowed with mechanisms that can convert DDT to DDA.[160]

Not only is DDT little metabolized, but it is excreted to a negligible extent. DDT is transported passively across cell walls and in this manner it acts like a lipophilic drug. The lipophilic substances that are filtered out of blood at glomerulus return to the blood stream by diffusing across cell membranes in the tubules and hence will not appear in the urine in significant quantities.[172] Elimination of the photoisomer of cis-chlordane by goldfish was faster than that of cis-chlordane and occurs mostly through the bile.[173] Trans-chlordane is more easily metabolized by fish than cis-chlordane.[174]

Elimination of residues upon transfer to uncontaminated water is usually reported to be biphasic, with an initial rapid phase followed by a slower, later phase. HCB, a recalcitrant chemical, was eliminated very slowly with a half-life of 7 months to several years.[175] The half-life of HCB was estimated by using a kinetic equation; body weight and lipid levels were found to affect considerably the kinetics of a compound.

Spacie and Hamelink[176] reviewed the various proposed models to explain the elimination of contaminants from fish — first-order, one-compartment model where the rate of elimination is directly proportional to the concentration in fish and first-order, two-compartment model, where elimination is rapid in the early phases (due to elimination from a faster, central compartment) and slower, later (due to a redistribution from a second, peripheral compartment). The authors explained that while first-order kinetics are useful, they hold good only when elimination occurs mainly through possible diffusion at the gill or some other membrane. Since elimination is a metabolic process involving enzyme activity, the rate of biotransformation is defined better by the Michaelis-Menten equation. Also, second-order elimination kinetics (i.e., the reciprocal of residue concentration in the body is proportional to the time of depuration) have been reported.[62] This excellent paper by Spacie and Hamelink[176] may be consulted for a detailed discussion of the various models.

VI. BIOCHEMICAL PATHWAYS OF DEGRADATION

Fish were once thought to be devoid of drug metabolizing enzymes and the lipophilic substances were supposed to be excreted at the gill surface, but subsequently, many biochemical pathways for detoxifying foreign compounds have been shown to occur in fish. Ever since Buhler and Rasmusson,[177] proved conclusively that fish possess enzyme systems comparable to the cytochrome p-450 of mammals, such systems have been studied extensively in fish. These pathways are similar in most respects to those reported from mammals, though the rate of their activity in fish is somewhat slower. A number of excellent reviews on the xenobiotic detoxification mechanisms in fish have appeared recently.[178-183]

In mammals, the oxidation of many foreign substances is catalyzed by a series of hepatic enzymes primarily residing in the smooth endoplasmic reticulum and associated with the microsomal fraction of the cell. They are part of the electron transport chain and their main function is in the intermediary metabolism. They require NADPH and free oxygen and are known as cytochrome p-450. Mason[184] introduced the term

Table 2
OVERVIEW OF METABOLIC
PROCESSES IN AQUATIC
FAUNA

Process

I. Primary Modifications of Chemicals

Oxidation
  Hydroxylation
    Aliphatic
    Aromatic
  Desulfurization
  Dealkylation
    On oxygen
    On nitrogen
  N-Oxidation
  Deamination
  Sulfoxidation
Reduction
  Azo and nitro
Methylation
    On oxygen
    On sulfur
Hydrolysis
    Carboxylic esters
    Organophosphates
    Epoxides
Bromination

II. Conjugation

Glucuronic acid
Glucose
Sulfuric acid
Glutathione
Glycine

From Zitko, V., in *Handbook of Environmental Chemistry,* Hutzinger, O., Ed., Springer-Verlag, Berlin, 1980, 220. With permission.

mixed function oxidase (MFO) for the enzyme system involved and these enzymes have also been called monooxygenases (MO).[183] Their presence in many other groups of living organisms is now well known and it is as though nature has ordained that the enzyme that is universally involved in the life-sustaining energy release process should also be involved fortuitously in the life-saving detoxification mechanisms.

In mammals, a certain amount of specificity to certain types of compounds is attributed to different forms of cytochrome p-450 and cytochrome p-448; at least six forms of these cytochromes are now known. An increase in the capacity to detoxify foreign compounds appears to be the result of an increase in the amount of enzyme protein — a process referred to as MFO induction — most often seen in mammals, and now known to also occur in fish, though to a limited extent.

Xenobiotic detoxification mechanisms comprise not only MFOs, but certain other enzymatic processes as well (Table 2). The oxidative biotransformation, mediated by the MFOs is one of the major metabolic processes available for handling foreign compounds, which along with other processes like reductions (carried out by enzymes similar to MFOs), methylation, hydrolysis, etc., represent only the first step in the detoxification process. The second step comprises the conjugation of the metabolites of the first step, with a molecule like glucuronic acid or amino acids provided by the body.[185] These biochemical pathways, although they often lead to detoxification, may sometimes result in the activation of a relatively nontoxic compound to a toxic form.

A. MFO Activity

Numerous substrates have been used to study the MFO activity in vitro. Among such substrates are aniline (aniline hydroxylase), para-nitroanisole (para-nitroanisole-demethylase), aminopyrine (aminopyrine-*N*-demethylase), ethylmorphine (ethylmorphine-*N*-demethylase), and benzo(a)pyrene (aromatic hydrocarbon hydroxylase). Besides, benzphetamine-*N*-demethylese (BEND), or ethoxy coumarin-*O*-deethylase (ECOD), or ethoxy resorufin-*O*-deethylase (EROD) activity has been used to characterize the different cytochrome p-450s.

Optimum temperature for fish MFOs is lower than that for mammals and is around 25°C. MFO activity is mainly confined to the liver and is negligible in other tissues. Seasonal variation in the activity was noted in wild fish populations but not in hatchery-reared fish. Aldrin epoxidase activity was higher in the bluegill fry compared to the adults.[186] Sex difference in the cytochrome p-450 levels in mature trout were reported.[187] The aminopyrine demethylase activity in liver and p-450 in liver and kidney of mature males were greater than those in females; the reverse was true in the case of benzo(a)pyrene hydroxylase activity.

1. OCs and Pyrethroids

The increased toxicity of some cyclodiene insecticide photoisomers was attributable to the oxidative dehydrochlorination of these compunds to their corresponding, more toxic, ketones by the MFO system.[188] In the carp and rainbow trout liver, microsomal esterases hydrolyzed trans-permethrin more extensively than cis-permethrin.[189]

Epoxidation of aldrin to the more toxic dieldrin is a well known MFO-mediated reaction,[178] and is considered an activation and not a detoxification process. Pretreatment with MFO inducers like sesamex or SKF-525A, however, reduced the amount of dieldrin formed in the mosquitofish, but did not alter the 48-h LC 50 of aldrin, indicating that epoxidation to dieldrin is not the activation process it is presumed to be.[190] Higher levels of MFO activity were reported in resistant strains of mosquitofish.[191] Among the different hepatic MFOs reported to be involved in xenobiotic detoxification, dieldrin, during a 30-day exposure of plaice, inhibited aminopyrine demethylase, but not aniline hydroxylase.[185]

2. OPs and Carbamates

The conversion of many OPs with a P=S group to P=O is another instance of activation by MFO, resulting in an increase in the toxicity.[192] This process explains the greater toxicity of metabolites like paraoxon, malaoxon, fenitrooxon, etc., than that of their parent compounds. Some species of fish can simultaneously activate and detoxify certain compounds, as has been reported in the case of metabolism of parathion and methyl parathion by sunfish.[193] The lesser toxicity of methyl parathion than that of parathion is due to the greater hydrolysis of methyl paraoxon than paraoxon (five times) by fish liver homogenates. Diazinon was degraded by the liver microsomal enzymes in fish.[194,195] Further, confirming the earlier report that marine fish were more susceptible to OP and carbamate compounds than freshwater fish, the MFO levels in the former were shown to be about half of those in freshwater fish.[194] On the other hand, in vitro aldrin epoxidation rates in the estuarine fish *Fundulus* sp. were reported to be comparable to those in the freshwater fish.[196]

Carbofuran was metabolized by the microsomal-NADPH system in fish, *Trichogaster pectoralis;* oxidative N-hydroxylation was the major route of metabolism of carbofuran.[197]

B. Other Biochemical Pathways

Reduction reactions are catalyzed by enzymes similar to the microsomal MFO system. The azo- and nitro-reductase activity and hydrolysis of esters (especially in the case of OP compounds) and amides by a variety of esterases have been reported from many species of fish.

While the first-phase reactions help increase polarity, conjugation reactions help in the elimination of xenobiotic compounds. PCA and PCP are conjugated with glucuronic acid and excreted, the latter directly and the former after methylation.[135] At the same concentration, the lampricide 3-trifluoromethyl-4-nitrophenol (TFM) is highly toxic to the lamprey, but not to the rainbow trout. In vitro studies showed that the sea lamprey had a lower rate of formation of TFM-glucuronide conjugate than trout, leading to the accumulation of more of the free compound in the former than in the trout — hence the higher toxicity of TFM to sea lamprey.[198] Likewise, glucuronide conjugation and subsequent elimination of the lampricide — Bayer® 73 — by rainbow trout was reported.[199]

Although increase in the polarity of the compound and consequent elimination is generally desirable, increased toxicity of such metabolites (as in the case of OP compounds) may render such a process not so desirable. An important pathway of degradation of HCB and PCB is hydroxylation, HCB to PCP and PCB to chlorobiphenylols.[200] In both these cases, the metabolites are more toxic than the parent compounds, hence the slow metabolism of some of these compounds or its lack in fish should be a welcome feature.

VII. MFO INDUCTION IN FISH

Induction of MFO in mammals is very well known and is the means of increased detoxification. Earlier studies in the fish were not definitive as to the inducibility of MFO system. Recent works have adequately demonstrated that MFO system in fish is inducible, especially by petroleum hydrocarbons. Since such elevated levels of MFOs can be used as markers in identifying previous exposure to xenobiotic contaminants, MFO systems are being increasingly used in biological monitoring of environmental contaminants.

Induction of microsomal MFOs leads to elevated rates of detoxification. Compounds like phenobarbital are inducers of MFOs and were employed to hasten the detoxification of dieldrin and its metabolites in lactating cows.[201] Following the observation of loss of fry from fish having higher levels of DDT, a study was conducted to examine whether phenobarbital could hasten the excretion of DDT in fish by the induction of MFO. Subsequent to the exposure of goldfish to DDT, a group of fish was exposed to phenobarbital and the level of DDT and its metabolites was monitored. Phenobarbital failed to hasten the excretion of DDT by goldfish.[201] In mammals and birds, DDT and DDE are known to be powerful inducers of MFO. In fish DDT failed to induce MFOs.[202] DDE also failed to induce liver microsome enzymes in bluegills.[202,203] It appears that the MFO system in fish is insensitive to induction by DDT-type compounds, in contrast to mammals. On the other hand, PCBs are inducers of the MFO system in fish.[204-209]

Fundulus collected from polluted waters had elevated levels of cytochrome p-450.[197]

Even hexane extracts of polluted waters, when injected i.p., could induce benzo(a) pyrene monoxygenase.[210,211] On the other hand, pike from polluted waters showed a reduced in vitro MFO activity; however, no change in the MFO activity of two species of *Salmo* was recorded under the same conditions.[212] Although some fish may have an effecient mechanism of oxidizing and excreting xenobiotic compounds, the induction of such enzymes does not ensure survival under conditions of continued stress that will be present in chronically polluted environments.

Discussing the nonspecificity of the cytochrome systems in vertebrates, Hodgson[179] examined the question of the likely selective pressures that would have caused the selection and universal preservation of such a system and also the functional significance of such a detoxification process. He pointed out that the food of animals contains many lipophilic substances of plant origin, such as terpenes, steroids, and methylene-dioxyphenyl compounds, that exert consistent low toxicity. In view of the nonspecificity of such a variety of compounds, it is understandable, according to Hodgson, that a universal detoxification process, with a low specificity to the target compund, arose and evolved, and was preserved.

VIII. BIOCONCENTRATION FACTORS AND QUANTITATIVE STRUCTURE-ACTIVITY RELATIONSHIP (QSAR) STUDIES

To satisfy the requirements of environmental protection laws in operation in different countries, the large number of existing and new chemicals have to be tested for their environmental safety and acceptability. Since it is an impossible task to test the persistence, mobility, toxicity, bioconcentration/bioaccumulation, metabolism, etc., of every suspected environmental contaminant, there is a need for a rapid and cost-efficient method of evaluation of the chemicals. Relating the chemical structure to the biological activity precisely serves that purpose and such studies have become an important part of the subject of environmental chemistry.

QSAR Studies for toxicological prediction have their roots in pharmacology where the molecular structure is used in correlating the known effects of a drug as part of a strategy to forecast the action of a new drug with a comparable structure. Such an approach helps reduce the cost and time taken to complete a battery of tests for evaluating a potentially useful new compound.[213]

In a classic paper in 1963, Hansch et al.[214] proposed an equation for correlating the effect of a given chemical substituent with the biological activity of phenoxyacetic acids (acting as plant growth regulators) and chloromycetin analogs. They assumed that the growth regulators penetrate to the site of action by partitioning between organic and aqueous phases and chose octanol-water as a model system. While emphasizing that living systems cannot be oversimplified and treated as two simple phases, Hansch et al. justified the use of octanol-water partition coefficients on the ground that it is not unreasonable to use the results from one set of solvents to predict results in a second set. Using this approach, they found a very high correlation between chemical structure and biological activity. Such QSAR Studies have found widespread use and acceptance in predictive toxicology and hazard assessment, both as a means of rapid evaluation of the possible risk that may result from the use of a new chemical and as a means of reducing the cost of such a prediction. Since chemical structure, lipophilicity, water solubility, and degree of ionization primarily influence the extent of bioconcentration of chemicals, attempts have been made to use one or more of these factors for such predictions.

A. BCF and Lipophilicity

Hamelink et al.[55] proposed that exchange equilibria control the degree of uptake of lipophilic compounds by the aquatic organisms. Subsequently, several simple relationships between the physicochemical properties of a compound and the extent of its bioconcentration/bioaccumulation in the aquatic ecosystem have been postulated. Neely et al.[147] held that the partition coefficient (P) of a pollutant would be the most logical parameter among its many properties to examine the extent of bioconcentration by aquatic organisms. To evaluate the relationship between octanol-water P (K_{ow}) and the uptake of a substance, Neely et al. plotted the experimentally determined BCFs against log octanol-water P (log K_{ow}, also called log P by some workers). A high degree of correlation was found between log octanol-water P and log BCF, (Figure 5). The relationship between the two was described by the following equation.

$$\text{Log BCF} = 0.542 \log (P) + 0.124$$

When the above equation was used to predict the BCF of other chemicals (endrin, chloropyrifos, and 3,5,6-trichloropyridinol) an excellent agreement was noticed between the experimental and predicted values.

The usefulness of correlation of a chemical property (P) with bioconcentration potential was further confirmed by Kanazawa[2] who found a satisfactory linear relationship between log octanol-water P of 15 pesticides and the experimentally obtained log BCF (employing topmouth gudgeon). A good agreement between the experimentally derived BCFs employing rainbow trout and those calculated on the basis of octanol-water Ps of phosphate ester hydraulic fluids has also been reported.[215] For one compound — NPDPP (nonylphenyl diphenyl phosphate) — however, the BCF obtained with rainbow trout was higher than the predicted value.

Mackay[216] suggested a direct relationship between BCF and K_{ow}, which is derived by the equation.

$$\log K_{B} = \log K_{ow} + \log A$$

where K_B is the ratio of uptake and depuration rate constants and A is the one-constant correlation. A correlation between log BCF and aqueous solubility was also suggested by Mackay.[216] The suggested correlation between BCF and K_{ow} fails in instances of high K_{ow}, i.e., 10^6 and above. He suggested that factors like membrane permeability may limit bioconcentration and chemicals that are bound to the protein may be consistently underestimated.

That the bioconcentration potential is dependent entirely on the chemical structure of the compound and its solubility in lipid is further confirmed by the comparison of the BCFs of several compounds obtained with fish with those obtained with cattle and swine. The BCFs of several chemicals in fish correlated well with those derived for cattle or swine, although the BCFs in beef and swine fat were lower by several orders of magnitude.[217] Further, despite the difference in the BCF in the fat of fish and cattle or swine (the difference being attributable to the different ways of administering the chemical), the absolute residue values in fish, cattle, and swine were similar in magnitude. The BCFs in cattle, swine and fish showed significant correlations with one another. BCFs obtained with cattle also significantly correlated with octanol-water P. Moreover, the octanol-water P has been useful in predicting the BCF of not only pesticides, but a number of other types of compounds like dyestuffs as well.[218]

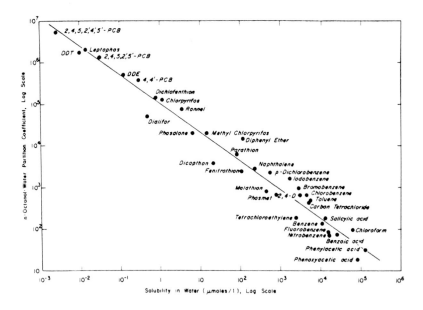

FIGURE 6.   Relationship between the partition coefficients and aqueous solubilities of various organic compounds. (Reprinted with permission from Chiou, C. T., Freed, V. H., Schmedding, D. W., and Kohnert, R. L., *Environ. Sci. Technol.*, 11, 475, 1977. Copyright 1977, American Chemical Society.)

B. BCF and Water Solubility

High octanol-water P indicates higher solubility in lipid and lower solubility in the aqueous phase. Hence, it is logical to expect a high P or K_{ow} value for compounds that have a poor water solubility. The extent of bioaccumulation of PCBs and DDE observed in model ecosystem studies was plotted against water solubility of those compounds by Metcalf et al.[42] and a good negative correlation was observed. They concluded that the water solubility (log_{ws}) and octanol-water P (log K_{ow}) appear to provide a realistic estimate of the extent of biological magnification [*sic*] of organic compounds. Further, a satisfactory linear relationship between log K_{ow} and log_{ws}, extending to more than eight orders of magnitude in aqueous solubility (10^{-3} to 10^4 mg/ℓ) and six orders of magnitude in partition coefficients (10 to 10^7) was found by Chiou et al.[219] (Figure 6). This relationship permits the assessment of log K_{ow} directly from water solubility. Extending the findings of Chiou et al., Mackay[220] emphasized that both P and aqueous solubility are functions of the aqueous phase activity coefficient of the compound. Freed et al.[221] plotted the log of water solubility against the log of n-octanol-water P and obtained an inverse linear relationship and a high negative correlation between the two. The relationship between water solubility (S) and K_{ow} of 35 compounds could be expressed by the equation Log K = -0.670 log S + 5.00 with a correlation coefficient of -0.985. The extent of accumulation of trifluralin under field conditions could be accurately predicted by using the empirical relationship between log BCF and log K_{ow} or log BCF and log S.[151] No influence of the species, body size, or feeding habits on the BCF was apparent. A simple inverse relationship and excellent correlation was reported between the S and bioconcentration of 34 chemicals, by the alga, Chlorella.[222] A linear relationship was also reported between log_{ws} and log_{BCF} in the case of 15 pesticides.[2]

The relationship between soil sorption (K_{oc}), octanol-water P (K_{ow}), BCF, and water solubility (K_{ws}) was discussed and the regression equations of all the 20 possible combinations of these 4 factors were reviewed.[223] Binary regression equations between the logarithms of these values gave significant correlations. The known values of any one of the four parameters could be used to calculate the average values of the other three with a reasonable degree of accuracy. A data base for 170 compounds was developed on all or several of the 4 factors mentioned above. Knowledge of any 2 factors would suffice for the assessment of the environmental hazard of a compound. Kenaga[224] calculated the BCF and K_{oc} for 358 chemicals from their water solubilities. These values are useful for predicting the partitioning of any compound in soil or in animal tissues and the consequent environmental hazard. Ellgehausen et al.[62] found a direct relationship between bioaccumulation and n-octanol-water P of a number of compounds in a model ecosystem comprising an alga (*Scenedesmus*, sp.), *Daphnia*, and catfish *(Ictalurus melas)*. The relationship could be described by

$$\log K \ alga = 0.70 \log P - 0.26 \ (r = 0.93)$$

$$\log K \ Daphnia = 0.71 \log P - 1.26 \ (r = 0.94)$$

$$\log K \ catfish = 0.83 \log P - 1.71 \ (r = 0.97)$$

They suggested that S of the compound may also be used to predict the bioaccumulation potential.

Banerjee et al.[225] measured the S and octanol-water P (K_{ow}) of 27 different chemicals and criticized the correlation suggested by Chiou et al.[219] which appears invalid in the case of solids with a high melting point. An alternate equation for arriving at K-S relationship was described

$$\log K = 6.5 - 0.89 \ (\log S) - 0.015 \ (mp) \ (r = 0.96)$$

Mackay et al.[226] discussed the relationship between aqueous solubility and K_{ow} and developed a new correlation that included a melting point (fugacity ratio) correlation. The correlation was found to be satisfactory for 45 organic compounds but was not applicable to organic acids. Also, substances with a high molecular weight deviate, in that they do not show linearity between lipophilicity and K_{ow}. When the molecular weight exceeds 290, log K_{ow} levels off, which is environmentally advantageous. If such substances do not bioconcentrate to the extent expected, they may prove to be less hazardous to the biota.

C. Molecular Structure and BCF

OPs are supposed to have little chronic toxicity owing to their limited uptake and rapid hydrolysis. Following a careful analysis of a number of physicochemical properties of selected OP compounds, including K_{ow}, Freed et al.[221] found that some of the OP compounds have K_{ow} values similar to those of many OCs and hence are likely to be bioaccumulated by the organisms. Contrary to this prediction, leptophos, which has a higher log K_{ow} value than even DDT (6.31 and 6.19, respectively),[219] was concentrated only 650 times by *Daphnia* and 146 times by bluegill.[10] Similarly, Ellgehausen et al.[62] reported that profenfos with a log K_{ow} of 4.68 was actually concentrated to less than half the value predicted by the regression equation between log BCF and log K_{ow}; the low BCF was attributable to a high clearance rate. Hence, in the case of OP compounds, although a high environmental hazard may be predicted on the basis of QSAR Studies, in practice, the risk appears somewhat less.

Aliphatic compounds, except those with chlorine substitution, are generally less accumulated. Degradation-resistant alcohols are also accumulated to a lesser extent by fish. Substitution by hydrophilic atomic groups like hydroxy-, carboxy-, nitro-, or sulfo-groups also reduces bioaccumulation potential.[155] On the other hand, chlorine substitution increases the bioaccumulation potential at an exponential ratio of the substituted number of chlorine atoms. QSAR Studies with 13 dinitrogen heterocyclic molecules revealed that both an increase in methyl substitution and increase in the number of aromatic rings per compound result in increased toxicity to the common ciliate, *Tetrahymena pyriformis.*[227]

D. Calculation of BCF

BCFs have been calculated using theoretically calculated or experimentally derived octanol-water Ps, S, the retention times of reversed phase HPLC (high performance liquid chromatography), kinetic models, or steady-state concentrations in relation to the concentration of a chemical in water. Various molecular descriptors have also been used for this purpose.

Originally, Hansch et al.[214] used octanol-water partitioning as a model system, stating that the Ps for a given compound in two different solvent systems (e.g., ether-water, octanol-water) are related as follows.

$$\log P_1 = a \log P_2 + b \text{ (a and b are constants)}$$

Hence, the results of one set of solvents can be used to predict results in a second set. At the same time, they emphasized that "one cannot hope for very high precision with the oversimplifying assumption that they can be treated as two simple phases." Yang and Sun[228] used benzene-water Ps and hexane-water Ps for relating p with the toxicity of OP and OC compounds (Figure 7). They also concluded that the use of a P with different solvents does not substantially alter the correlation. Likewise, no consistent variation in the solubility of a number of organic compounds in different types of lipids was found.[4] Hence, it appears that octanol-water Ps, to the extent they are dependable (see Section F), may serve as well as any other solvent system for predicting the BCFs.

One word of caution regarding the use of theoretically calculated K_{ow} is in order. Recently, Tulp and Hutzinger[229] have shown that at least in the case of PCBs, the calculated K_{ow} values would be wrong if the differences in the position of the chlorine atoms (ortho-, meta-, or para- to the phenyl-phenyl bond) are not taken into account. Hence they recommended the use of reversed phase HPLC retention times instead of "log P" values to predict BCFs. HPLC retention times correlated well with S and hence also with K_{ow}.

Neely et al.[147] measured the uptake (K_1) and clearance (K_2) rates of various chemicals in trout muscle under steady-state conditions and calculated the BCF as the ratio of log K_1/K_2. Since some compounds may reach equilibrium conditions only after several months of continuous exposure, Branson et al.[148] described an accelerated kinetic method of calculation of the BCF. The rate constants of uptake and depuration were calculated using a nonlinear regression analysis. The calculated rate constants following the exposure of rainbow trout to a compound for 42 days agreed closely with the values predicted by the accelerated test. Hence it was suggested that the accelerated tests can provide the same information, faster, and at a lesser cost than a routine bioconcentration test. The relationship at steady-state is expressed by

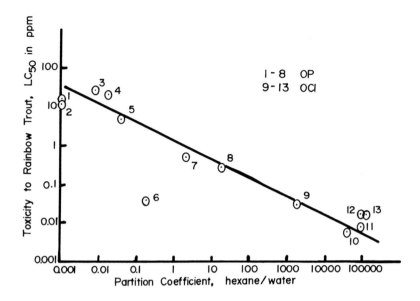

FIGURE 7. Correlation between partition coefficient (hexane/water) and toxicity to rainbow trout of organophosphorus and OC insecticides: 1 = dicrotophos, 2 = monocrotophos, 3 = trichlorofon, 4 = dimethoate, 5 = phosphamidon, 6 = mevinphos, 7 = dichlorvos, 8 = naled, 9 = lindane, 10 = dieldrin, 11 = DDT, 12 = aldrin, and 13 = heptachlor. (From Yang, C. F. and Sun, Y. P., *Arch. Environ. Contam. Toxicol.,* 6, 325, 1977. With permission.)

$$\frac{C_f}{C_w} = \frac{k_1}{k_2} = K_{BCF}$$

where C_f is concentration in fish, C_w is concentration in water, K_1 is uptake rate, K_2 is clearance rate and K_{BCF} is the BCF at steady-state.

Veith et al.[14] considered the kinetic method of calculation of BCF proposed by Branson et al.[148] as an uncertain method, as it takes into consideration only the initial uptake rate constant, which may later change with time, and the depuration rate may not remain constant. Veith et al. exposed fathead minnows, green sunfish, and rainbow trout for 32 days in continuous-flow water and calculated the extent of bioconcentration from water (concentration in fish ÷ concentration in water). The relation between log BCF and log K_{ow} (P) was expressed by Veith et al. as

$$\log BCF = 0.85 \log P - 0.70$$

$$r^2 = 0.897$$

They recommended the simultaneous testing of many chemicals to reduce the time and cost of calculating the BCF, since the extent of uptake of one compound was not in any way influenced by the uptake of another. Recently Esser and Moser[230] reviewed the different proposals for calculating the BCF.

E. Molecular Descriptors for QSAR

The octanol-water P is one of the molecular descriptors, related to lipophilicity or hydrophobicity, used for formulating QSARs. Another broad class of molecular descriptors is based on quantitation of the chemical structure. The observed biological activity is expressed as a function of descriptors assigned either to substituent groups or to portions of the parent molecule or both.[231] Schultz et al.[231] examined the relationship between cellular response and molecular connectivity indexes for a series of 24 mono- and dinitrogen heterocyclic compounds and showed that the toxicity of the compounds increased with an increase in the number of atoms and the degree of methylation per compound; toxicity decreased with an increase in nitrogen substitution. Matsuo[232-235] used the i/o (inorganic/organic)* characters and established linear relationships between Σ i; Σ o or Σ i/Σ o and bioaccumulation of OP compounds in model ecosystems. The derived relationship was expressed as

$$\log BR = a \, \Sigma \, i + b \, \Sigma \, o \text{ and}$$
$$\log BR = c \, \Sigma \, i/\Sigma \, o + d$$

where BR is equivalent to bioaccumulation through food chain at equilibrium and a,b,c, and d are constants. On the basis of i/o analysis, Matsuo[232-235] concluded that bioconcentration of chemicals in fish is the result of interactions between the polar and nonpolar parts of the compounds and tissues of fish, which could also explain the deviations from the expected BCF values. It has also been pointed out that bioaccumulation of PCBs in fish is entirely controlled by a large positive entropic change.[235]

F. Exceptions to Predicted BCFs

Although relating molecular structure to biological activity has proved to be a very useful means of predicting environmental behavior and associated risks of a compound even before it is marketed, and although such studies have helped not only to reduce the cost of evaluation of every new chemical but also to indentify the chemicals that should undergo further testing (see Chapter 12), QSAR predictions have certain limitations. First, either K_{ow} or K_{ws} predicts a single BCF value, but different organisms are capable of metabolizing the same compound to a different extent. Within the same species, metabolic activity is a function of age, stage of growth, level of feeding, reproductive stage, season, etc. Second, the chemical structure may predict and facilitate high lipid solubility, but in practice, certain chemical substituents may decelerate uptake or accelerate excretion. The largeness of the size of the molecule itself may impede membrane permeability. Finally, the degree of accuracy of prediction itself is dependent on the degree of accuracy with which the various factors chosen to predict BCF are determined.

Southworth et al.[237] emphasized that in general, uptake and bioconcentration are well correlated with the octanol-water Ps. Although this relationship is often useful in estimating the bioconcentration potential, such predictions provide only an estimate of the degree of bioconcentration attained, the difference between the predicted and observed value being attributable to detoxification and elimination of the compound; the latter are not taken into account in such predictions. For example, predicted BCF of quinoline and dibenz(a,h)acridine by *Daphnia* and fathead minnows (derived by using the relationship developed by Veith et al.[14]) differed from the experimental BCFs. In the fathead minnow, bioconcentration of compounds differing in their octanol-water Ps was similar, whereas in *Daphnia* the BCF increased steadily with increasing K_{ow}. Thus, lipophilicity played a more important role in *Daphnia* than in the fathead min-

---

*   The parameters i and o were developed by Fujita[236] to characterize the physicochemical properties of chemicals; i represents the number and strength of polar group units and o, the nonpolar ones.

nows, bioconcentration being overestimated on the basis of K_{ow} in the latter. Similarly, interspecific variation in the extent of bioconcentration has to be taken into account, even though the log K_{ow} or K_{ws} predicts only one value for the BCF. When killifish and goldfish were exposed to 1 mg/ℓ TDCPP (tris [1,3-dichlorisopropyl] phosphate), a phosphate ester, the former concentrated the compound 79 times, whereas the latter concentrated it only 3.5 times in 24 hr.[238] Readily biodegradable compounds are bioaccumulated less and cleared faster as is shown in the case of EHDP (2-ethylhexyl diphenyl phosphate), a widely used flame retardant. The experimental BCF is less than that predicted by the equation of Veith et al., the experimental BCF with rainbow trout fry being 1147 to 1481, whereas the calculated BCF was 3548.[18] Rainbow trout took up less fluridone than that predicted from S, using the equations of Chiou et al.[219] or Kenaga and Goring;[223] experimental BCF for terbutryn was somewhat higher than that predicted from S, which may be the result of oversimplification of the initial uptake rates in the prediction. Also the higher, experimental BCF may be attributed to the measuring of the total ^{14}C-content of the whole fish, including the metabolites, instead of the parent compound alone, as was explained by the authors.[239] While Kenaga and Goring predicted a BCF of 16 for PCP, experimental BCFs were 200 and 240 at low and high exposure levels (35 ± 6 and 660 ± 220 ng/ℓ).[240]

Another reason for the discrepancy in predicted BCFs may be the K_{ow} value used and the method by which it is calculated. Platford[241] reported that the K_{ow} of lindane varied depending primarily on the amount of octanol present in the system. For instance, log K_{ow} of lindane is 3.2; if octanol is in the form of a lens floating on water, log K_{ow} is 3.9, whereas between a monolayer of octanol and underlying water, the log K_{ow} is 4.5.

Further, the BCF is not dependent on fat solubility of a compound alone. Dobbs and Williams[4] studied the solubility of several organic compounds in different types of lipids. No close relation between fat solubility and BCF was noted. Also, the log lipid solubility vs. log K_{ow} had a very low correlation (−0.40 for 31 data points). They concluded that fat solubility is not a reliable predictor of BCF or K_{ow}. The activity coefficient of the chemical seems to be the predominant factor governing bioconcentration, and solibility in fat is only of secondary importance. Substances with low S, and hence a high K_{ow} may also have a low BCF.

The various regression equations developed to indicate the relationship between BCF and K_{ow}, BCF and K_{ws}, or K_{ow} and K_{ws}, are as accurate as the values of K_{ow} and K_{ws} used. It is well known that it is extremely difficult to assess the S of hydrophobic compounds, and the solubility values assigned to some of the poorly water-soluble compounds range over two to three orders of magnitude. Likewise, as has already been pointed out, Tulp and Hutzinger[229] have shown that at least in the case of PCBs, values of log P generated by the "Hansch-approach", would be erroneous if the different values for different positions of the chlorine (ortho-, meta-, or para-) substituents are not taken into consideration. Hence a discrepancy is often observed between the calculated and measured "P" values. Further, analyzing the limitations of the suggested relationship between log_{BCF} and log K_{ow} or log $_{ws}$, Tulp and Hutzinger stressed that such a relationship does not hold good indefinitely and higher lipophilicity (as expressed by a higher "P" value) cannot be equated with a higher tendency for bioconcentration/bioaccumulation. Citing the instance of chlorinated paraffins which do not bioaccumulate to the extent predicted by log K_{ow}, they postulated that there is an optimal lipophilicity for bioaccumulation and steric factors may be responsible for the observed upper limit for the uptake. They also suggested that a quadratic relationship between BCF and various physicochemical properties may give a better fit than a simple linear relationship. Molar volume or Molar refractivity index or parachor is an important steric parameter that may correlate better with BCF. Parachor, especially, gave an excellent correlation with log BCF when the data of Neely et al.[147] were replotted (log BCF vs.

parachor). The overestimation of bioconcentration may also be due to the fact that the hydrophobic and steric factors cannot denote the negative influence of metabolism on bioaccumulation. Hence Tulp and Hutzinger proposed a model that can take into consideration all the above parameters and predict the bioconcentration more accurately than the other relationship proposed.

Sugiura et al.[242] reported that accumulation of mono-, di-, and tetrachlorobiphenyls and di-, tri-, and tetrabromobiphenyls by the killifish was linear to octanol-water P and log K_{ow} was $\leqslant$ 6, but not when it was > 6. They suggested that movement of compounds in tissues may be difficult when log K_{ow} > 6 and hence BCF will be smaller at higher log K_{ow} values.

Shaw and Connell[243] examined the effect of steric factors and substitution patterns of chlorine atoms in PCBs that caused lower accumulation of some PCB isomers in the sea mullet relative to that of the other isomers, although the former had similar physical and chemical properties. They are (1) three or four chlorine atoms in positions ortho- to the phenyl-phenyl bond, (2) three or four chlorines adjacent to one another on a phenyl ring, and (3) two chlorines in 3,5 positions. These substitutions either distort the molecule or increase the width of the molecule. Steric effect coefficients have been developed and very high correlation (r = 0.97) between them and BCF was noted.

Könemann and Leeuwen[5] also observed a sharp decline in the uptake rate when log P is more than 5.4 and the uptake rate constant could be better related to the P by a parabolic curve rather than a straight line. The bioaccumulation of chlorobenzenes increased with log K_{ow} with an optimum at about 6.5. At higher log K_{ow}, a reduction in bioaccumulation and a deviation from a linear behavior was noted.

Since the correlation between log P (K_{ow}) and BCF is nonlinear for compounds that have a very low log P value (< 2) or a very high log P value (> 6.5), Spacie and Hamelink[176] proposed an alternate sigmoidal model, representing the drug transport model of Yalkowsky and Morozowich,[244] which reasonably described the transport of chemicals across membranes. This model predicts a linearity when log P = 2 to 5, with an inflection at the lower end of the curve to account for a poor uptake of low molecular weight, high polarity compounds, and an inflection at the upper end where the uptake is not influenced by log P, but by S and diffusion at the membrane boundaries (Figure 8). The authors suggested that a model of this type would permit optimization of the design of the bioconcentration experiments, as it is possible to estimate the rate constants K_1 and K_2 from correlations with log P and such a model would lead to better predictions for a wider variety of chemicals.

Zitko[245] reported that the accumulation of PBBs (polybrominated biphenyls) by juvenile Atlantic salmon decreased with increasing molecular weight and increasing number of chlorine substituents (> 4 chlorine atoms). Juvenile Atlantic salmon accumulated very little or no chlorinated parrafins, whereas they readily took up PCBs from suspended solids; low uptake may be limited by the higher molecular weight of these compounds.[246] Similarly, hexabromobenzene was not taken up from water or food by juvenile Atlantic salmon. Also, isopropyl PCBs were taken up to a lesser extent although they are more lipid soluble than PCBs and hence fish should accumulate more of the former than the latter; in practice, the reverse was true. Zitko and Carson[247] suggested that the presence of isopropyl groups renders this class of compounds more prone to oxidation and hence these compounds are metabolized and excreted. Summing up the knowledge on the usefulness of QSAR studies, Kawasaki[155] remarked "It is still difficult to generalize theoretically structure-activity correlations of chemical substances and to find sufficient physical-chemical parameters which can predict the biodegradability or bioaccumulation potential of chemicals."

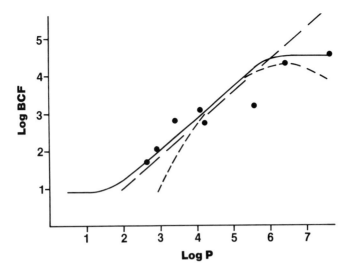

FIGURE 8.   Relationship between BCF for whole fish and *n*-oc-tanol-water partition coefficient (solid line). (From Spacie, A. and Hamelink, J. L., *Environ. Toxicol. Chem.*, 1, 309, 1982. With permission. Copyright 1982, Pergamon Press.)

IX. CONCLUSIONS

QSAR Studies have proved to be very useful in assessing the environmental hazards of xenobiotic chemicals. Since it is an impossible task to attempt to test the persistence, mobility, toxicity, uptake, and metabolism of every chemical in existence and all the new chemicals that are being continuously added, the need for rapid and cost-efficient predictive tools cannot be overemphasized. Relating the chemical structure to biological activity precisely serves that purpose, and in general, has proved to be dependable in predictive toxicology. Measures of hydrophobicity like octanol-water P, aqueous solubility, or better still, aqueous phase activity coefficient, molecular descriptors like molecular connectivity, molecular volume, and parachor, have all proved to be useful in predicting BCFs. It should also be emphasized that such predictions have certain limitations. For instance the relationship between BCF and K_{ow} seems to hold good when log K_{ow} is less than 6.5, beyond which the bioconcentration/bioaccumulation levels off, which may be due to the increased number of certain types of substituents.

REFERENCES

1. Ware, G. W., Effects of pesticides on nontarget organisms, *Residue Rev., 76*, 173, 1980.
2. Kanazawa, J., Measurement of the bioconcentration factors of pesticides by freshwater fish and their correlation with physico-chemical properties or acute toxicities, *Pestic. Sci., 12*, 417, 1981.
3. Anderson, R. L. and DeFoe, D. L., Toxicity and bioaccumulation of endrin and methoxychlor in aquatic invertebrates and fish, *Environ. Pollut., 22*, 111, 1980.
4. Dobbs, A. J. and Williams, N., Fat solubility — a property of environmental relevance?, *Chemosphere, 12*, 97, 1983.
5. Könemann, H. and Leeuwen, K. V., Toxicokinetics in fish: accumulation and elimination of six chlorobenzenes by guppies, *Chemosphere, 9*, 3, 1980.
6. Khan, H. M. and Khan, M. A. Q., Biological magnification of photodieldrin by food chain organisms, *Arch. Environ. Contam. Toxicol., 2*, 289, 1974.
7. Brungs, W. A. and Mount, D. I., Introduction to a discussion of the use of aquatic toxicity tests for evaluation of the effects of toxic substances, in *Estimating the Hazard of Chemical Substances to Aquatic Life*, ASTM STP 657, Cairns, J., Jr., Dickson, K. L., and Maki, A. W., Eds., American Society for Testing and Materials, Philadelphia, 1978, 15.
8. Anon., Ambient water quality criteria for DDT, US EPA 440/5-80-038, Office of Water Regulations and Standards Criteria and Standards Division, United States Environmental Protection Agency, Washington, D.C., 1980.
9. Fujiwara, K., Japanese law on new chemicals and the methods to test the biodegradability and bioaccumulation of chemical substances, in *Analyzing the Hazard Evaluation Process*, Dickson, K. L., Maki, A. W., and Cairns, J., Jr., Eds., American Fisheries Society, Washington, D.C., 1979.
10. Macek, K. J., Petrocelli, S. R., and Sleight, B. H., III, Considerations in assessing the potential for, and significance of biomagnification of chemical residues in aquatic food chains, in *Aquatic Toxicology*, ASTM STP 667, Marking, L. L. and Kimerle, R. A., Eds., American Society for Testing and Materials, Philadelphia, 1979, 392.
11. Mayer, F. L., Mehrle, P. M., and Sanders, H. O., Residue dynamics and biological effects of polychlorinated biphenyls in aquatic organisms, *Arch. Environ. Contam. Toxicol., 5*, 501, 1977.
12. Ernst, W., Factors affecting the evaluation of chemicals in laboratory experiments using marine organisms, *Ecotoxicol. Environ. Saf., 3*, 90, 1979.
13. Frederick, L. L., Comparative uptake of a polychlorinated biphenyl and dieldrin by the white sucker *(Catostomus commersoni), J. Fish. Res. Board Can., 32*, 1705, 1975.
14. Veith, G. D., DeFoe, D. L., and Bergstedt, B. V., Measuring and estimating the bioconcentration factor of chemicals in fish, *J. Fish. Res. Board Can., 36*, 1040, 1979.
15. Sasaki, K., Suzuki, T., Takeda, M., and Uchiyama, M., Bioconcentration and excretion of phosphoric acid triesters by killifish, *(Oryzeas latipes), Bull. Environ. Contam. Toxicol., 28*, 752, 1982.
16. DeFoe, D. L., Veith, G. D., and Carlson, R. W., Effects of Aroclor® 1248 and 1260 on the fathead minnow *(Pimephales promelas), J. Fish. Res. Board Can., 35*, 997, 1978.
17. Muir, D. C. G. and Grift, N. P., Environmental dynamics of phosphate esters. II. Uptake and bioaccumulation of 2-ethylhexyl diphenyl phosphate by fish, *Chemosphere, 10*, 847, 1981.
18. Hattula, M. L., Reunanen, H., and Arstila, A. U., The toxicity of MCPA to fish, light and electron microscopy and the chemical analysis of the tissue, *Bull. Environ. Contam. Toxicol., 19*, 465, 1978.
19. Schimmel, S. C., Patrick, J. M., Jr., and Forester, J., Toxicity and bioconcentration of BHC and lindane in selected estuarine animals, *Arch. Environ. Contam. Toxicol., 6*, 355, 1977.
20. Schimmel, S. C. and Wilson, A. J., Jr., Acute toxicity of Kepone® to four estuarine animals, *Chesapeake Sci., 18*, 224, 1977.
21. Reinert, R. E., Stone, L. J., and Willford, W. A., Effect of temperature on accumulation of methylmercuric chloride and p,p'-DDT by rainbow trout *(Salmo gairdneri), J. Fish. Res. Board Can., 31*, 1649, 1974.
22. Spigarelli, S. A., Thommes, M. M., and Prepejchal, W., Thermal and metabolic factors affecting PCB uptake by adult brown trout, *Environ. Sci. Technol., 17*, 88, 1983.
23. Schimmel, S. C., Patrick, J. M., Jr., and Forester, J., Uptake and toxicity of toxaphene in several estuarine organisms, *Arch. Environ. Contam. Toxicol., 5*, 353, 1977.
24. Goodman, L. R., Hansen, D. J., Manning, C. S., and Faos, L. F., Effects of Kepone® on the sheepshead minnow in an entire life-cycle toxicity test, *Arch. Environ. Contam. Toxicol., 11*, 335, 1982.
25. Spacie, A., Landrum, P. F., and Leversee, G. J., Uptake, depuration, and biotransformation of anthracene and benzo(a)pyrene in bluegill sunfish, *Ecotoxicol. Environ. Saf., 7*, 330, 1983.
26. Kobylinski, G. J. and Livingston, R. J., Movement of mirex from sediment and uptake by the hogchoker, *Trinectes maculatus, Bull. Environ. Contam. Toxicol., 14*, 692, 1975.

27. Halter, M. T. and Johnson, H. E., A model system to study the desorption and biological availability of PCB in hydrosoils, *Aquatic Toxicology and Hazard Evaluation, ASTM STP 634,* Mayer, F. L. and Hamelink, J. L., Eds., American Society for Testing and Materials, Philadelphia, 1977, 178.

28. Courtney, W. A. M. and Langston, W. J., Accumulation of polychlorinated biphenyls in turbot *(Scophthalmus maximus)* from sea water sediments and food, *Helgol. Meeresforsch.,* 33, 333, 1980.

29. Murray, H. E., Ray, L. E., and Giam, C. S., Analysis of marine sediment, water and biota for selected organic pollutants, *Chemosphere,* 10, 1327, 1981.

30. Kent, J. C. and Johnson, D. W., Organochlorine residues in fish, water and sediment of American Falls Reservoir, Idaho, 1974, *Pestic. Monit. J.,* 13, 28, 1979.

31. Fay, R. R. and Newland, L. W., Organochlorine insecticide residues in water, sediment and organisms, Aransas Bay, Texas, September 1969—June 1970, *Pestic. Monit. J.,* 6, 97, 1972.

32. Hannon, M. R., Greichus, Y. A., Applegate, R. L., and Fox, A. C., Ecological distribution of pesticides in Lake Poinsett, South Dakota, *Trans. Am. Fish. Soc.,* 99, 496, 1970.

33. Smith, G. N., Watson, B. S., and Fischer, F. S., The metabolism of (^{14}C) O,O-diethyl O-(3,5,6-trichloro-2-pyridyl) phosphorothioate (Dursban) in fish, *J. Econ. Entomol.,* 59, 1464, 1966.

34. Terriere, L. C., Kiigemagi, U., Gerlach, A. R., and Borovicka, R. L., The persistence of toxaphene in lake water and its uptake by aquatic plants and animals, *J. Agric. Food Chem.,* 14, 66, 1966.

35. Kapoor, I. P., Metcalf, R. L., Nystrom, R. F., and Sangha, K., Comparative metabolism of methoxychlor, methiochlor and DDT in mouse, insects, and in a model ecosystem, *J. Agric. Food Chem.,* 18, 1145, 1970.

36. Metcalf, R. L., Sangha, G. K., and Kapoor, I. P., Model ecosystem for the evaluation of pesticide biodegradability and ecological magnification, *Environ. Sci. Technol.,* 5, 709, 1971.

37. Sanborn, J. R. and Yu, C. C., The fate of dieldrin in a model ecosystem, *Bull. Environ. Contam. Toxicol.,* 10, 340, 1973.

38. Coats, J. R., Metcalf, R. L., and Kapoor, I. P., Metabolism of the methoxychlor isostere, dianisylneopentane, in mouse, insects and a model ecosystem, *Pestic. Biochem. Physiol.,* 4, 201, 1974.

39. Yu, C. C. and Sanborn, J. R., The fate of parathion in a model ecosystem, *Bull. Environ. Contam. Toxicol.,* 13, 543, 1975.

40. Virtanen, M., Hattula, L. M., and Arstila, A. U., Behavior and fate of 4-chloro-2-methylphenoxyacetic acid (MCPA) and 4,6-dichloro-O-cresol as studied in an aquatic-terrestrial model ecosystem, *Chemosphere,* 8, 431, 1979.

41. Virtanen, M. T., Roos, A., Arstila, A. U., and Hattula, M. L., An evaluation of model ecosystem with DDT, *Arch. Environ. Contam. Toxicol.,* 9, 491, 1980.

42. Metcalf, R. L., Sanborn, J. R., Lu, P. Y., and Nye, D., Laboratory model ecosystem studies of the degradation and fate of radiolabeled tri-, tetra-, and pentachlorobiphenyl compared with DDE, *Arch. Environ. Contam. Toxicol.,* 3, 151, 1975.

43. Södergren, A., Transport distribution, and degradation of chlorinated hydrocarbon residues in aquatic model ecosystems, *Oikos,* 24, 30, 1973.

44. Reinert, R. E., Accumulation of dieldrin in an alga *(Scenedesmus obliquus), Daphnia magna,* and the guppy *(Poecilia reticulate), J. Fish. Res. Board Can.,* 29, 1413, 1972.

45. Hansen, P. D., Uptake and transfer of the chlorinated hydrocarbon lindane (γ-BHC) in a laboratory freshwater food chain, *Environ. Pollut.,* 21, 97, 1980.

46. Johnson, B. T., Laboratory procedure for estimating residue dynamics of xenobiotic contaminants in a freshwater food chain, Technical paper No. 103, Fish and Wildlife Service, U.S. Department of the Interior, Washington, D.C., 1980, 1.

47. Skaar, D. R., Johnson, B. T., Jones, J. R., and Huckins, J. N., Fate of Kepone and mirex in a model aquatic environment: sediment, fish and diet, *Can. J. Fish. Aquat. Sci.,* 38, 931, 1981.

48. Eberhardt, L. L., Meeks, R. L., and Peterle, T. J., Food chain model for DDT kinetics in a freshwater marsh, *Nature,* 230, 60, 1971.

49. Macek, K. J., Walsh, D. F., Hogan, J. W., and Holz, D. D., Toxicity of the insecticide Dursban® to fish and aquatic invertebrates in ponds, *Trans. Am. Fish. Soc.,* 101, 420, 1972.

50. Woodwell, G. M., Wurster, C. F., Jr., and Isaacson, P. A., DDT residues in an east coast estuary: a case of biological concentration of a persistent insecticide, *Science,* 156, 821, 1967.

51. Butler, P. A., Pesticides in the estuary, *Proc. Marsh Estuary Management Symp.,* Louisiana State Univ., Newsom, D., Ed., Moran Publishing, Baton Rouge, La., 1968, 120.

52. Finley, M. T., Ferguson, D. E., and Ludke, J. L., Possible selective mechanisms in the development of insecticide resistant fish, *Pestic. Monit. J.,* 3, 212, 1970.

53. Bulkley, R. V., Leung, S. T., and Richard, J. J., Organochlorine insecticide concentrations in fish of the Des Moines River, Iowa, 1977—78, *Pestic. Monit. J.,* 15, 86, 1981.

54. Rees, G. A. V. and Au, L., Use of XAD-2 macroreticular resin for the recovery of ambient trace levels of pesticides and industrial organic pollutants from water, *Bull. Environ. Contam. Toxicol.,* 22, 561, 1979.

55. Hamelink, J. L., Waybrant, R. C., and Ball, R. C., A proposal: exchange equilibria control the degree chlorinated hydrocarbons are biologically magnified in lentic environments, *Trans. Am. Fish. Soc.,* 100, 207, 1971.

56. Hamelink, J. L. and Waybrant, R. C., DDE and lindane in a large scale model lentic ecosystem, *Trans. Am. Fish. Soc.,* 105, 124, 1976.

57. de la Cruz, A. A. and Lue, K. Y., Mirex incorporation in estuarine animals, sediment, and water, Mississippi Gulf coast — 1972—74, *Pestic. Monit. J.,* 12, 40, 1978.

58. Paz, J. D., Preliminary study of the occurrence and distribution of DDT residues in the Jordan watershed, 1971, *Pestic. Monit. J.,* 10, 96, 1976.

59. Ginn, T. M. and Fisher, F. M., Jr., Studies on the distribution and flux of pesticides in waterways associated with a ricefield-marshland ecosystem, *Pestic. Monit. J.,* 8, 23, 1974.

60. Harrison, H. L., Loucks, O. L., Mitchell, J. W., Parkhurst, D. F., Tracy, C. R., Watts, D. G., and Yannacone, V. J., Jr., Systems studies of DDT transport, *Science,* 170, 503, 1970.

61. Bloom, S. G. and Menzel, D. B., Decay time of DDT, *Science,* 172, 213, 1971.

62. Ellgehausen, H., Guth, J. A., and Esser, H. D., Factors determining the bioaccumulation potential of pesticides in the individual components of aquatic food chains, *Ecotoxicol. Environ. Saf.,* 4, 134, 1980.

63. Macek, K. J. and Korn, S., Significance of the food chain in DDT accumulation by fish, *J. Fish. Res. Board Can.,* 27, 1496, 1970.

64. Holden, A. V., A study of the absorption of ^{14}C-labelled DDT from water by fish, *Ann. Appl. Biol.,* 50, 467, 1962.

65. Premdas, F. M. and Anderson, J. M., The uptake and detoxification of ^{14}C-labelled DDT in Atlantic salmon, *Salmo salar, J. Fish. Res. Board Can.,* 20, 827, 1963.

66. Ferguson, D. E. and Goodyear, C. P., The pathway of endrin entry in black bullheads, *Ictalurus melas, Copeia,* 1967, 467, 1967.

67. Chadwick, G. G. and Brocksen, R. W., Accumulation of dieldrin by fish and selected fish-food organisms, *J. Wildl. Manage.,* 33, 693, 1969.

68. Murphy, P. G., The effect of size on the uptake of DDT from water by fish, *Bull. Environ. Contam. Toxicol.,* 6, 20, 1971.

69. Moriarty, F., The effects of pesticides on wildlife: exposure and residues, *Sci. Total Environ.,* 1, 267, 1972.

70. Hunt, E. G. and Bischoff, A. I., Inimical effects on wildlife of periodic DDD applications to Clear Lake, *Calif. Fish Game,* 46, 91, 1960.

71. Meeks, R. L., The accumulation of ^{36}Cl ring-labeled DDT in a freshwater marsh, *J. Wildl. Manage.,* 32, 376, 1968.

72. Ernst, W., Accumulation and metabolism of DDT ^{14}C (dichloro-diphenyl-trichloro-ethane) in marine organisms, in *Marine Pollution and Sea Life,* Ruivo, M., Ed., Fishing News (Books), London, 1972, 260.

73. Argyle, R. L., Williams, G. C., and Dupree, H. K., Endrin uptake and release by fingerling channel catfish *(Ictalurus punctatus), J. Fish. Res. Board Can.,* 30, 1743, 1973.

74. Lock, R. A. C., Uptake of methylmercury by aquatic organisms from water and food, in *Sublethal Effects of Toxic Chemicals on Aquatic Animals,* Koeman, J. H. and Strik, J. J. T. W. A., Eds., Elsevier, Amsterdam, 1975, 61.

75. Gruger, E. H., Jr., Karrick, N. L., Davidson, A. I., and Hurby, T., Accumulation of 3,4,3',4'-tetrachlorobiphenyl and 2,4,5,2',4',5'- and 2,4,6,2',4',6'-hexachlorobiphenyl in juvenile coho salmon, *Environ. Sci. Technol.,* 9, 121, 1975.

76. Shannon, L. R., Accumulation and elimination of dieldrin in muscle tissue of channel catfish, *Bull. Environ. Contam. Toxicol.,* 17, 637, 1977.

77. Jarvinen, A. W., Hoffman, M. J., and Thorslund, T. W., Long-term toxic effects of DDT food and water exposure on fathead minnows, *J. Fish. Res. Board Can.,* 34, 2089, 1977.

78. Jarvinen, A. W. and Tyo, R. M., Toxicity to fathead minnows of endrin in food and water, *Arch. Environ. Contam. Toxicol.,* 7, 409, 1978.

79. Lockhart, W. L., Metner, D. A., and Solomon, J., Methoxychlor residue studies in caged and wild fish from the Athabasca River, Alberta, following a single application of blackfly larvicide, *J. Fish. Res. Board Can.,* 34, 626, 1977.

80. Fowler, S. W. and Elder, D. L., PCB and DDT residues in the Mediterranean pelagic food chain, *Bull. Environ. Contam. Toxicol.,* 19, 244, 1978.

81. Berry, W. O. and Fisher, J. W., Transfer of ^{14}C-toluene from mosquito larvae to bluegill sunfish, *Bull. Environ. Contam. Toxicol.,* 23, 733, 1979.

82. Tulp, M. Th. M., Haya, K., Carson, W. G., Zitko, V., and Hutzinger, O., Effect of salinity on uptake of ^{14}C-2,2',4,5,5'-pentachlorobiphenyl by juvenile Atlantic Salmon, *Chemosphere,* 8, 243, 1979.

83. Canton, J. H., Wegman, R. C. C., Vulto, T. J. A., Verhoef, C. H., and Esch, G. J. V., Toxicity-, accumulation- and elimination studies of α-hexachlorocyclohexane (α-HCH) with saltwater organisms of different trophic levels, *Water Res.,* 12, 687, 1978.

84. Pastel, M., Bush, B., and Kim, J. S., Accumulation of polychlorinated biphenyls in American shad during their migration in the Hudson River, Spring, 1977, *Pestic. Monit. J.,* 14, 11, 1980.

85. Scura, E. D. and Theilacker, G. H., Transfer of the chlorinated hydrocarbon PCB in a laboratory marine food chain, *Marine Biol.,* 40, 317, 1977.

86. Dobroski, C. J., Jr. and Epifanio, C. E., Accumulation of benzo(a)pyrene in a larval bivalve via trophic transfer, *Can. J. Fish. Aquat. Sci.,* 37, 2318, 1980.

87. Monod, G. and Keck, G., PCBs in Lake Geneva (Lake Leman) fish, *Bull. Environ. Contam. Toxicol.,* 29, 570, 1982.

88. Frank, R., Holdrinet, M. V. H., Desjardine, R. L., and Dodge, D. P., Organochlorine and mercury residues in fish from Lake Simcoe, Ontario, 1970—76, *Environ. Biol. Fish.,* 3, 275, 1978.

89. Reinert, R. E., Stone, L. J., and Bergman, H. L., Dieldrin and DDT: accumulation from water and food by lake trout *(Salvelinus namaycush)* in the laboratory, *17th Conf. Great Lakes, Res.,* International Association for Great Lakes Research, Ann Arbor, Mich., 1974, 52.

90. Wedemayer, G., Role of intestinal microflora in the degradation of DDT by rainbow trout *(Salmo gairdneri), Life Sci.,* 7, 219, 1968.

91. Reinert, R. E. and Bergman, H. L., Residues of DDT in lake trout *(Salvelinus namaycush)* and coho salmon *(Oncorhynchus kisutch)* from the Great Lakes, *J. Fish. Res. Board Can.,* 31, 191, 1974.

92. Bjerk, J. E. and Brevik, E. M., Organochlorine compounds in aquatic environments, *Arch. Environ. Contam. Toxicol.,* 9, 743, 1980.

93. Holden, A. V., Organochlorine insecticide residues in salmonid fish, *J. Appl. Ecol.,* 3, 45, 1966.

94. Neely, W. B., Estimating rate constants for the uptake and clearance of chemicals by fish, *Environ. Sci. Technol.,* 13, 1506, 1979.

95. Rodgers, D. W. and Beamish, F. W. H., Uptake of water borne methylmercury by rainbow trout *(Salmo gairdneri)* in relation to oxygen consumption and methylmercury concentration, *Can. J. Fish. Aquat. Sci.,* 38, 1309, 1981.

96. Addison, R. F., Organochlorine compounds and marine lipids, *Prog. Lipid Res.,* 21, 47, 1982.

97. McKim, J., Schmieder, P., and Veith, G., Absorption dynamics of organic chemical transport across trout gills as related to octanol-water partition coefficient, *Toxicol. Appl. Pharmacol.,* 77, 1, 1985.

98. Norstrom, R. J., McKinnon, A. E., deFreitas, A. S. W., and Miller, D. R., Pathway definition of pesticide and mercury uptake by fish, in *Environmental Quality and Safety,* Suppl. Vol 3, Coulston, F. and Corte, F., Eds., Georg Thieme Verlag, Stuttgart, 1975, 11.

99. Harding, G. C., Peter Vass, W., and Drinkwater, K. F., Importance of feeding, direct uptake from seawater, and transfer from generation to generation in the accumulation of an organochlorine (*p,p'*-DDT) by the marine planktonic copepod *Calanus finmarchicus, Can. J. Fish. Aquat. Sci.,* 38, 101, 1982.

100. Zitko, V. and Hutzinger, O., Sources, levels and toxicological significance of PCB in hatchery-reared Atlantic salmon, *Am. Chem. Soc. Div. Water, Air, Waste Chem.,* 12, 157, 1972.

101. Addison, R. F., Organochlorine compounds in aquatic organisms: their distribution, transport and physiological significance, in *Effects of Pollutants on Aquatic Organisms,* Lockwood, A. P. M., Ed., Cambridge University Press, London, 1976.

102. Plack, P. A., Skinner, E. R., Rogie, A., and Mitchell, A. I., Distribution of DDT between the lipoproteins of trout serum, *Comp. Biochem. Physiol.,* 62, 119, 1979.

103. Dvorchik, B. H. and Maren, T. H., The fate of *p,p'*-DDT (2,2-BIS (P-chlorophenyl), 1,1,1-trichloroethane) in the dog fish *Squalus acanthias, Comp. Biochem. Physiol.,* 42, 205, 1972.

104. Olson, K. R., Bergman, H. L., and Fromm, P. O., Uptake of methyl mercuric chloride and mercuric chloride by trout: a study of uptake pathways into the whole animal and uptake by erythrocytes in vitro, *J. Fish. Res. Board Can.,* 30, 1293, 1973.

105. Gakstatter, J. H. and Weiss, C. M., The elimination of DDT-C^{14}, dieldrin-C^{14}, and lindane-C^{14} from fish following a single sublethal exposure in aquaria, *Trans. Am. Fish. Soc.,* 96, 301, 1967.

106. Buhler, D. R., Rasmusson, M. E., and Shanks, W. E., Chronicoral DDT toxicity in juvenile coho and chinook salmon, *Toxicol. Appl. Pharmacol.,* 14, 535, 1969.

107. Ernst, W. and Goerke, H., Anreischung, Verteilung, Umwandlung und Ausscheidung von DDT-^{14}C bei *Solea solea* (Pisces: Soleidae), *Mar. Biol.,* 24, 287, 1974.

108. Murphy, P. G. and Murphy, J. V., Correlation between respiration and direct uptake of DDT in the mosquito-fish *Gambusia affinis, Bull. Environ. Contam. Toxicol.,* 6, 581, 1971.

109. Edgren, M., Olsson, M., and Renberg, L., Preliminary results on uptake and elimination at different temperatures of *p,p'*-DDT and two chlorobiphenyls in perch from brackish water, *Ambio,* 8, 270, 1979.

110. Crawford, R. B. and Guarino, A. M., Effects of DDT in *Fundulus:* studies in toxicity, fate and reproduction, *Arch. Environ. Contam. Toxicol.,* 4, 334, 1976.

111. Mitchell, A. I., Plack, P. A., and Thomson, I. M., Relative concentrations of ^{14}C-DDT and of two polychlorinated biphenyls in the lipids of cod tissues after a single overdose, *Arch. Environ. Contam. Toxicol.,* 6, 525, 1977.

112. Bathe, R., Ullmann, L., Sachsse, K., and Hess, R., Relationship between toxicity to fish and to mammals: a comparative study under defined laboratory conditions, *Excerpta Med. Int. Congr. Ser.,* 376, 351, 1975.

113. Darrow, D. C. and Addison, R. F., The metabolic clearance of ^{14}C-*p,p'*-DDT from plasma and its distribution in the thorny skate, *Raja radiata, Environ. Physiol. Biochem.,* 3, 196, 1973.

114. Agarwal, H. C. and Gupta, B., Distribution and metabolism of DDT in the catfish *Heteropneustes fossilis* in relation to the signs of poisoning, *Toxicol. Appl. Pharmacol.,* 29, 204, 1974.

115. Gakstatter, J. H., Rates of accumulation of ^{14}C-dieldrin residues in tissues of goldfish exposed to a single sublethal dose of ^{14}C-aldrin, *J. Fish. Res. Board Can.,* 25, 1797, 1968.

116. Grzenda, A. E., Taylor, W. J., and Paris, D. F., The uptake and distribution of chlorinated residues by goldfish *(Carassius auratus)* fed a ^{14}C-dieldrin contaminated diet, *Trans. Am. Fish. Soc.,* 100, 215, 1971.

117. Khan, H. M., Neudorf, S., and Khan, M. A. Q., Absorption and elimination of photodieldrin by *Daphnia* and goldfish, *Bull. Environ. Contam. Toxicol.,* 13, 582, 1975.

118. Shannon, L. R., Equilibrium between uptake and elimination of dieldrin by channel catfish, *Ictalurus punctatus, Bull. Environ. Contam. Toxicol.,* 17, 278, 1977.

119. Sugiura, K., Matsumoto, N., Washino, T., Muhara, Y., and Goto, M., Accumulation of organo-chlorine compounds in fishes. Distribution of 2,4,5-T, α-HCH, β-HCH and 2,4,6, 2',4',6'-hexachlorobiphenyl in tissues, *Chemosphere,* 8, 365, 1979.

120. Jackson, G. A., Biological half-life of endrin in channel catfish tissues, *Bull. Environ. Contam. Toxicol.,* 16, 505, 1976.

121. Schimmel, S. C., Patrick, J. M., Jr., and Forester, J., Heptachlor: uptake, depuration, retention, and metabolism by spot, *Lepomis xanthurus, J. Toxicol. Environ. Health,* 2, 169, 1976.

122. Skea, J. C., Simonin, H. J., Jackling, S., and Symula, J., Accumulation and retention of mirex by brook trout fed a contaminated diet, *Bull. Environ. Contam. Toxicol.,* 27, 79, 1981.

123. Iwie, G. W., Gibson, J. R., Bryant, H. E., Begin, J. J., Barnett, J. R., and Dorough, H. W., Accumulation, distribution and excretion of mirex-^{14}C in animals exposed for long periods to the insecticide in diet, *J. Agric. Food Chem.,* 22, 646, 1974.

124. Niimi, A. J. and Cho, C. Y., Uptake of hexachlorobenzene (HCB) from feed by rainbow trout *(Salmo gairdneri), Bull. Environ. Contam. Toxicol.,* 24, 834, 1980.

125. Sanborn, J. R., Childers, W. F., and Hansen, L. G., Uptake and elimination of (^{14}C) hexachlorobenzene (HCB) by the green sunfish *Lepomis cyanellus* Raf., after feeding contaminated food, *J. Agric. Food Chem.,* 25, 551, 1977.

126. Gruger, E. H., Jr., Hruby, T., and Karrick, N. L., Sublethal effects of structurally related tetrachloro-, pentachloro-, and hexachlorobiphenyl on juvenile coho salmon, *Environ. Sci. Technol.,* 10, 1033, 1976.

127. Hansen, L. G., Wiekhorst, W. B., and Simon, J., Effects of dietary Aroclor® 1242 on channel catfish *(Ictalurus punctatus)* and the selective accumulation of PCB components, *J. Fish. Res. Board Can.,* 33, 1343, 1976.

128. Braun, F. and Meyhofer, B., Untersuchungen zur Anreicherung polychlorierter Biphenyl (Clophen C) in Fish Organen unter Laborbedingungen, in *Fish and Umwelt,* Reichenback-Klinke, H. H., Ed., Gustav Fischer Verlag, Stuttgart, 1977, 1.

129. Lockhart, W. L., Metner, D. A., and Grift, N., Biochemical and residue studies on rainbow trout *(Salmo gairdneri)* following field and laboratory exposures to fenitrothion, *Manit. Entomol.,* 7, 26, 1973.

130. Seguchi, K. and Asaka, S., Intake and excretion of diazinon in freshwater fishes, *Bull. Environ. Contam. Toxicol.,* 27, 244, 1981.

131. Gray, C. and Knowles, C. O., Uptake of propamocarb fungicide by bluegills and channel catfish, *Chemosphere,* 9, 329, 1980.

132. Gray, C. and Knowles, C. O., Metabolic fate and tissue residues of propamocarb in bluegills and channel catfish, *Chemosphere,* 10, 469, 1981.

133. Kanazawa, J., Uptake and excretion of organophosphorus and carbamate insecticides by freshwater fish, Motsugo, *Pseudorasbora parva, Bull. Environ. Contam. Toxicol.,* 14, 346, 1975.

134. Ernst, W. and Weber, K., The fate of pentachlorophenol in the Weser Estuary and the German Bight, *Veroeff. Inst. Meeresforsch. Bremerhaven,* 17, 45, 1978.

135. Glickman, A. H., Statham, C. N., Wu, A., and Lech, J. J., Studies on the uptake, metabolism, and disposition of pentachlorophenol and pentachloroanisols in rainbow trout, *Toxicol. Appl. Pharmacol.,* 41, 649, 1977.

136. Virtanen, M. T. and Hattula, M. L., The fate of 2,4,6-trichlorophenol in an aquatic continuous-flow system, *Chemosphere*, 11, 641, 1982.

137. Pruitt, G. W., Grantham, B. J., and Price, R. H., Accumulation and elimination of pentachlorophenol by the bluegill, *Lepomis Macrochirus, Trans. Am. Fish. Soc.*, 106, 462, 1977.

138. Schultz, D. P., Dynamics of a salt of (2,4-dichlorophenoxy) acetic acid in fish, water and hydrosoil, *J. Agric. Food Chem.*, 21, 186, 1973.

139. Rodgers, C. A., Uptake and elimination of simazine by green sunfish (*Lepomis cyanellus* Raf.), *Weed Sci.*, 18, 134, 1969.

140. Sikka, H. C., Appleton, H. T., and Gangstad, E. O., Uptake and metabolism of dimethylamine salt of 2,4-dichlorophenoxyacetic acid by fish, *J. Agric. Food Chem.*, 25, 1030, 1977.

141. Sikka, H. C., Ford, D., and Lynch, R. S., Uptake, distribution and metabolism of endothall in fish, *J. Agric. Food Chem.*, 23, 849, 1975.

142. Knowles, C. O., Benezet, H. J., and Mayer, F. L., Jr., Thidiazuron uptake, distribution and metabolism in bluegills and channel catfish, *J. Environ. Sci. Health*, 15, 351, 1980.

143. Olson, L. E., Allen, J. L., and Hogan, J. W., Biotransformation and elimination of the herbicide dinitramine in carp, *J. Agric. Food Chem.*, 25, 554, 1977.

144. Kanazawa, J. and Tomizawa, C., Intake and excretion of 2,4,6-trichlorophenyl-4'-nitrophenyl ether by topmouth gudgeon, *Pseudoresbora parva, Arch. Environ. Contam. Toxicol.*, 7, 397, 1978.

145. Schaefer, C. H., Dupras, E. F., Jr., Stewart, R. J., Davidson, L. W., and Colwell, A. E., The accumulation and elimination of diflubenzuron by fish, *Bull. Environ. Contam. Toxicol.*, 21, 249, 1979.

146. Tooby, T. E. and Durbin, F. J., Lindane residue accumulation and elimination in rainbow trout (*Salmo gairdneri* Richardson) and roach (*Rutilus rutilus* Linnaeus), *Environ. Pollut.*, 8, 79, 1975.

147. Neely, W. B., Branson, D. R., and Blau, G. E., Partition coefficient to measure bioconcentration potential of organic chemicals in fish, *Environ. Sci. Technol.*, 8, 1113, 1974.

148. Branson, D. R., Blau, G. E., Alexander, H. C., and Neely, W. B., Bioconcentration of 2,2',4,4'-tetrachlorobiphenyl in rainbow trout as measured by an accelerated test, *Trans. Am. Fish. Soc.*, 104, 785, 1975.

149. Krzeminski, S. F., Gilbert, J. T., and Ritts, J. A., A pharmacokinetic model for predicting pesticide residues in fish, *Arch. Environ. Contam. Toxicol.*, 5, 157, 1977.

150. Eberhardt, L. L., Some methodology for appraising contaminants in aquatic systems, *J. Fish. Res. Board Can.*, 32, 1852, 1975.

151. Spacie, A. and Hamelink, J. L., Dynamics of trifluralin accumulation in river fishes, *Environ. Sci. Technol.*, 13, 817, 1979.

152. Norstrom, R. J., McKinnon, A. E., and deFreitas, A. S. W., A bioenergetics-based model for pollutant accumulation by fish. Simulation of PCB and methylmercury residue levels in Ottawa River yellow perch *(Perca flavescens)*, *J. Fish. Res. Board Can.*, 33, 248, 1976.

153. Griesbach, S., Peters, R. H., and Youakim, S., An allometric model for pesticide bioaccumulation, *Can. J. Fish. Aquat. Sci.*, 39, 727, 1982.

154. Roberts, J. R. deFrietas, A. S. W., and Gidney, M. A. J., Influence of lipid pool size on bioaccumulation of the insecticide chlordane by northern redhorse suckers *(Mixostoma macrolepicdotum)*, *J. Fish. Res. Board Can.*, 34, 89, 1977.

155. Kawasaki, M., Experiences with the test scheme under the chemical control law of Japan: an approach to structure-activity correlations, *Ecotoxicol. Environ. Saf.*, 4, 444, 1980.

156. Statham, C. N., Melancon, M. J., Jr., and Lech, J., Bioconcentration of xenobiotics in trout bile: a proposed monitoring aid for some waterborne chemicals, *Science*, 193, 680, 1976.

157. Greer, G. L. and Paim, U., Degradation of DDT in Atlantic salmon *(Salmo salar)*, *J. Fish. Res. Board Can.*, 25, 2321, 1968.

158. Addison, R. F. and Zinck, M. E., The metabolism of some DDT-type compounds by brook trout *(Salvelinus fontinalis)*, in *Environmental Quality and Safety,* Suppl. Vol. 3, Coulston, F. and Korte, F., Eds., Georg Thieme Verlag, Stuttgart, 1975, 500.

159. Addison, R. F., Zinck, M. E., and Leahy, J. R., Metabolism of single and combined doses of ^{14}C-aldrin and ^{3}H-*p,p'*-DDT by Atlantic salmon (*Salmo salar*) fry, *J. Fish. Res. Board Can.*, 33, 2073, 1976.

160. Addison, R. F. and Willis, D. E., The metabolism by rainbow trout *(Salmo gairdneri)* of *p,p'*-(^{14}C) DDT and some of its possible degradation products labeled with ^{14}C, *Toxicol. Appl. Pharmacol.*, 43, 303, 1978.

161. Cairns, T. and Parfitt, C. H., Persistence and metabolism of TDE in California Clear Lake fish, *Bull. Environ. Contam. Toxicol.*, 24, 504, 1980.

162. Cherrington, A. D., Pairm, U., and Page, O. T., In vitro degradation of DDT by intestinal contents of Atlantic salmon *(Salmo salar)*, *J. Fish. Res. Board Can.*, 26, 47, 1969.

163. Anon., Ambient Water Quality Criteria for Endosulfan, US EPA 440/5-80-046, Office of Water Regulations and Standards Criteria and Standards Division, United States Environmental Protection Agency, Washington, D.C., 1980.

164. Rao, D. M. R., Devi, A. P., and Murty, A. S., Toxicity and metabolism of endosulfan and its effect on oxygen consumption and total nitrogen excretion of the fish *Macrognathus aculeatum, Pestic. Biochem. Physiol.*, 15, 282, 1981.

165. Feroz, M. and Khan, M. A. Q., Metabolism of ^{14}C-heptachlor in goldfish *(Carassius auratus), Arch. Environ. Contam. Toxicol.*, 8, 519, 1979.

166. Casida, J. E., Veda, K., Gaughan, L. C., Jao, L. T., and Soderlund, D. M., Structure-biodegradability relationships in pyrethroid insecticides, *Arch. Environ. Contam. Toxicol.*, 3, 491, 1976.

167. Cook, G. H. and Moore, J. C., Determination of malathion, malaoxon, and mono- and dicarboxylic acids of malathion in fish, oyster, and shrimp tissue, *J. Agric. Food Chem.*, 24, 631, 1979.

168. Moore, R., Toro, E., Stanton, M., and Khan, M. A. Q., Absorption and elimination of ^{14}C alpha- and gamma chlordane by a freshwater alga, daphnid, and goldfish, *Arch. Environ. Contam. Toxicol.*, 6, 411, 1977.

169. Sudershan, P. and Khan, M. A. Q., Metabolic fate of (^{14}C) endrin in bluegill fish, *Pestic. Biochem. Physiol.*, 14, 5, 1980.

170. Melancon, J. M. and Lech, J. J., Uptake, metabolism and elimination of ^{14}C-labeled 1,2,4-trichlorobenzene in rainbow trout and carp, *J. Toxicol. Environ. Health*, 6, 645, 1980.

171. Pritchard, B. J., Karnaky, K. J., Jr., Guarino, A. M., and Kinter, W. B., Renal handling of the polar DDT metabolite DDA (2,2-bis (P-chlorophenyl) acetic acid) by marine fish, *Am. J. Physiol.*, 233, 126, 1977.

172. Surak, J. G. and Bradley, R. L., Jr., Transport of organochlorine chemicals across cell membranes, *Environ. Res.*, 11, 343, 1976.

173. Ducat, D. A. and Khan, M. A. Q., Absorption and elimination of ^{14}C-cis-chlordane and ^{14}C-photo-cis-chlordane by goldfish *Carassius auratus, Arch. Environ. Contam. Toxicol.*, 8, 409, 1979.

174. Feroz, M. and Khan, M. A. Q., Fate of ^{14}C-cis-chlordane in goldfish, *Carrassius auratus* (L.), *Bull. Environ. Contam. Toxicol.*, 23, 64, 1979.

175. Niimi, A. J. and Cho, C. Y., Elimination of hexachlorobenzene (HCB) by rainbow trout *(Salmo gairdneri)* and an examination of its kinetics in Lake Ontario salmonids, *Can. J. Fish. Aquat. Soc.*, 38, 1350, 1981.

176. Spacie, A. and Hamelink, J. C., Alternative models for describing the bioconcentration of organics in fish, *Environ. Toxicol. Chem.*, 1, 309, 1982.

177. Buhler, D. R. and Rasmusson, M. E., The oxidation of drugs by fishes, *Comp. Biochem. Physiol.*, 25, 223, 1968.

178. Chambers, J. E. and Yarbrough, J. D., Xenobiotic biotransformation systems in fishes, *Comp. Biochem. Physiol.*, 55, 77, 1976.

179. Hodgson, E., Comparative studies of cytochrome p-450 and its interaction with pesticides, in *Survival in Toxic Environments,* Khan, M. A. Q. and Bederka, J. P., Eds., Academic Press, New York, 1974.

180. Adamson, R. H. and Sieber, S. M., The disposition of xenobiotics by fishes, in *Survival in Toxic Environments,* Khan, M. A. Q. and Bederka, J. P., Eds., Academic Press, New York, 1974.

181. Lech, J. L. and Bend, R., Relationship between biotransformation and the toxicity and fate of xenobiotic chemicals in fish, *Environ. Health Perspectives*, 34, 115, 1980.

182. Zitko, V., Metabolism and distribution by aquatic animals, in *Handbook of Environmental Chemistry,* Hutzinger, O., Ed., Springer-Verlag, Berlin, 1980, 221.

183. Lech, J. J., Vodicnik, M. J., and Elcombe, C. R., Induction of monooxygenase activity in fish, in *Aquatic Toxicology,* Weber, L. J., Ed., Raven Press, New York, 1982, 107.

184. Mason, H. S., Mechanisms of oxygen metabolism, *Science*, 125, 1185, 1957.

185. Vink, G. J., Uptake of dieldrin and dieldrin-induced changes in the activities of microsomal liver enzymes the marine flatfish *Pleuronectes platessa* L., in *Sublethal Effects of Toxic Chemicals on Aquatic Animals,* Koeman, J. H. and Strik, J. J. T. W. A., Eds., Elsevier, Amsterdam, 1975, 234.

186. Stanton, R. H. and Khan, M. A. Q., Mixed function oxidase activity toward cyclodiene insecticides in bass and bluegill sunfish, *Pestic. Biochem. Physiol.*, 3, 351, 1973.

187. Stegman, J. J. and Chevion, M., Sex differences in cytochrome p-450 and mixed function oxygenase activity in gonadally mature trout, *Biochem. Pharmacol.*, 29, 553, 1980.

188. Khan, M. A. Q., Stanton, R. H., Sutherland, D. J., Rosen, J. D., and Maitra, N., Toxicity-metabolism relationship of the photoisomers of certain chlorinated cyclodiene insecticide chemicals, *Arch. Environ. Contam. Toxicol.*, 1, 159, 1973.

189. Glickman, A. H., Shono, T., Casida, J. E., and Lech, J. J., *In vitro* metabolism of permethrin isomers by carp and rainbow trout liver microsomes, *J. Agric. Food Chem.*, 27, 1038, 1979.

190. Ludke, J. L., Gibson, J. R., and Lusk, C. I., Mixed function oxidase activity in freshwater fishes: aldrin epoxidation and parathion activation, *Toxicol. Appl. Pharmacol.*, 21, 89, 1972.

191. Wells, M. R., Ludke, J. L., and Yarbrough, J. D., Epoxidation and fate of ^{14}C aldrin in insecticide-resistant and susceptible populations of mosquito-fish *(Gambusia affinis), J. Agric. Food Chem.,* 21, 428, 1973.

192. Potter, J. L. and O'Brien, R. D., Parathion activation by livers of aquatic and terrestrial vertebrates, *Science,* 144, 55, 1964.

193. Benke, G. M., Cheever, K. L., Mirer, F. E., and Murphy, S. D., Comparative toxicity, anticholinesterase action and metabolism of methyl parathion and parathion in sunfish and mice, *Toxicol. Appl. Pharmacol.,* 28, 97, 1974.

194. Fujii, Y. and Asaka, S., Metabolism of diazinon and diazoxon in fish liver preparations, *Bull. Environ. Contam. Toxicol.,* 29, 455, 1982.

195. Hogan, J. W. and Knowles, C. O., Metabolism of diazinon by fish liver microsomes, *Bull. Environ. Contam. Toxicol.,* 8, 61, 1972.

196. Burns, K. A., Microsomal mixed function oxidases in an estuarine fish, *Fundulus heteroclitus,* and their induction as a result of environmental contamination, *Comp. Biochem. Physiol.,* 53, 443, 1976.

197. Gill, S. S., *In vitro* metabolism of carbofuran by liver microsomes of the paddifield fish *Trichogaster pectoralis, Bull. Environ. Contam. Toxicol.,* 25, 697, 1980.

198. Lech, J. J. and Statham, C. N., Role of glucuronide formation in the selective toxicity of 3-trifluoromethyl-4-nitrophenol (TFM) for the sea lamprey: comparative aspects of TFM uptake and conjugation in sea lamprey and rainbow trout, *Toxicol. Appl. Pharmacol.,* 31, 150, 1975.

199. Allen, J. L., Dawson, V. K., and Hunn, J. B., Excretion of the lampricide Bayer 73 by rainbow trout, in *Aquatic Toxicology,* ASTM STP 667, Marking, L. L. and Kimerle, R. A., Eds., American Society for Testing and Materials, Philadelphia, 1979, 392.

200. Ketchum, B. H., Zitko, V., and Saward, D., Aspects of heavy metal and organohalogen pollution in aquatic ecosystems, in *Ecological Toxicology Research,* McIntyre, A. D. and Mills, C. F., Eds., Plenum Press, New York, 1975.

201. Young, R. G., John, L. St., and Lisk, D. J., Degradation of DDT by goldfish, *Bull. Environ. Contam. Toxicol.,* 6, 351, 1971.

202. Addison, R. F., Zinck, M. E., and Willis, D. E., Mixed function oxidase enzymes in trout *(Salvelinus fontinalis)* liver: absence of induction following feeding of p,p'-DDT or p,p'-DDE, *Comp. Biochem. Physiol.,* 57, 39, 1977.

203. Spiegel, P. A. and Cranmer, M. F., The influence of p,p'-DDE, a model liver microsomal enzyme stimulation, of p,p'-DDT toxicity in the bluegill, *Lepomis macrochisus* (Rafinesque), *Toxicol. Appl. Pharmacol.,* 12th Annu. Meet. 471.

204. Addison, R. F., Zinck, M. E., Willis, D. E., and Darrow, D. C., Induction of hepatic mixed function oxidases in trout by polychlorinated biphenyls and butylated monochlorodiphenyl ethers, *Toxicol. Appl. Pharmacol.,* 49, 245, 1979.

205. Addison, R. F., Zinck, M. E., and Willis, D. E., Induction of hepatic mixed-function oxidase (MFO) enzymes in trout *(Salvelinus fontinalis)* by feeding Aroclor 1254 or 3-methylcholanthrene, *Comp. Biochem. Physiol.,* 61, 323, 1978.

206. Addison, R. F., Zinck, M. E., Willis, D. E., and Wrench, J. J., Induction of hepatic mixed function oxidase activity in trout (*Salvelinus fontinalis)* by Aroclor 1254 and some aromatic hydrocarbon PCB replacements, *Toxicol. Appl. Pharmacol.,* 63, 166, 1982.

207. Hansen, P. D., Addison, R. F., and Willis, D. E., Hepatic microsomal O-de-ethylases in cod *(Gadus morhua):* their induction by Aroclor 1254 but not Aroclor 1016, *Comp. Biochem. Physiol.,* 74, 173, 1983.

208. Franklin, R. B., Vodicnik, M. J., Ekobe, C. R., and Lech, J. L., Alterations in hepatic mixed function oxidase activity of rainbow trout after acute treatment with polybrominated biphenyl isomers and firemaster BP-6, *J. Toxicol. Environ. Health,* B7, 817, 1981.

209. Narbonne, J. F. and Gallis, J. L., *In vivo* and *in vitro* effect of phenochlor DP 6 on drug metabolizing activity in mullet liver, *Bull. Environ. Contam. Toxicol.,* 23, 338, 1979.

210. Kurelec, B., Matijasevic, Z., Rijavec, M., Alacevic, M., Britivic, S., Muller, W. E. G., and Zahn, R. K., Induction of benzo(a)pyrene monooxygenase in fish and the salmonella test as a tool for detecting mutagenic/carcinogenic xenobiotics in the aquatic environment, *Bull. Environ. Contam. Toxicol.,* 21, 799, 1979.

211. Kurelec, B., Protic, M., Britivic, M., Kezic, S. N., Rijavec, M., and Zahn, R. K., Toxic effects in fish and the mutagenic capacity of water from the Sava River in Yugoslavia, *Bull. Environ. Contam. Toxicol.,* 26, 179, 1981.

212. Ahokas, J. T., Karki, N. T., Oikari, A., and Soivio, A., Mixed function monooxygenase of fish as an indicator of pollution of aquatic environment by industrial effluent, *Bull. Environ. Contam. Toxicol.,* 16, 270, 1976.

213. Josephson, J., Is predictive toxicology coming?, *Environ. Sci. Technol.,* 15, 379, 1981.

214. Hansch, C., Muir, R. M., Fujita, T., Maloney, P. P., Geiger, F., and Streich, M., The correlation of biological activity of plant growth regulators and chloromycetin derivatives with Hammett constants and partition coefficients, *J. Am. Chem. Soc.*, 85, 2817, 1963.

215. Mayer, F. L., Adems, W. J., Finley, M. T., Michael, P. R., Mehrle, P. M., and Saeger, V. W., Phosphate ester hydraulic fluids. An aquatic environmental assessment of pydrauls 50E and 115E, in *Aquatic Toxicology and Hazard Assessment: 4th Conf.*, ASTM STP 737, Branson, D. R. and Dickson, K. L., Eds., American Society for Testing and Materials, Philadelphia, 1981, 103.

216. Mackay, D., Correlation of bio-concentration factors, *Environ. Sci. Technol.*, 16, 274, 1982.

217. Kenaga, E. E., Correlation of bioconcentration factors of chemicals in aquatic and terrestrial organisms with their physical and chemical properties, *Environ. Sci. Technol.*, 14, 553, 1980.

218. Anliker, R., Clarke, E. A., and Moser, P., Use of the partition coefficient as an indicator of bioaccumulation tendency of dyestuffs in fish, *Chemosphere*, 10, 263, 1981.

219. Chiou, C. T., Freed, V. H., Schmedding, D. W., and Kohnert, R. L., Partition coefficient and bioaccumulation of selected organic chemicals, *Environ. Sci. Technol.*, 11, 475, 1977.

220. Mackay, D., Comment on the paper of Chiou et al., *Environ. Sci. Technol.*, 11, 1219, 1977, from Chiou, T., Freed, V. H., Schmedding, D. W., and Kohnert, R. L., Partition coefficient and bioaccumulation of selected organic chemicals, *Environ. Sci. Tech.*, 11, 475, 1977.

221. Freed, V. H., Chiou, C. T., Schmedding, D., and Kohnert, R., Some physical factors in toxicological assessment tests, *Environ. Health Perspect.*, 30, 75, 1979.

222. Geyer, H., Viswanathan, R., Freitag, D., and Korte, F., Relationship between water solubility of organic chemicals and their bioaccumulation by the alga *Chlorella*, *Chemosphere*, 10, 1307, 1981.

223. Kenaga, E. E. and Goring, C. A. I., Relationship between water solubility, soil sorption, octanol-water partitioning, and concentration of chemicals in biota, in *ASTM STP 707*, Eaton, J. G., Parrish, P. R., and Hendricks, A. C., Eds., American Society for Testing and Materials, Philadelphia, 1980, 78.

224. Kenaga, E. E., Predicted bioconcentration factors and soil sorption coefficients of pesticides and other chemicals, *Ecotoxicol. Environ. Saf.*, 4, 26, 1980.

225. Banerjee, S., Yalkowsky, S. H., and Valvani, C., Water solubility and octanol/water partition coefficients of organics, limitations of the solubility-partition coefficient correlation, *Environ. Sci. Technol.*, 14, 1227, 1980.

226. Mackay, D., Bobra, A., and Shiu, W. Y., Relationships between aqueous solubility and octanol-water partition coefficients, *Chemosphere*, 9, 701, 1980.

227. Schultz, T. W. and Quezada, M. C., Structure-toxicity relationships of selected nitrogenous heterocyclic compounds. II. Dinitrogen molecules, *Arch. Environ. Contam. Toxicol.*, 11, 353, 1982.

228. Yang, C. F. and Sun, Y. P., Partition distribution of insecticides as a critical factor affecting their rates of absorption from water and relative toxicities to fish, *Arch. Environ. Contam. Toxicol.*, 6, 325, 1977.

229. Tulp, M. Th. M. and Hutzinger, O., Some thoughts on aqueous solubilities and partition coefficients of PCB, and the mathematical correlation between bioaccumulation and physio-chemical properties, *Chemosphere*, 7, 849, 1978.

230. Esser, H. O. and Moser, P., An appraisal of problems related to the measurement and evaluation of bioaccumulation, *Ecotoxicol. Environ. Saf.*, 6, 131, 1982.

231. Schultz, T. W., Kier, L. B., and Hall, L. H., Structure toxicity relationships of selected nitrogenous heterocyclic compounds. III. Relations using molecular connectivity, *Bull. Environ. Contam. Toxicol.*, 28, 373, 1982.

232. Matsuo, M., The i/o-characters to describe ecological magnification of some organophosphorous insecticides in fish, *Chemosphere*, 8, 477, 1979.

233. Matsuo, M., The i/o-characters to relate accumulation factors of some halogenated biphenyls in fish, *Chemosphere*, 9, 61, 1980.

234. Matsuo, M., The i/o-characters to correlate bioaccumulation of some chlorobenzenes in guppies with their chemical structures, *Chemosphere*, 9, 409, 1980.

235. Matsuo, M., A thermodynamic interpretation of bioaccumulation of Aroclor 1254 (PCB) in fish, *Chemosphere*, 9, 671, 1980.

236. Fujita, A., *Pharm. Bull.*, 2, 163, 1954, in Matsuo, M., The i/o-characters to describe ecological magnification of some organophosphorous insecticides in fish, *Chemosphere*, 8, 477, 1979.

237. Southworth, G. R., Keffer, C. C., and Beauchamp, J. J., Potential and realized bioconcentration. A comparison of observed and predicted bioconcentration of azaarenes in the fathead minnow *(Pimephales promelas)*, *Environ. Sci. Technol.*, 14, 1529, 1980.

238. Sasaki, K., Takeda, M., and Uchiyama, M., Toxicity, absorption and elimination of phosphoric acid triesters by killifish and goldfish, *Bull. Environ. Contam. Toxicol.*, 27, 775, 1981.

239. Muir, D. C. G., Grift, N. P., Townsend, B. E., Metner, D. A., and Lockhart, W. L., Comparison of the uptake and bioconcentration of fluridone and terbutryn by rainbow trout and *Chironomus tetans* in sediment and water systems, *Arch. Environ. Contam. Toxicol.,* 11, 595, 1982.

240. Niimi, A. J. and McFadden, C. A., Uptake of sodium pentachlorophenate (NaPCP) from water by rainbow trout *(Salmo gairdneri),* exposed to concentrations in the ng/*l* range, *Bull. Environ. Contam. Toxicol.,* 28, 11, 1982.

241. Platford, R. F., The environmental significance of surface films. II. Enhanced partitioning of lindane in thin films of octanol on the surface of water, *Chemosphere,* 10, 719, 1981.

242. Sugiura, K., Ito, N., Matsumoto, N., Michara, Y., Murata, K., Tsukakoshi, Y., and Goto, M., Accumulation of polychlorinated biphenyls and polybrominated biphenyls in fish: limitation of "correlation between partition coefficients and accumulation factors", *Chemosphere,* 7, 731, 1978.

243. Shaw, G. R. and Connell, D. W., Relationship between steric factors and bioconcentration of polychlorinated biphenyls (PCB's) by the sea mullet *(Mugil cephalus* Linnaeus), *Chemosphere,* 9, 731, 1980.

244. Yalkowsky, S. H. and Morozowich, W., A physical chemical basis for the design of orally active prodrugs, in *Drug Design,* Ariens, E. J., Ed., Vol 9, Academic Press, New York, 1980, 121.

245. Zitko, V., The accumulation of polybrominated biphenyls by fish, *Bull. Environ. Contam. Toxicol.,* 17, 285, 1977.

246. Zitko, V., Uptake of chlorinated paraffins and PCB from suspended solids and food by juvenile Atlantic salmon, *Bull. Environ. Contam. Toxicol.,* 12, 406, 1974.

247. Zitko, V. and Carson, W. G., A comparison of the uptake of PCB's and isopropyl-PCB's *(Chloralkylene* 12) by fish, *Chemosphere,* 6, 133, 1977.

248. Courteny, C. H. and Reed, J. K., Accumulation of DDT from food and from water by golden shiner minnows, *Notemigonus crysoleucas. Proc. 25th Annu. Conf. Southeastern Assoc. Game Fish Comm.,* 1972, 426.

249. Sanborn, J. R., Childers, W. F., and Metcalf, R. L., Uptake of three polychlorinated biphenyls, DDT, and DDE by the green sunfish, *Lepomis cyanellus* Raf., *Bull. Environ. Contam. Toxicol.,* 13, 209, 1975.

250. Hansen, D. J. and Wilson, A. J., Significance of DDT residues in fishes from the estuary near Pensacola, Fla., *Pestic. Monit. J.,* 4, 51, 1970.

251. Crosby, D. G. and Tucker, R. K., Accumulation of DDT by *Daphnia magna, Environ. Sci. Technol.,* 5, 714, 1971.

252. Lorio, W. J., Jenkins, J. H., and Huish, M. T., Deposition of dieldrin in four components of two artificial aquatic systems and a farm pond, *Trans. Am. Fish. Soc.,* 105, 695, 1976.

253. Schimmel, S. C., Patrick, J. M., Jr., and Forester, J., Heptachlor: toxicity to and uptake by several estuarine organisms, *J. Toxicol. Environ. Health,* 1, 955, 1976.

254. Tagatz, M. E., Effect of mirex on predator-prey interaction in an experimental estuarine ecosystem, *Trans. Am. Fish. Soc.,* 105, 546, 1976.

255. Parrish, P. R., Schimmel, S. C., Hansen, D. J., Patrick, J. M., Jr., and Forester, J., Chlordane: effects on several estuarine organisms, *J. Toxicol. Environ. Health,* 1, 485, 1976.

256. Giam, C. S., Murray, H. E., Ray, L. E., and Kira, S., Bioaccumulation of hexachlorobenzene in killifish *(Fundulus similis), Bull. Environ. Contam. Toxicol.,* 25, 891, 1980.

257. McLeese, D. W., Metcalf, C. D., and Zitko, V., Lethality of permethrin, cypermethrin and fenvalerate to salmon, lobster and shrimp, *Bull. Environ. Contam. Toxicol.,* 25, 950, 1980.

258. Hattula, M. L., Wasenius, V. M., Reunanen, H., and Arstila, A. V., Acute toxicity of some chlorinated phenols, catechols and cresols to trout, *Bull. Environ. Contam. Toxicol.,* 26, 295, 1981.

259. Trujillo, D. A., Ray, L. E., Murray, H. E., and Giam, C. S., Bioaccumulation of pentachlorophenol by killifish *(Fundulus similis), Chemosphere,* 11, 25, 1982.

260. Bull, C. J., The Effects of Sumithion, an Organophosphate Insecticide, on the Behaviour of Juvenile Coho Salmon, *Oncorhynchus kisutch,* Walbaum, M.Sc. thesis, University of Victoria, Victoria, British Columbia, 1971, 73; in Bull, C. J. and McInerey, J. E., Behaviour of juvenile coho salmon *(Oncorhynchus kisutch),* exposed to sumithion (Fenitrothion), an organophosphate insecticide, *J. Fish. Res. Board Can.,* 21, 1867, 1974.

261. Kanazawa, J., Bioconcentration ratio of diazinon by freshwater fish and snail, *Bull. Environ. Contam. Toxicol.,* 20, 613, 1978.

262. Muir, D. C. G., Grift, N. P., Blouw, A. P., and Lockhart, W. L., Persistence of fluridone in small ponds, *J. Environ. Qual.,* 9, 151, 1980.

263. Sigmon, C., Oxygen consumption in *Lepomis macrochirus* exposed to 2,4-D or 2,4,5-T, *Bull. Environ. Contam. Toxicol.,* 21, 826, 1979.

264. Han, J. C. Y., Residue studies with (^{14}C) fosamine ammonium in channel catfish, *J. Toxicol. Environ. Health,* 5, 957, 1979.

265. Schmeider, P. W., Jr., Gibson, J. R., Cramm, G. C., and Shrivastava, S. P., Uptake, depuration and toxicity of hexamethylphosphoramide in aquatic organisms, in *Aquatic Toxicology,* ASTM STP 667, Marking, L. L. and Kimerle, R. A., Eds., American Society for Testing and Materials, Philadelphia, 1979, 181.
266. Sanders, H. O. and Hunn, J. B., Toxicity, bioconcentration, and depuration of the herbicide Bolero 8EC in freshwater invertebrates and fish, *Bull. Jpn. Soc. Sci. Fish.,* 48, 1139, 1982.

Chapter 4

TOXICITY TESTS AND TEST METHODOLOGY

I. INTRODUCTION

A. Definition

In the first chapter it was established that all man-made chemicals eventually find their way into the aquatic environment, where they may prove to be toxic to many nontarget organisms. Generally, the potential impact of the pollutants is more on the aquatic organisms than on the terrestrial organisms, because, in the hydrosphere, pesticides and such other substances are transported to a greater distance and hence many more nontarget organisms are likely to be exposed to them than in the terrestrial environment. Moreover, unlike in the terrestrial environment, in the aquatic environment, the body of the organism is bathed by the medium containing the toxicant. Ever since the use of synthetic organic pesticides began, many reports on the hazards of pesticides to the aquatic organisms have appeared. As early as 1944 the greater toxicity of DDT to fish than to mammals[1] and the vulnerability of fish in laboratory tests, were reported.[2] Odum and Sumerford[3] reported that DDT was highly toxic to goldfish and mosquitofish and that mosquito pupae were more resistant than mosquitofish to DDT. Since then, the increasing awareness of the environmental hazards of pesticides has necessitated the testing of the toxicity of different pesticides to diverse aquatic organisms. As has been aptly pointed out by Cairns,[4] no instrument ever designed by man — notwithstanding the tremendous strides made in designing and perfecting very sensitive analytical instruments — can measure the toxicity; only a test organism can be used for this purpose. In the young science of aquatic toxicology, fish play as important a role in toxicity testing and hazard evaluation as do the white rat and guinea pig in mammalian toxicology.[5]

The purpose of a toxicity test is to determine how toxic an agent is to the test species. In this context, it is necessary to emphasize that toxicity tests differ from bioassays. Unfortunately, in the recent past, these two terms have been used as though they are synonymous. Perhaps the confusion arose because of a certain amount of similarity between the two tests, but as was pointed out by Stephan[6] and Brown,[7] the two types of tests are distinct and serve different purposes. In a bioassay, the effect used is either a beneficial or an adverse one, whereas in toxicity tests only an adverse effect is measured. A bioassay test is similar to a chemical test and is a tool for determining the amount of concentration of a specific agent. When the known response of an organism is used to measure the concentration or amount of a chemical or an effluent, it ought to be called a bioassay. Bioassays are based on the principle of parallelism and are conducted to compare relative potencies or concentrations. Mount[8] also emphasized this distinction, stating that bioassay tests measure only the potency or strength of a substance and as long as the response is sensitive enough, the test organism — bacteria, invertebrates, or fish — can be substituted one for the other. In toxicity test, the effect of a toxicant — may it be death or physiological, biochemical or behavioral change, or long term effects on growth and reproduction — on a specific organism is tested. Most of the tests in the realms of aquatic toxicology, incorrectly called bioassays, strictly speaking should be styled toxicity tests. In the following discussion, the term "toxicity test" is used to denote all types of tests that are conducted to measure some adverse effect caused by pesticides.

Different types of toxicity tests serve different purposes. The 96-hr toxicity test or the short-term or acute toxicity test is one of the most commonly employed tests in the evaluation of toxicity. Chronic toxicity tests conducted over a period of 30 days to several months, life cycle or partial life cycle tests, embryo-larval tests, bioconcentration/bioaccumulation tests, avoidance and other behavioral tests, biochemical/physiological tests, and histological/histochemical tests are some other tests that have been employed during the last 35 years of toxicity testing with pesticides.

The modern aquatic toxicity test protocols in use are the result of a series of attempts at the standardization of the test methodology. The earliest and one of the most useful of these test methods is that of Doudoroff et al.,[9] which forms the basis of all other attempts. In the standard methods of the American Public Health Association (APHA),[10] bioassay and toxicity test procedures are described in detail. Sprague[11-13] reviewed the state of the art up to 1970 and emphasized the need for having a clear concept of the different aspects of toxicity testing. The United States Environmental Protection Agency (USEPA) committee on the methods for toxicity tests with aquatic organisms[14] published a comprehensive review on the methods for conducting acute aquatic toxicity test. Later, this committee was replaced by the American Society for Testing and Materials (ASTM) Committee on Pesticides and the Subcommittee on Safety to Aquatic Organisms. The recommendations of this Committee[15] along with those of the "OECD Guidelines for Testing Chemicals"[16] are the most recent attempts at adopting a world-wide uniform methodology to test the toxicity of xenobiotic chemicals.

B. Early Toxicity Tests

The earliest toxicity tests traced by the author date back to 1944.[1] Odum and Sumerford[3] tested the toxicity of DDT to fish. Pielou[17] exposed fish to DDT dissolved in paraffin and reported that at a dilution of 1 in 18 million parts of water, all the test fish *(Tilapia kaufensis)* died within 24 hr. Cottam and Higgins[18] summarized the data on the acute toxicity of DDT to fish and other nontarget species. Langford[19] tested the toxicity of DDT to several species of fish and concluded that the toxicity threshold ranged from less than 1 $\mu g/\ell$ to speckled trout fry, to 5 to 10 $\mu g/\ell$ for speckled trout yearlings and the creek chub. These early reports on the toxicity of DDT and a few other pesticides were sporadic attempts at alerting other researchers to the possible side-effects of what was then believed to be the panacea for pest problems all over the world. The need for adopting uniform and standard methods of testing — to the extent possible and necessary — culminated in the recommendations of Doudoroff et al.[9] References to the then-existing methods can be found in this work. For an interested reader there can be no better source of information on toxicity test methodology than the recommendations of Doudoroff et al., the APHA Standard Methods,[10] the ASTM Subcommittee on Safety to Aquatic Organisms,[15] and the excellent reviews by Sprague.[11-13] In the following pages, besides briefly outlining the salient points of these works, some additional aspects of toxicity testing (mostly concerned with acute aquatic toxicity tests) are reviewed.

II. TEST CONDITIONS

A. Physical Conditions
1. Holding and Test Tanks

The materials used for the construction of the tanks should not remove residues by sorption or leach any undesirable products into the test medium, or in general, interfere with or alter the desired test conditions. The ASTM Committee reviewed in detail the types of materials that may be used, the care to be taken in constructing the holding chambers, and special requirements for certain types of test. Glass, stainless steel, or fluoroplastics were recommended for use. After proper conditioning, concrete or unplasticized plastic tanks may be used for holding and acclimation of the test organisms, but test tanks should be of stainless steel or glass. The depth and the smallest horizontal dimension of the test chamber, must be, respectively, at least 1.5 times the average height and the average horizontal dimension of the test organism. The test solution should be 150 mm deep for organisms over 0.5 g and at least 50 mm deep for the smaller organisms.[15]

Polyethylene-lined fiber glass tanks were used as holding[20] and test chambers,[21] and 200 ℓ polyethylene drums were used for preparing large quantities of the test medium, which was later delivered to the test tanks in a continuous flow.[22] When sprayed on three polyethylene-lined artificial ponds, Dursban®, Reldan®, and Abate® rapidly disappeared from water and were adsorbed to polyethylene, whence they were later desorbed.[23] Tygon tubing, rubber tubing, and polyethylene tubing, often used for toxicant delivery, and neoprene stoppers, have all been reported either to adsorb the test chemicals or desorb other toxic products into the test medium.[24,25] Hence, it is advisable to avoid, to the extent possible, the use of any of the above materials.

2. Physical Factors

It is important that water temperature be maintained at a constant and acceptable level. Doudoroff et al.[9] recommended a water temperature of 20 to 25°C for the warm water species and 12 to 18°C for the cold water species. Recommended temperatures for the American species have been listed by the ASTM Subcommittee.[15] The U.S. National Technical Advisory Committee on Water Quality Criteria recommended that the temperature increase for freshwater organisms should not be more than 3°C higher than the average monthly minimum temperature of the stream usually inhabited by the test organisms.[26] The actual test temperature should not deviate from the selected test temperature by more than 1°C at any time during the test.[15] In order to test the effect of temperatures other than those at which the fish live under natural conditions, the fish should be slowly and gradually acclimated to the test temperatures, never changing the acclimation temperature too drastically. A device to maintain a constant temperature in the test tanks was described.[27] It is also necessary to maintain proper hours of daylight and darkness as many responses of fish, including spawning, are known to be stimulated and controlled by appropriate photoperiods. It is advisable to employ the photoperiods approriate to the season of the test. An inexpensive method for simulating diel patterns of light was described.[28]

B. Chemical Conditions

Lee[29] reviewed the various chemical aspects that should be carefully monitored while conducting toxicity and bioassay tests. Unless constant and acceptable chemical conditions of the water are maintained, the results of toxicity testing will not be reproducible and acceptable. It was suggested that some of the earlier works on the toxicity of 3-trifluoromethyl-4-nitrophenol (TFM) to aquatic organisms cannot be compared with later works as the former did not include the data on the quality of water used for the tests.[30]

1. Toxicity of Chlorine to Fish

In the absence of other direct sources of water, city or municipal tap water is often used in conducting toxicity tests with freshwater fish. Several studies indicated that chlorine, used as a disinfectant, is highly toxic to fish. Chlorine in water induced hyperventilation, and increased coughing and bradycardia in trout; blood lactate and hematocrit values were significantly elevated over that of the controls.[31] Sensitivity of salmonids[32] and other fish[33] to chlorine was reported and the toxicity of chlorine to freshwater fish was reviewed.[34] Chloramines, formed by the reaction of free chlorine with organic nitrogenous compounds are more toxic than free chlorine itself. The formation of 1,1,1-trichloroacetone and chloroform by the reaction of free chlorine with water was reported.[35] The possible mechanism of toxicity of chlorine to fish was discussed.[36] All these studies emphasize that chlorine in the free and combined states is highly toxic to aquatic organisms. Hence, it is imperative to remove any free chlorine that is present and as far as practicable, avoid the use of chlorinated water for conducting toxicity tests.

Free chlorine can be removed by treatment with sodium thiosulfate, approximately 7 mg of the latter being required to remove 1 mg of chlorine.[37] The ASTM Committee recommended that dechlorinated water should be used only as a last resort, that sodium bisulfite is a better agent than sodium sulfite for removing free chlorine, and that the concentration of residual chlorine should not exceed 3 $\mu g/\ell$. Traditionally, residual chlorine is removed by carbon filters, which are prone to fail owing to clogging. Although by itself it is not toxic to fish, sodium thiosulfate is reported to interfere with metal toxicity. Armstrong and Scott[38] reported that 1200 W high pressure or 40 W low pressure cool mercury vapor lamps could be used to dechlorinate city supply water photochemically. The efficiency of removal was not affected by temperature, but decreased with increasing pH. With eight 40-W lamps, up to 13 ℓ/min could be dechlorinated with 90% efficiency of chlorine removal; two 1200-W lamps operating in tandem could treat up to 50 ℓ/min. Such photochemically dechlorinated water is harmless to fish.

2. Dilution Water

To minimize variation in experimental conditions between one test and another, apart from ensuring minimal variation between batches of test fish, it is necessary to minimize variation in the quality of water used for tests. If natural freshwater is used as a source of dilution water, it should be of constant quality and devoid of contaminants, and preferably be from a well or a spring.[39] The minimal criteria for acceptable natural dilution water were listed by Doudoroff et al.[9] and the ASTM Committee.[15]

Occasionally, standard dilution water, prepared by the addition of reagent grade chemicals to distilled or deionized water, is employed. The preparation and characteristics of such standard dilution water, variously termed reconstituted water, synthetic dilution water, dilution water, standard reference water, etc., has been described.[40-45] Marking[46] described the different constituents needed to prepare four types of reconstituted water, viz., very soft, soft, hard, and very hard water and the resultant pH, hardness, and alkalinity (Table 1). Courtright et al.[47] described the formulation of synthetic sea water for conducting experiments with marine organisms.

3. pH

A system for regulating and recording the pH of the test medium was described by Lillie and Klaverkamp.[48] The ASTM Subcommittee listed the different proportions of buffers that have to be mixed to obtain a test medium with a pH in the range of 6 to 10.[15] Choice and maintenance of the proper pH may be critical in tests conducted with readily ionizable compounds.

4. Oxygen

Dissolved oxygen level is a critical factor that has to be carefully controlled. In order to maintain adequate oxygen levels, the test medium is often aerated.[49,50] However, the recovery of dieldrin from tanks that were aerated was low, the percent of the initial concentration recovered after 24, 36, 48, and 72 hr from two aerated tanks being 12.8, 6.6, 7.9, and 5 in one tank and 15.5, 9.7, 10.9, and 5.6 in the other.[51] On the whole, it appears that it is not advisable to aerate the test tanks and when the oxygen concentra-

Table 1

QUANTITIES OF SALTS AND CHARACTERISTICS OF RECONSTITUTED
WATERS

| Water type | Salts added in mg/ℓ | | | | pH range | Total as ppm CaCO$_3$ | |
	NaHCO$_3$	CaSO$_4$	MgSO$_4$	KCl		Hardness	Alkalinity
Very soft	12	7.5	7.5	0.5	6.4—6.8	10—13	10—13
Soft [a]	48	30.0	30.0	2.0	7.2—7.6	40—48	30—35
Hard	192	120.0	120.0	8.0	7.6—8.0	160—180	110—120
Very hard	384	240.0	240.0	16.0	8.0—8.4	280—320	225—245

[a]   Routine bioassay water.

From Marking, L. L., *Bull. Wildl. Dis. Assoc.*, 5, 291, 1969. With permission.

tion is likely to be a critical factor, continuous flow system should be employed to maintain adquate oxygen concentration (usually at 60 to 100% saturation at the chosen temperature). Mount[52] described a system for controlling the dissolved oxygen content which can be used for holding tanks.

5. Carrier Solvents

The homogenous dispersal of the toxicant in the test medium is a problem in conducting aquatic toxicity tests. This problem assumes larger dimensions when the toxicity of very poorly water-soluble compounds is tested. The use of a carrier solvent to enhance the solubility of poorly water-soluble compounds was recommended. For instance, the APHA Standard Methods[10] recommended the use of acetone, dimethylformamide, ethanol, methanol, isopropanol, dimethylacetamide, acetonitrile, or ethylene glycol to prepare the stock solutions of poorly water-soluble toxicants. A surfactant like Triton® X-100 has also been recommended. The concentration of the solvent in the test medium should not exceed 0.5 mℓ/ℓ in static and 0.1 mℓ/ℓ in flow-through tests. Similarly, the ASTM Subcommittee recommended diemthylformamide and triethylene glycol, (not exceeding 0.5 mℓ/ℓ in the test medium) as good solvents for preparing solutions, but also considered methanol, acetone, and ethanol as equally suitable. To ensure that the solvent itself does not have any toxic effect, it was recommended that the toxicity of the solvent also should be tested simultaneously by adding the solvent alone to the control tank at the highest level used to introduce the toxicant.[15] However, Lee[29] rightly pointed out that the addition of a solvent to the control tanks does not help in determining the interaction between the carrier solvent and the toxicant.

The recommendation of the use of a carrier solvent by various standardization committees implies that the carrier solvent is expected to enhance water-solubility of the hydrophobic compounds. In a recent review on aquatic toxicity testing, Buikema et al.[53] stated "Toxicity tests conducted with water insoluble chemicals, e.g., many biocides usually use a solvent to enhance solubility." Fujiwara[54] stated that according to the Chemical Substances Control Act of Japan, a suitable solubilizer may be used in conducting the 48 hr toxicity test whenever the toxicants are poorly water-soluble. Whether a carrier solvent can enhance the solubility of hydrophobic compounds has been examined only recently. Herzel and Murty[55] tested the water-solubility of dieldrin, nitrofen, and captan in the presence of acetone, at three concentrations within the range recommended for aquatic toxicity tests, i.e., 10, 100, and 500 $\mu\ell$/ℓ, and also in the absence of the carrier solvent. No difference in the solubility of dieldrin and nitrofen in the presence or absence of acetone was found; in the case of captan, a 41%

Table 2

SOLUBILITY (μg/ℓ) OF THREE PESTICIDES IN WATER, WITH OR
WITHOUT ACETONE

Compound	Solubility in the presence of acetone at a concentration of			Solubility without acetone
	10 μℓ/ℓ	100 μℓ/ℓ	500 μℓ/ℓ	
Dieldrin	252 ± 3	252 ± 6	256 ± 2	250 ± 4
Nitrofen	593 ± 19	594 ± 35	565 ± 27	609 ± 22
Captan	5328 ± 274	5992 ± 337	6526 ± 319	4642 ± 144

Note: All values are correlated to the nearest whole number; each value is a mean of five determinations with the standard deviation indicated.

Data from Herzel, F. and Murty, A. S., *Bull. Environ. Contam. Toxicol.,* 32, 53, 1984. With permission.

increase in its solubility in the presence of the highest concentration of acetone was noticed (Table 2). It was pointed out that the small influence of acetone in increasing the water solubility of captan, however, is of little practical significance except in rare instances where the slope of the dose mortality regression line is very steep.

Another point to consider is the usefulness of the LC 50 values of compounds of poor water solubility, for which the reported LC 50 value exceeded the water solubility of the compound. For example, Buccafusco et al.[56] stated that the acute toxicity of most of the chmicals tested by them was at a concentration above their water-solubility, and therefore, the test material or one or more of the constituents precipitated or formed a slick on the water surface. They opined: "Therefore, most of the LC 50 values reported . . . are high and do not reflect the actual concentrations of the chemical which were in solution in the diluent." Similarly Heitmuller et al.[57] reported that many of the chemicals they tested were insoluble in sea water, and either floated on the surface or formed globules at the bottom of the test container. In both cases, the amount of the toxicant to which the test organism was exposed remains unknown, as was emphasized by Herzel and Murty.[55] It is interesting to note that the ASTM Subcommittee recommended: "If necessary concentrations above solubility in water should be used because organisms are sometimes exposed to concentrations above solubility and because solubility is often not well known." The justification that " . . . because organisms are sometimes exposed to concentrations above solubility . . . ," for the recommendation " . . . concentrations above solubility should be used . . . " is somewhat tenuous. The ASTM Subcommittee, however, was of the view that the use of concentrations 10 times that of the water-solubility is probably not worthwhile. When an organic chemical is added to water above its water-solubility, the quantity in excess of its saturation limit does not remain in true solution, but precipitates out, adheres to the walls, or evaporates. Hylin[58] emphasized that only that part that is in true solution is bioavailable. This point was also illustrated by Brungs and Bailey,[59] who found that the amount of endrin in solution and in adsorption to activated carbon was 26 μg/ℓ, but of this only 0.62 μg/ℓ was biologically active in killing the test fish. The latter value was not significantly different from the concentration of endrin in controls (without any suspended particles). When an organism is exposed to an unknown concentration, the resultant LC 50 value is not meaningful. The extent to which the insoluble material goes into solution subsequent to the absorption of the original amount in true solution remains unknown. In the absence of such information, it is not proper to rely on 96-h LC 50 values that exceed the water solubility of the test compounds.

Another important aspect in the use of carrier solvents is the interaction, if any, between the solvent and the toxicant, and the possible alteration of the membrane permeability. Even though direct evidence is scanty, it has been suggested on occasion that the carrier solvent may interfere with the uptake of the toxicant. Bioconcentration of tris (2,4-di-ter-butylphenyl)phosphite by the killifish was increased in the presence of the surfactant, Tween 20® at concentration up to 5 mg/ℓ but decreased thereafter.[60] Mac and Seelye[61] reported that the uptake of PCB (polychlorinated biphenyl) increased in the presence of acetone. From the methodology described by them, it appears that in their experiments, the fry were exposed to a greater amount of the toxicant over a period of 52 days in the presence of acetone. Hence it would be logical to expect higher residue concentrations in the presence of acetone than in its absence. Majewski et al.[62] reported that high concentrations of acetone induced increased ventilation rate and buccal pressure amplitude, while ethanol produced an opposite effect in the test fish. Lest one misinterprets these results and concludes that the carrier solvents are toxic to the test organisms, they pointed out that the concentrations of the carrier solvents chosen by them were much higher than those usually employed in the aquatic toxicity tests. Besides, the noninterference of the carrier solvent (at recommended concentrations) with the results of the toxicity tests was reported.[63,64] Murty and Hansen[65] studied the uptake of HCB (hexachlorobenzene) in the presence of either of two carrier solvents and reported that rainbow trout absorbed the same quantity of HCB in the presence or absence of carrier solvents. The bioconcentration of HCB by rainbow trout in 4 days or 30 days was not significantly altered by acetone or ethylene glycol monoethyl ether. However, the available evidence would not permit one to conclude either way about the interaction of the carrier solvent with the toxicant. There has not been any work on the uptake of the toxicant in the presence of ethanol, dimethylformamide, or a number of other solvents.

Since it has been suggested or suspected that the carrier solvent may interact with the toxicant, several attempts have been made to conduct toxicity tests without the use of a carrier solvent by generating saturated water solutions of different types of test compounds. Chadwick and Kiigemagi[66] packed glass columns of various dimensions (1.2 to 1.5 m long and 2.5 to 5 cm wide) with dieldrin (or HEOD) and a saturated solution of this compound in water was generated. After an initial stabilization period of about 3 weeks, the concentration of the compound in water was almost constant over a period of several months. Subsequently, several other devices have been reported for generating saturated solutions of toxicants in water.[67-70]

C. Biological Conditions
1. Test Species
Doudoroff et al.[9] recommended the use of native fish, common to unpolluted parts of the ecosystem. Laboratory tests with species like goldfish, harlequin fish, zebra fish, and goldorfe have been justified on the basis of the easy availability of the species throughout the year or the ease of handling, care, and culturing of such fish. Apart from the criticism that such species do not represent the populations that are likely to be affected by pesticide residues in nature, a serious objection to the use of such fish is their excessive or poor sensitivity to many test chemicals. Goldfish was once a frequently employed experimental fish; now it is seldom employed in pesticide toxicity tests. The ASTM Committee recommended 8 North American freshwater species and 14 salt water species. These species were chosen to promote uniformity and comparability of results and with a view to obtaining much information about a few species, rather than a little information about many species. The desirable test species for European countries are listed in the OECD (Organization for Economic Cooperation and Development) guidelines.[16] In Japan, the orange-red killifish *(Oryzias latipes)* and the carp *(Cyprinus carpio)* are used for many types of tests.[54,71]

When available, species that have been reared in the laboratory are best suited because the population is somewhat homogenous. Many reports on the care needed in maintaining and culturing many useful species of test fish are now available.[44,72,73] The care needed in collecting and handling fish for purposes of conducting toxicity tests has been dealt with by the APHA Standard Methods. Labor-saving devices for use in tests with fish were described.[74] When laboratory or hatchery-reared fish are not available, wild populations of fish without previous history of exposure to pesticides and other toxicants may be used.[75] In the case of marine and estuarine species, owing to the difficulties in rearing the species in the laboratory, one is forced to use fish caught in nature; e.g., Baltic Sea bleaks *(Alburnus alburnus)* were used for evaluating the toxicity of 78 chemicals to estuarine organisms.[76] While using marine and estuarine fish, one cannot always be sure of the lack of any previous exposure to pollutants.

Fish weighing 0.5 to 5 g[15] or measuring less than 3 in. in length[9] are used in toxicity tests. All the fish in a particular test should be of the same age and size. Doudoroff et al. recommended that the length of the largest fish should not be more than 1.5 times that of the smallest fish. Uniformity in size and age is recommended because larger fish are more tolerant to pesticides. However, Adelman et al.[77] reported little difference in the LC 50 of pentachlorophenol (PCP) to large and small goldfish.

It is necessary to avoid any type of handling stress while transferring the fish from container to container or during the period of acclimation as well as testing. Handling stress has been reported to induce many biochemical changes.[78,79] Such changes could be easily mistaken for toxic responses resulting from exposure to a pollutant. Even disturbance during counting or removing the dead fish in tests is likely to cause increased mortality and hemorrhaging.[80] In hematological, and occasionally other types of studies, it is customary to anesthetize fish. Caution should be exercised in using certain types of anesthetics, as quinaldine sulfate, tricaine,[81] or MS 222[82] as an anesthetic was reported to reduce the in vitro hydroxylation of benzo(a)pyrene. Hence, it cannot be overemphasized that the fish should be least-disturbed both during acclimation and testing, and the use of anesthetics should be avoided as far as possible.

If the fish are cultured or maintained in the laboratory before employing them in toxicity tests, the rearing density may determine their size and susceptibility to toxicants. Tadpoles reared at a density of 50/ℓ were significantly smaller than those reared at a density of 10/ℓ.[83] When both varieties were exposed to 0.1 mg/ℓ DDT, at the end of 2 days there was more DDT in the former although their lipid content was less.

2. Acclimation and Feeding

a. Acclimation

The fish should be well acclimated to the laboratory conditions and to the water that will be used in the test. Doudoroff et al.[9] recommended an acclimation period of at least 1 week. Sprague[11] concluded that it may be necessary to use longer acclimation periods. However, tests have been conducted after acclimating the fish for as few as 24[75] or 48 hr.[84]

b. Feeding

During the period of acclimation, the fish must be fed with natural uncontaminated diet or pelleted feed. Fish are usually fed at 2 to 3% of their wet weight per day.[85] Diet plays an important role in determining the degree of susceptibility. For example, low dietary protein increased the susceptibility of rainbow trout to chlordane — the 96-h LC 50 value for fish that were given a diet with 23 or 45% protein was 29 and 47 μg/ℓ, respectively.[86] The quality of protein was also an important factor, fish fed with commerical diets with a higher protein content had LC 50 values similar to those fed 23% protein in synthetic diet with casein as the main source of protein. Albino rats fed for 28 days from the date of weaning on diets containing lower-than-normal casein content had a lower LD 50 value. The decrease in LD 50 was directly proportional to the casein content of the diet. Undue increase in protein content of the diet was again detrimental; when the casein content was increased to three times the normal amount, the LD 50 decreased.[87]

In another study, rainbow trout were fed one of four commercial diets or either of two diets with a low (23%) or a high (45%) protein content. The fish that were fed the high protein content were significantly more tolerant to chlordane than those that were fed other types of diet. Similarly, rainbow trout, bluegill, or channel catfish that were fed a diet containing casein or gelatin as protein were more tolerant to PCBs than those fish which had fish meal or soybean meal as the main source of protein. Increasing the content of the amino acid, methionine, from 0.9 to 2.2% resulted in increased susceptibility to DDT, but it also led to a decreased toxicity of dieldrin. Fish that were fed higher methionine content had higher DDT but lower dieldrin residues in the adipose tissue than those fed a lower methionine content. Fish that were fed a vitamin C content of 63 mg/kg in the diet had significantly-reduced growth when exposed to 106, 218, or 475 ng/ℓ toxaphene in comparison with those fish fed a vitamin C content of 670 or 5000 mg/kg diet and exposed to similar concentration of toxaphene.[88] Studies with mammals showed that the quality of the diet influences the microsomal mixed function oxidase (MFO) activity. It is likely that decreased protein content of the diet leads to a decreased MFO activity and hence a decreased ability to metabolize the toxicants.

Several workers have reported the contamination of pelleted feed with organochlorine (OC) pesticide residues and industrial organic chemical residues.[89-92] For instance, dry pelleted feed and Oregon moist pellets were contaminated with heptachlor, heptachlor epoxide, δ-HCH (hexachlorocyclohexane) and methoxychlor derivatives, DDE, and Aroclor® 1254; concentration of methoxychlor was the highest among all the OC compounds, and from 20.5 to 57.7 mg/kg (wet weight). Lake trout raised on this diet concentrated various OC compounds to a considerable extent.[93] The uptake of HCB from feed by rainbow trout, and consequently the body burden, increased in direct relation to the HCB content of the diet.

Since OC residues have become ubiquitous, it is really difficult to obtain feeds completely devoid of contamination. The ASTM Committee[15] recommended that a batch of feed shall not be used when the total concentration of OC pesticide plus PCB residues exceeds 0.3 μg/g (wet weight). Stober and Payne[95] described a method for preparing pesticide-free pelleted feed.

In most of the standard methods for conducting toxicity tests, it is recommended that the fish shall not be fed for 2 days prior to the commencement of the test. To test whether the duration of elapsed time between last feeding and the commencement of toxicity tests has any effect on the tolerance of a fish to a toxicant, Cairns et al.[96] exposed goldfish to a lethal concentration of zinc at 0, 1, 2, 4, 6, 12, 24, and 72 hr after feeding. Time until death was recorded for individual fish. The results indicated no significant difference in the survival time of fish exposed to zinc at different time intervals after feeding. It was concluded that there appears to be no support for the standard requirement that the fish may not be fed for 24 to 48 hr prior to their exposure to a toxicant. This may be so with metals and other nonlipophilic compounds, but the results of studies with pesticide residues are at variance with the above conclusions. Phillips and Buhler[97] noted that fish fed higher rations of diet accumulated higher concentrations of dieldrin. Increased absorption of the toxicant in those fish fed higher rations was supposed to be the result of a larger storage reservoir (lipid) owing to increased food consumption. Hence, the time when feeding is stopped and also the quality of the diet seem to influence the extent of uptake of residues, especially in those

Table 3
OBSERVATIONS OF ABNORMAL FISH BEHAVIOR AND SOME
COMMON CAUSES FOR THIS BEHAVIOR [a]

Observation	Possible causes	Explanation of the problem
Surfacing and swimming with mouth half emerged	1, 2, 3, 4	1. Insufficient oxygen; toxic chemicals; high NH_3
Scraping against sides of tanks[b]	2, 4, 6	2. Parasitism of skin or gills
Erratic swimming	1, 2, 3	3. Rapid temperature changes; parasitism of nervous system; virus disease
Crowding around water inflow	1, 2	4. Parasitism of intestine; bacterial disease
Distended abdomen and difficulty in swimming	4, 5, 6	5. Diet consistency
Refusal to feed actively	1, 3, 4, 5, 6	6. Nutrition deficiency
Listlessness, emaciation	2, 3, 4, 5, 6	

[a]   Several observations may be caused by a combination of two or more problems.
[b]   Normal fathead minnow courtship behavior includes coloration change and display near tank sides.

From Brauhn, J. L. and Schoettger, R. A., in EPA-660/3-75-011, U.S. Environmental Protection Agency, Duluth, Minn. With permission.

tests where the fish is exposed to the residue through food. Undigested food in the gut may act as a source of a lipid pool that favors increased absorption of lipophilic residues. Lennon and Walker[44] reported that after the last feeding an interval of about 36 to 84 hr is needed in different species to empty the gut (36 hr in rainbow trout, 48 hr in goldfish, 60 hr in green sunfish, 72 hr in longear sunfish, and 84 hr in bluegill). They suggested that food be withheld for as long as 96 hr before screening the fish and exposing it to the toxicant.

3. Treatment of Unhealthy Fish

Prevention of disease and treatment of affected fish are very important aspects of toxicity testing. Prophylactic and therapeutic treatments of freshwater fish are listed in the recommendations of the ASTM methods.[15] Fish should be carefully screened to weed out all specimens that appear stressed, mutilated, or abnormal. While most of the recommendations suggested that mortality during holding and acclimation should not exceed 10%, the ASTM Committee recommended that a batch of fish should not be used if more than 3% die during the 48 hr immediately preceding the test. The possible causes for certain types of abnormal fish behavior are listed in Table 3.

4. Loading

The total amount of biomass in the test tanks should be optimal and never so high as to cause conditions of overcrowding and stress or depletion of the desired toxicant concentration. It is recommended that the loading shall not exceed 0.8 g/ℓ at 17°C or below and 0.5 g/ℓ at higher temperatures, in static tests. For flow-through tests, the total biomass shall not exceed 1 g/ℓ of test medium passing through the tank in 24 hr or 10 g/ℓ at any time, at 17°C or below. At higher temperatures, the recommended loading is 0.5 g/ℓ/day, or 5 g/ℓ at any time. Occasionally, higher loadings have been reported in the literature,[98-100] with the system being sometimes aerated.[49,50] In the former condition, the physiological and biochemical changes induced by stress due to hypoxia and overloading cannot be distinguished from toxicant-induced changes; in the latter, the dissolved oxygen concentration may be maintained satisfactorily, but as stated previously, aeration leads to a rapid loss of the toxicant. While testing the toxicity of a compound to larger fish, or employing a larger sample, the problem of inadequate oxygen concentration can be circumvented by using larger tanks and continuous flow systems with a faster replacement time, as was employed by Iwama and Greer.[101] Employing 25 times the recommended loading and a continuous flow system with a 90% water replacement time of 1.5 hr (Section II.C.6), they obtained 96-h LC 50 values of sodium pentachlorophenate to chinook salmon that compared favorably with earlier reports where normal loading was employed.

5. Optimal Size of the Test Sample and Randomization
a. Size of the Test Sample

Doudoroff et al. and the APHA Standard Methods recommended a minimum of 10 animals in each concentration. The ASTM Subcommittee recommended that at least 10 organisms in static tests and at least 20 organisms in flow-through tests should be exposed to each concentration. Jensen[102] investigated the relationship between the relative error and sample size, both empirically and theoretically. On the basis of tests conducted with instant increase in temperature as the lethal agent, he concluded that an increase of the sample size significantly reduces the standard error of the LC 50 until the sample size reaches 30. Increasing the sample size from 10 to 20 decreases the standard error of the LC 50 by 29%; a further increase from 20 to 30 decreases the standard error by 13%. Keeping in mind the additional costs involved in testing a larger sample and the precision achieved, Jensen concluded that for practical purposes, a sample of 20 fish at each test level or concentration would be optimal.

b. Randomization of Test Fish

Randomization of test tanks, as well as random distribution of test fish among different test tanks is highly desirable. Although the APHA Standard methods recommended the distribution of fish among all test tanks as if dealing a pack of cards among players, Sprague,[11] quoting personal communication from Dr. C. E. Stephan of the National Water Quality Laboratory, at Duluth, Minn., recommended that fish may be distributed randomly to the different test tanks, using random numbers from standard tables.

6. Replacement Time

Sprague[11] aptly pointed out that in continuous flow tests, replacement time is not equal to the time taken to empty a full tank, but it is the time required to displace every molecule in the test chamber. He developed a graph to calculate the time required for 50 to 90% replacement of the water in a test tank, which is reproduced in Figure 1. Sprague recommended a 90% replacement time of 8 to 12 hr. Shorter replacement times (i.e., faster flow rate) may be called for while testing highly volatile substances or larger fish.

7. Duration of the Test

Prior to the adoption of uniform procedures, short-term or acute toxicity tests were conducted over a period of 24 to 96 hr. As recently as 1980, 72-h LC 50 value was reported.[103] Alabaster[40] reported the 48-h LC 50 values of 164 compounds to the harlequin fish. The choice of 96-hr test duration is quite arbitrary but seems to have served well. From time to time there have been doubts whether a 96-hr duration is adequate for conducting toxicity tests. Following exposure of rainbow trout to methyl parathion for 96 hr and transfer of the fish to clean water, significant additional mortality was recorded during a further 30-day period of observation.[104] A change in the relative

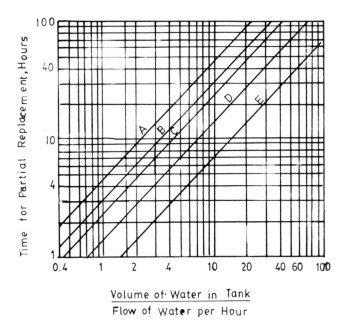

FIGURE 1. Approximate times required for partial replacement of
water in tanks for constant flow situations. A — 99% replacement; B
— 95% replacement; C — 90% replacement; D — 75% replacement;
E — 50% replacement. Example: for a tank containing 30 ℓ, with a
flow of 10 ℓ/hr, there would be 50% replacement of water in the tank
in about 2 hr, 75% in about 4 hr, 90% in 7 hr, and 95% replacement
in 9 hr. Another time-period could replace hours, but the same time
must be used for volume and flow. (Based on information supplied
by Alfred Heusner, after Sprague, J. B., *Water Res.,* 3, 793, 1969.
With permission. Copyright 1969, Pergamon Press.)

sensitivity of flagfish and trout to picloram was noted depending on the length of
exposure. In the first 96 hr of the test, trout was more sensitive than the flagfish, but
when the exposure was prolonged to the 10th day, the reverse was true.[105] Similar
observations led to the questioning of the choice of 96-hr as the test duration. Kaila
and Saarikoski[106] reported 8-day LC 50 values of PCP and 2,3,6-trichlorophenol.
Phipps et al.[107] not only calculated the 96-h LC 50 of a number of phenolic compounds
to the fathead minnows, but continued the tests for four more days to determine
whether there is any increase in the toxicity after the traditionally determined 96-h LC
50. The threshold indexes calculated (TI = $\frac{\text{192-h LC 50}}{\text{96-h LC 50}}$) showed that the 192-h LC
50 of PCP was the same as 96-h LC 50, but in the case of a few other compounds (2-
chlorophenol and 2,4,6-trichlorophenol) the TI indicated continued increase of toxicity
beyond 96-hr. The OECD Guidelines[16] recommended a prolonged toxicity test of at
least 14 days to determine the LC 50 at several intervals in order to establish a threshold
concentration. Termed lethal threshold concentration, LTC is the concentration lethal
to 50% of the individuals exposed for periods sufficiently long for the acute lethal
action to cease (see Sprague[11]). Alexander et al.[108] examined whether LTC can provide
more useful information than the 96-hr acute toxicity test that would justify the extra
expenditure entailed by the prolongation of the test. Using the data for 10 years, they
tested for significant correlation between LC 50 and LTC of toxicants, for which both
values had been reported. The fitted regression (Figure 2) line showed a strong correlation (r = 0.99) between observed and predicted LTC values and a simple linear regression equation LTC = 0.774 × LC 50 described the relationship between the two. The

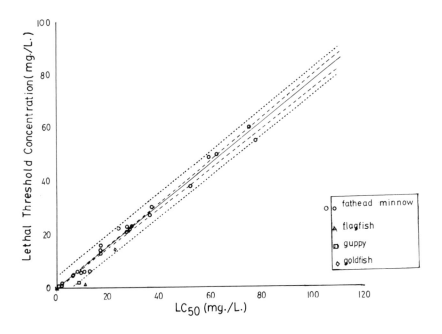

FIGURE 2.   Observed and predicted lethal threshold concentration (LTC), confidence and prediction limits for the regression of LTC on LC 50. The regression line is indicated by the solid line (—), the 95% confidence limits by the broken line (---), and the 95% prediction limits by the dotted line (...). (Reprinted with permission from Alexander, H. C., et al., *Chemosphere*, 12, 415, 1983. Copyright 1983, Pergamon Press.)

authors concluded that prolonged toxicity study of at least 14 days, as recommended by the OECD Guidelines,[16] does not provide more useful and meaningful information than the traditionally conducted 96-hr toxicity test.

8. Static and Flow-Through Tests

Acute toxicity tests are conducted in one of four ways.[14,15]

1.   In the static technique, the test medium, after its preparation and introduction of the fish, is left undistrubed for the duration of the test.
2.   In the recirculation technique, rarely used, the test medium is prepared at the beginning of the test and the medium is recirculated through an apparatus wherein it is aerated, filtered, and sterilized before being returned to the test tank.
3.   In the static renewal technique, the medium is renewed periodically, usually once in 24 hr.
4.   In the continuous flow systems, fresh test solution passes through the test chamber continuously.

a. Static Tests

Whether or not static systems or continuous flow systems should be employed has been widely discussed. Static tests are useful for short-term exposures and serve as first checks to evaluate the acute toxicity of a chemical to a number of organisms.[109]

Static tests have sometimes been criticized because of decline in toxicant concentration due to its absorption by the test organisms, adsorption to the container walls or surfaces and chemical alteration of the toxicant. One of the objections to the static tests is that the LC 50 estimated by this method is always higher than the one obtained with continuous flow systems. For instance, there was a difference in the LC 50 of malathion when the water was not changed during the 96-hr experimental period, or when it was changed on alternate days or once a day.[110] In another study, fish were exposed to a number of pesticides under static conditions and the effect of increasing temperature was studied. With the exception of methoxyclor, toxicity increased with temperature. This effect was pronounced in the first 24 hr and was negligible in the next 72 hr. The decrease in the effect of temperature may not be real, but may be due to the decrease in the concentration of the pesticide itself with time.[111] Decrease in the toxicity of tetraethyl diphosphate (TEPP), parathion, malathion, systox, O-ethyl-O-(p-nitrophenyl) phenyl phosphorothioate (EPN), between 24 and 96 hr under static conditions was the result of rapid hydrolysis and degradation of the test compound.[112] The LC 50 of Guthion® to goldfish was 14 times that to fathead minnows under static conditions, but in continuous flow system the 11-day LC 50 to both species was almost identical.[112] The effect of phosphate ester mixtures on the behavior of aquatic organisms was more pronounced under flow-through conditions than in static tests.[113] The 96-h LC 50 value of chlordecone to 30-day-old fathead minnows was 420 $\mu g/\ell$ under static conditions and 340 $\mu g/\ell$ under flow-through conditions, indicating the reduction in the concentration of the toxicant in the former.[114] Lincer et al.[115] reported lower 96-h LC 50 of endrin to fathead minnows in flow-through tests. Field grade TFM was more toxic to *Gammarus* and crayfish in flow-through conditions than in the static tests.[30] Further, Applegate et al.[116] found that the toxic effects of mononitrophenols were considerably less under conditions that simulated treatment of a stream than under static conditions. While noting that the toxicity of field grade TFM to several species of fish was similar under static and flow-through conditions, it was recommended that flow-through conditions should be employed to evaluate the chronic toxicity.[117] Reduced toxicity under static conditions was also reported in the case of PCP,[118] four volatile organic solvents,[119] endosulfan,[120] and PCBs.[63] Holden[121] exposed brook trout to ^{14}C-DDT in duplicate tanks (510 to 530 g of biomass in 10 ℓ of water) and reported that 80 to 90% of the added DDT was lost within 10 hr. Synthetic pyrethroids and natural pyrethrum were about 2 to 5 times more toxic under flow-through conditions than in static tests owing to the deactivation of the toxicant under static conditions.[122] When mirex-incorporated sediment was flooded and fish were introduced, the toxicant concentration in water was more under static conditions, but the fish bioconcentrated the compound three times more under flow-through conditions.[123]

Static tests are also criticized because it is difficult to maintain an adequate level of dissolved oxygen concentration under static conditions. The oxygen demand created by dead fish can be high and detrimental to the other fish in the test tank in static systems. For instance, a combination of two live and three dead fish at 25°C reduced the oxygen levels overnight, from near-saturation levels to less than 1 mg/ℓ.[124] Moreover, metabolites like ammonia, if allowed to accumulate in the test tanks, would prove to be toxic by themselves. Low dissolved oxygen also increases the toxicity of ammonia;[125] both these conditions are met with in the static systems. Further, the toxicant itself may remove oxygen from the system, as was noticed in tests with coal synfuel blends.[126]

Normally, bioconcentration increases with time until equilibrium concentrations are achieved, whereafter steady state is maintained as long as the organism is exposed to the toxicant. The residue load starts to decline only with the transfer of the organisms to clean water. In an experiment on the bioconcentration of phosphoric acid esters by goldfish and killifish under static conditions, it was found that even as the test fish was supposed to be exposed to the toxicant, the bioconcentration factor began decline, indicating the rapid disappearance of the toxicant from the 20th hr onward, thus simulating conditions of depuration in clean water.[127] In a similar study, white crappies

Table 4

CONCENTRATION OF
METHOXYCHLOR IN 30 ℓ OF WATER
DURING THE EXPOSURE OF FIVE
YELLOW PERCH (APPROXIMATELY
50 G TOTAL WEIGHT) FOR 96 HR

Time (hr)	Conc	Methoxychlor ($\mu g/\ell$)		
0	Nominal conc	40	30	20
4	Measured conc	35.4	21.4	15.5
24	Measured conc	15.4	12.3	8.3
48	Measured conc	5.1	2.1	2.2
96	Measured conc	2.0	1.3	1.0

From Merna, J. W., Bender, M. E., and Novy, J. R., *Trans. Am. Fish. Soc.,* 101, 298, 1972. With permission.

were exposed to 10 $\mu g/\ell$ diflubenzuron which was concentrated 822, 533, and 613 times the ambient water concentration; after 24, 48, and 72 hr exposure, respectively, under static conditions, there were indications that there was onset of conditions of depuration even before the end of 48 hr, although the fish were supposed to be continuously exposed to the toxicant even thereafter. When the water was changed daily, with slightly larger fish than in the previous experiment but with the same concentration of diflubenzuron, the bioconcentration factors were 158, 306, and 268 after 24, 48, and 72 hr, respectively.[128] The concentration of methoxychlor decreased with time under static conditions; at the end of 24 hr about 40% remained; at the end of 96 hr only 5 to 6% remained[129] (Table 4). In a static system, about 92% of the radioactive chlordane added to water (25.94 $\mu g/\ell$ as ^{14}C-cis-chlordane in 18 ℓ) was lost during the initial 6 hr.[130]

It is felt that static systems are still useful if the test material enters the environment only once or periodically as slugs.[39] If on the other hand, the material is being continuously discharged, flow-through systems may be more appropriate. If the test material is degradable, volatile, high in oxygen demand, or rapidly detoxifying, static systems are unsuitable.

Notwithstanding the fact that the results of static tests may be different from those of the flow-through tests, the former serve a useful purpose. Ferguson et al.[131] emphasized that the results with static systems are reproducible when the conditions are specified. Since pesticide concentration usually increases rapidly as the toxicant enters the aquatic ecosystem and then quickly declines as the toxicant moves downstream, they felt that static toxicity tests may be more realistic than the continuous flow systems in simulating natural conditions. Sprague[132] considered that continuous flow test is not greatly superior to a well done static test but has some advantages. Mount[133] emphasized that exposure under constant concentrations as practised in standard toxicity test procedures is very unnatural. He considered that such tests consistently over- or underestimate the toxicity. The tendency is to overestimate the likely toxicity of a compound.

The USEPA and other groups favor continuous flow systems in which the test solution is constantly renewed to maintain a constant concentration of the toxicant. Cairns and Gruber[134] pointed out that in nature, constancy is an exception rather than the rule. A 1-year series of tests conducted on an industrial effluent by the Aquatic Ecology Group of Virginia Polytechnic Institute disclosed variations of a thousandfold in the toxicity of one waste line. Further, constant test conditions may not always yield meaningful data. For instance, if a chemical reaches the aquatic environment as intermittent pulses or gradations resulting from a single dose as in accidental spills, classical testing procedure with a constant concentration may not provide meaningful data.[135] In such a case, a static test may be more appropriate.

b. *Flow-Through Tests and Toxicant Delivery Systems*

A constant concentration of the toxicant can be maintained by employing flow-through conditions. Sometimes variation in the concentrations of the toxicant is observed even under flow-through conditions, and is attributable to the variation induced by the dosing system.[136]

A serial diluter, consisting of water delivery and toxicant feed systems, and based on an apparatus devised by Warner in 1962, was described by Mount and Warner.[137] In this model, the toxicant feed system is coupled with the main water delivery system; if for any reason, the latter slows down or fails, the toxicant injection also slows down or is stopped, thereby preventing the exposure of the test organisms to unusually high concentration of the toxicant that may be detrimental. Also, the serial dilution system can deliver a series of concentrations with a dilution factor equal to or greater than 50% between each concentration. Mount and Brungs[138] further modified and improved the system of Mount and Warner.[137] The resulting device, called the proportional diluter, is based on simultaneous dilution of one concentration so that it can deliver up to five or more dilutions, each as much as 90% of the preceding concentration, with a maximum flow rate of 400 mℓ/min. Brungs and Mount[139] further modified their 1967 proportional diluter to suit small fish-holding tanks. This device is free from clogging caused by suspended solids and living organisms and can deliver 500 mℓ to each of six holding tanks as often as every 2 min. Brungs and Mount[140] described a device, which is a modification of the water-metering cell of Mount and Warner,[137] to deliver a calibrated volume to introduce a known amount of chemical into the holding chamber to treat diseases or parasites of fish that require continuous treatment. McAllister et al.,[141] while essentially retaining the water delivery and the serial diluter components of Mount and Brungs, improved upon the toxicant metering device. This device is devoid of moving parts and hence free of evaporation losses of the toxicant, especially if the latter is a volatile substance. Abram[142] described a pneumatically operated apparatus that circumvents the problem of electrical control in the wet environment of a fish laboratory. While other devices permit no variation in test conditions, this device incorporated arrangement for providing a controlled variation for dosing different poisons alternately, or for delivering a variable mixture. Granmo and Kollberg[143] described a simple water flow system that can deliver a toxicant volume ranging from milliliters to liters accurately and is easy to handle. Benoit and Puglisi[144] described a simplified apparatus which can be used with the proportional diluter of Mount and Brungs and can deliver water in four ways. Subsequently, Chandler et al.[145] described a simple low cost accurate metering device that is free of moving parts. Delivery of small or large volumes is made possible by a simple variation of the volume of the device. DeFoe[146] described a mechanical multichannel toxicant injection system that can be coupled with the proportional diluter of Mount and Brungs. This device dispenses equal amounts of toxicant dispersants like carrier solvents, wetting agents, etc., to all toxicant concentrations and to a control. This system permits the changing of one toxicant concentration independent of others, and also permits the calculation of the amount of toxicant injected and the volume of water used, on which basis the toxicant concentration can be calculated. This system is mechanically operated and in the event of failure of the water flow, the operation of the injector also ceases. Solon et al.[147] described a continuous flow automatic device for conducting short-term toxicity tests. This device is inexpensive, very simple in design, and requires little maintenance.

Although the proportional diluter of Mount and Brungs is the most often-used dosing apparatus for conducting flow-through toxicity tests, one disadvantage of this device is that it cannot give a dilution greater than 50%. DeFoe[146] overcame this problem through a mechanical multichannel injector, which gave a dilution of more than 50%. Smith et al.[148] considered that a pneumatic dosing apparatus with a multichannel injection system developed by them has advantage over the mechanical method of toxicant injection like that of DeFoe because return springs, counter-balances, and other mechanical devices were completely eliminated. Only one initial toxicant concentration is required and there is no need to make use of several stock solutions. Further, in the pneumatic type of dosing apparatus, the syringe-reloading is fully automatic. Burke and Ferguson[149] described a flow-through apparatus for maintaining constant concentration of toxicant in aquatic toxicity tests. This system is devoid of any electrically operated parts and there are no moving parts, either, hence the danger of over- or under-flow is eliminated. Moreover, this device is also inexpensive. Boling[150] described a computer-controlled toxicant injection system which can inject up to 85 mℓ/min into the system. This device consists of a digitally controlled injector, that can be interfaced with any digital computer.

Benoit et al.[151] described a continuous flow minidiluter system for conducting toxicity tests with early life stages of small organisms, and can be used in the laboratory as well as in the field. This system operates by gravity and permits the testing of the toxicity of hazardous, volatile chemicals. Novac et al.[152] devised a continuous flow device that can be used for testing the toxicity of chemicals to small animals, and can be scaled up to test larger animals. This device operates on the principle of continuously emptying the test container as opposed to filling it up, by using a peristaltic pump. Another advantage of this system is the avoidance of contact with anything but inert and nontoxic materials; screens, walls, flexible tubing, syringe pumps, etc. are made of glass, Teflon®, or polyethylene; heat welding and sleeving replace gluing at every connection. Smith and Hargreaves[153] also described a small continuous flow system for exposing small organisms. Brenniman et al.[154] pointed out that none of the various types of continuous flow devices described until then can handle highly volatile toxicants, especially those that are poorly water-soluble. Hence they designed a continuous flow device that can overcome these problems.

D. Toxicant Concentration

The concentration that one wishes to maintain in the test tanks and the actual concentration maintained are different. The terms "nominal" and "actual concentrations" are used to denote these two concentrations. The difference between these two concentrations amounts to about 30 to 45%.[155] Continuous flow systems are supposed to maintain a constant concentration. In the static systems, the toxicant concentration falls with time. It is also known that toxicity changes with aging. Marking and Olson[156] proposed the "Deactivation Index" (which is the ratio of the LC 50 values of the aged and unaged solutions under corresponding test conditions) as a measure of the reduction in the toxicity of an aged toxicant. If the index is approximately 1, the aged solution is as toxic as the fresh solution; if it is greater than 1, the aged solution is considerably deactivated; if it is less than 1, the solution had increased in activity.[157] Jarvinen and Tanner[158] observed that with aging the toxicity of the solutions of technical grade methyl parathion, diazinon, and a formulation — Penncap-M® — increased. The toxicity of technical grade Dursban® and Knox out® 2FM remained constant with time, whereas that of Dursban® 10 CR decreased with time. The increase of toxicity in the first three cases was due to the accumulation of the degradation products that are more toxic than the parent compounds. Only traces of methyl paraoxon were present in the case of technical grade and formulated methyl parathion, the increased toxicity being attributable to the accumulation of *p*-nitrophenol. The oxygen analog of diazinon, viz., diazoxan, which is more toxic than diazinon, accounted for the greater toxicity of the aged solution of diazinon. The encapsulated formulation of methyl parathion was 45 to 60% less toxic than technical grade under static conditions, whereas it was only 22% less toxic under flow-through conditions, because of the lower build-up of more toxic degradation products in the latter. The increased toxicity of aged solution of mexacarbate, owing to the increased toxicity of the initial hydrolysis product, was reported.[157] Upon standing for four more weeks, the toxicity of the latter lessened as a result of further degradation.

Many synthetic pyrethroids and natural pyrethrum extracts were deactivated with age; however, allethrin and S-Bioallethrin® were not deactivated, whereas the toxicity of trans-allethrin appeared to increase with age.[122] On the other hand, in the case of solutions of TFM, no appreciable reduction in their toxicity was noticed even after 1 week.[156]

Normally the concentration in the test tank is determined by extracting grab samples of the test medium with a suitable solvent and subsequent quantification. Sometimes, it may be difficult to quantify the amount of the compound present, as in the case of toxaphene; then the concentration delivered to each test tank is determined by the calibration of the effective dilution of the diluter system by using a dye.[159] Galassi and Vighi[160] proposed to calculate the concentration of five chlorobenzenes in algal culture media on the basis of their physical characteristics. Zitko et al.[161] proposed a formula for calculating the average concentration of a toxicant in the static tests, i.e.,

$$\bar{c} = \frac{ac_N}{t} \int_0^t e^{-bt} \, dt = -c_N \frac{a}{b\,t} (e^{-bt} - 1)$$

where $\bar{c}$, c_N = average and nominal concentration, respectively, a, b = empirical coefficients, t = exposure time of LT 50, h.

In accepting the results of static tests, it is believed that the amount of toxicant absorbed or metabolized by the test organism is insignificant compared with the total amount available, and secondly, the toxicant is evenly distributed in the medium from the start to the finish of the test. One of these assumptions, and often both, would be invalid in a majority of tests and therein lies the shortcoming of the static tests. To overcome this difficulty, Gillespie et al.[162] developed a model in which the amount of the toxicant is monitored during the test period and the data are fitted to a model to obtain constants for the system. This model, according to the authors, permits the estimation of the actual concentration to which the test organism is exposed.

Volatilization also contributes to significant losses of the compound from the test tanks. Even for relatively nonvolatile compounds, volatilization has been shown to be a major pathway of loss.[163] Only flow-through tests should be attempted in such instances. The decisive factors that determine the amount that remains in test tanks are the true water-solubility and the amount present in the test tanks. With those compounds with very low water-solubility, the loss of compounds owing to evaporation is very high, especially when aerated, while no such effect was observed when the aqueous solubility was high. It was also shown that very poorly water-soluble compounds have high activity coefficients in aqueous solutions. The resultant high equilibrium vapor partial pressures lead to high evaporation rates.[164] Mackay and Wolkoff[165] showed that the half-life of poorly soluble chlorinated hydrocarbons can be as low as a few minutes to a few hours and hence transfer from the aqueous phase to the atmosphere can be very rapid and substantial. The calculated half-lives of DDT, Aroclor® 1242, and Aroclor® 1260 were 3 to 7 days, 5 to 9 hr, and 0.5 hr. Hence low-solubility compounds like DDT and HCB, when present near their saturation limits in water, evaporate very quickly. These studies also underscore the futility of attempts to conduct toxicity tests with hydrophobic compounds, with the amounts in test tanks at or above the saturation limits. To circumvent this problem, Ernst[166] conducted preliminary tests with 12 compounds in sea water to determine the amounts that remained in water after specified periods of time and subsequently conducted tests with those concentrations.

In tests with HCB and PCB, employing algae, Södergren[167] found that large quantities of these compounds accumulated in the surface films. The compounds were transferred to the surface film even when the movement of the organisms to the top layer was prevented. Adsorbtion to container walls, sediments, and surface layers also contributed significantly to reduction of the toxicant concentration. When ^{14}C-di-2-ethylhexyl phthalate was added to water under static conditions, less than 0.02% of the total quantity initially introduced remained in water after 27 days, whereas 62% of the added compound was recovered from the various surfaces. Such an accumulation at interfaces seems to be a special problem with compounds of low water-solubility and high lipid partition coefficient.[168] Sharom and Solomon[169] reported that considerable amounts of permethrin were adsorbed to the container walls. PCBs have been reported to adsorb strongly to glass and plastic surfaces during experimentation.[170] Not only the container walls and such other surfaces adsorb the residues, but even dead fish remove the toxicant from the medium.[171] Murphy and Murphy[172] considered that the amount of DDT absorbed by dead fish in their experiments was negligible.

III. REPORTING THE RESULTS

A. Terminology

The median lethal concentration or the LC 50 value is the most-often-used measure of short-term toxicity. This is the concentration that kills 50% of the test population in a given time and was variously termed TLM, LD 50,[173] etc. Since only the concentration in the test tanks, and not the amount absorbed by the aquatic organism, is known, the concentration of the toxicant in water that kills 50% of the test animals in a given period of time is taken as a measure of its toxicity. In this context, it is necessary to draw the attention of the aquatic toxicologists to the wrong practice of writing LC 50 with a subscript, i.e., as LC_{50}. Sprague[11] correctly pointed out that Trevan, who first used the expression LD 50, wrote all symbols on the same line and not as LD_{50}. Subsequently, all major writers in pharmacology followed Trevan. Since LC 50 is a modified notation of LD 50, it is wrong to write LC 50 or any other LC (say 10 or 90, etc.,) with a subscript.

Sometimes the term "threshold LC 50" is used. This is the LC 50 that is attained when there is no mortality during a 48-hr period in any of the test tanks.[105] If the threshold LC 50 is not reached within 10 days, the test is terminated and it is concluded that no definite acute threshold LC 50 exists for that chemical. According to Fogels and Sprague[105] threshold LC 50 values should be preferred as end points as they represent time-independent measures of tolerance. Sprague[11] explained that terms like "incipient threshold concentration" denote the concentration at which toxic action ceases. He suggested that the term "incipient lethal level" has an advantage over other terms as it is part of a general scheme of classifying environmental factors and is defined as "That level of the environmental entity beyond which 50% of the population cannot live for an indefinite time." Cairns et al.[174] also used the term "threshold concentration" and defined it as the maximum concentration at which 100% of the population will survive for the duration of the experiment, which in most cases is several days. Incipient LC 50 is also defined as the concentration at which 50% of the population will survive indefinitely. TILC 50 or the time-independent concentration is also defined as the concentration at which 50% of the population will survive indefinitely.[122] Lloyd and Tooby[175] opined that in static tests, the initial concentration is not maintained for more than a few hours and hence it is wrong to use the term LC 50. They proposed a new term LC(I) 50 for static tests (I is the initial concentration), in which the concentration of the medium during the entire test period does not remain within 10% of the starting concentration.

B. Calculation of LC 50

Stephan[6] reviewed the various methods of calculation of the LC 50; he not only discussed the merits of the various methods of calculation in vogue, but tried to clear several misconceptions regarding the significance of LC 50 values. He examined the various premises on which toxicity tests are conducted and pointed out many wrong assumptions, as well as the contradiction between the greater number and closeness of the partial kills and the smaller spread of the confidence limits. Parametric methods of calculation of LC 50 do not permit the estimation of confidence limits in the event of one or no partial kills, whereas such a calculation is possible with nonparametric methods. He stressed that the importance of the slope of the regression curve is greatly exaggerated by the aquatic toxicologists because of the prevailing confusion and failure to distinguish between toxicity tests and bioassays. Since the latter are tests that depend on the principle of parallelism, the slope of the regression curve is very important for comparing the known response with the unknown response; there need be no such emphasis on the slope of the regression curve in the case of the toxicity tests.

After carefully examining the arguments in favor of two or more partial kills for calculating the LC 50, Stephan[6] stated that test results with less than two partial kills need not be discarded. The test concentrations need not be close to one another and a dilution factor of 0.6 would be enough between successive test concentrations. He also pointed out that graphical interpolation methods, as those recommended in the APHA Standard methods, cannot be used to calculate the confidence limits. The method of Litchfield and Wilcoxon,[176] an approximate probit method, is somewhat subjective and is partly graphical. If the criterion is to use all the toxicity tests, including those in which there were no kills, the moving average method is suitable with more sets of data than any other method. With no partial kills, this method provides only an estimate of the LC 50 and not its confidence limits. Further, in the absence of partial kills, it is useful in calculating only the LC 50 and not any other LC (say LC 10 or LC 20). The 95% confidence limits, which are in the same units as the LC 50, are often used and preferred to fiducial limits, although fiducial and confidence limits are numerically the same. The confidence limits calculated from one test do not give any indication of the reproducibility of the test or its precision. This is an important point which aquatic toxicologists should keep in mind. Other methods like the Spearman-Karber and logit methods have also been used to calculate LC 50 values. Hamilton et al.[177] developed a trimmed Spearman-Karber method for calculating the LC 50.

C. Control Mortality and Variable Test Results

Mortality of control fish during experimentation is a problem every aquatic toxicologist faces at one time or other. Abbott's formula, quoted by Finney,[178] is often used for correcting the control mortality. Stephan pointed out the futility of correcting the experimental data for control mortality. While suggesting that a species should not be tested until suitable techniques for maintaining it in the laboratory with minimal mortality are developed, Stephan stressed "Abbott's formula cannot make valid the results of test conducted with unhealthy or stressed organisms . . . correction of the LC 50 for this mortality would seem to be a meaningless exercise."

It is also quite common to observe higher mortality in lower concentration and vice versa. Lee et al.,[179] while testing the toxicity of mirex, noted 26.9 and 32.1% mortality at the end of 96 hr in 0.1 and 1 mg/ℓ concentration of mirex, but in the case of 0.01 and 10 mg/ℓ concentrations, the mortality was, respectively, 6.4 and 9%. Van Valin et al.[180] also noted that no relationship existed between the concentration of mirex and the mortality of bluegills. Henderson et al.[181] noted that in replicate tests with HCH, the results were highly variable, which according to them might have been due to the quantities of HCH, present far in excess of its water-solubility. Sprague and Fogels[136] also reported that during a period of 2 years, when 81 batches of effluents were tested, there was a wide variation in the results. There was greater mortality in the controls and in the lower concentrations than in the higher concentrations. In one batch, the control mortality was 45%; mortality with 12.5, 25, and 100% concentrated effluent was 25, 0, and 80%, respectively. In yet another study, they found that at a concentration of the effluent of 0, 12.5, 25, 50, and 100%, the mortality was 40, 20, 30, 10, and 0%, respectively.

Macek and Sanders[182] reported inherent biological variation in the susceptibility of different stocks belonging to the same species. The variability may be due to genetic factors or difference in the physiological conditions of the fish. Among five species of fish, viz., rainbow trout, fathead minnow, bluegill, largemouth bass and channel catfish, variation in their susceptibility to DDT was highest in fathead minnows. In general, the variation in fish species was more than that in invertebrates. Test-to-test variation in tests with DDT and fathead minnows was reported.[183] Similarly, in successive tests, among different batches of fish from the same stock, the 48-h LC 50 of zinc, ammonia, and phenol to rainbow trout varied by a factor of 2.5. The causes for this variation could not be identified.[184] Variation in the toxicity observed under apparently similar test conditions may be attributable to seasonal changes, circadian rhythms, or the differences in age, size, nutritional status, animal strain, and so on. Another possible source of such a variation is the reproductive state of the test fish.[185]

Singh and Narain[186] reported seasonal variations in the toxicity of endosulfan to the freshwater catfish *Heteropneustes fossilis*. For smaller fish (10 ± 0.7 cm in length), the LC 50 was 7.4 to 7.8 μg/ℓ in June to September and 12 to 13 μg/ℓ in the December to January period. Comparable values for larger fish (19.9 ± 0.4 cm) were 14 to 15 μg/ℓ during June to August, and 23 μg/ℓ in December to January. The toxicity of H_2S to goldfish was found to vary and was suggested to be a seasonal effect.[187]

How to deal with such anomalous and stray values is a vexatious question. Stephan[6] addressed himself to this question from yet another angle. Many authors perform tests in duplicate or triplicate to test the reproducibility of the results and pool the data from the replicates. Stephan questioned the very purpose of replicate tests if the data were to be pooled and suggested that only when the results are identical may replicate data be pooled. When the data differ, it is better to calculate the LC 50 values and their confidence limits separately and report them as such.

Sprague[11-14] suggested that two different LC 50 values could be compared for significant difference by using the LC 50 values and their fiducial limits. Sprague and Fogels[136] further elaborated on this point and suggested that the LC 50 values obtained over a period of time should be compared for significant difference; if they are not different, the weekly ups and downs may be forgotten; if, on the other hand, they are significantly different, the cause for this variation should be sought and attended to.

IV. STANDARD TEST FISH AND REFERENCE TOXICANTS

A. Standard Test Fish

To compare the test results of one laboratory with those of another and also the results obtained at different times in the same laboratory, it was suggested that a standard reference test fish and reference toxicant may be useful. For the selection of a standard fish, Adelman and Smith[118] listed the following criteria: (1) must have a constant response to a broad range of toxicants, tested under similar conditions, (2) be available in large quantities, (3) be easy to handle, (4) be easy to transport, (5) must be available all through the year and the desired age must be readily available, and (6) such a species should complete its life cycle within 1 year or less. The flagfish is recommended as a useful laboratory species for conducting chronic toxicity studies. The advantages with this species are (1) it breeds when it is 6 to 8 weeks old, (2) it spawns all through the year, (3) the sexes can easily be distinguished, and (4) the chronic test can be completed in as little as 3 to 4 months.[188]

Earlier, statistical treatment was employed to compare the relative tolerance of several species of fish to the same compound and to class them as more or less tolerant species.[105] According to Fogels and Sprague,[105] such statistical comparisons are of little practical value as they do not take into account the known variability of the response of some species to a compound at different times. In their laboratory, the response of rainbow trout to copper at different times, under identical conditions, varied fivefold. Davis and Hoos[189] found a twofold variation in the responses of rainbow trout to sodium pentachlorophenate in a carefully controlled interlaboratory attempt at standardization. Fogels and Sprague[105] concluded "The results of short-term bioassays should therefore be regarded as only estimates, within approximately one order of magnitude of the acute toxicity of a substance." Because the values were within one order of magnitude of each other and comparable for rainbow trout, zebrafish, and flagfish, they suggested that the latter two may be acceptable as standard species, especially because of the ease with which they can be maintained and bred in the laboratory.

Comparison of the toxicity curves was suggested as a better means of comparing the toxicity of compound to two species or the relative tolerance of a number of species.[105] Cairns[190] expressed the same opinion and stated that the difference in the response between one species and another is often substantially less than is thought. He opined that the data generated on the toxicity of one compound or a group of compounds in one country can be used as a starting point to assess the priorities of testing and toxicity evaluation in another country. He suggested that the use of an "aquatic white rat" is highly advisable, as it permits the comparison and standardization of toxicity test methods in a new place, new laboratory, or by new personnel, against a well-established standard. In another study to compare the variability of the response of a species of fish to a broad range of toxicants, acute toxicity tests with two species of fish were conducted over a 2-year period.[118] Tests with sodium chloride were the least variable at all times and hence this compound meets the criterion of minimum variability; PCP ranked second in variability. The ability of such tests in detecting abnormal fish by their deviant response is rather limited. On the basis of the tests conducted, neither goldfish nor fathead minnow was found superior and the variability was dependent on the toxicant, rather than the species. Although both species can be handled with ease in the laboratory and can be transported easily, fathead minnows may be considered as the better experimental fish, as the goldfish cannot be bred easily.[118]

In choosing a test fish, Sprague[12] suggested that one of three approaches is possible. The first is to test the most important sensitive species, the second is to test the most important local fish, and the third is to use a standard species. The standard species can be a fish like the harlequin fish or the guppy, which can easily reproduce in the laboratory; or it can be a widespread species like the rainbow trout, representing the cooler waters; or *Phoxinus laevis,* which represents the warmer European waters. The unsuitability of rainbow trout was explained by Sprague and Fogels.[136] Inexplicable mass die-offs in the holding tanks, the touchy and temperamental nature of the fish, and aggression among the fingerlings were major problems with rainbow trout. Even though mortality was low in holding tanks, as soon as the trout were placed in doughnut-shaped growth tanks with a current, they set up territories and fought vehemently with one another and started killing one another. Besides, there was the problem of very peculiar and inexplicable results, with higher mortality in the lower concentrations and vice versa. Another problem was that as trout grew, it was difficult to obtain small fish at certain times of the year, and larger trout could not be used because of the problem of maintaining the proper loading relative to the volume of the water used. Lastly, rainbow trout would not reproduce under laboratory conditions. As the chronic toxicity tests should be conducted through one reproductive cycle, it is difficult to conduct long-term toxicity tests with rainbow trout. Hence, Sprague and Fogels opined that rainbow trout is the least suitable of all the species, even though it is a widely distributed cool water fish. They considered *Jordanella floridae* as a suitable standard test fish.

Newsome[191] examined the suitability of several species of fish for use in a multi-generation toxicity test. He rejected the harlequin fish *Rasbora heteromorpha* because of its exacting water quality requirements, the American flagfish *Jordanella floridae* because of the failure of adult flagfish to spawn successfully, the goldfish because of the long time taken to attain maturity, and the zebra danio, *Brachydanio rario,* because of the high incidence of skeletal deformities. Newsome considered the convict cichlid *Cyclosoma nigrofasciatum* to be the most suitable as it breeds readily in the laboratory, has a relatively short maturation period, and has no exacting water quality requirements and diet. Further, it is small and genetically stable. Schimmel and Hansen[192] considered the sheepshead minnow, *Cyprinodon variegatus* as a suitable estuarine fish for chronic (entire life cycle) toxicity test.

B. Reference Toxicants

As with a standard test fish, the use of reference toxicants has also been recommended to compare the results from time to time within the same laboratory or between laboratories. A reference toxicant, explained Fogels and Sprague,[105] is used to provide a base line for comparing results from different laboratories. Klaverkamp et al.[193] listed six criteria for choosing a suitable reference toxicant: the lethality should be low, i.e., in the milligram per liter range; it should be easy to measure the concentrations of the toxicant in the test medium from time to time; the toxicant should be easily available in its purest form; it should be highly soluble in water; in the case of ionizable compounds the pKa should be at least one unit away from the normal pH range of the test medium; and it should have a known mode and site of action in the fish. In addition to these six criteria, Fogels and Sprague[105] added two more, viz., that the primary reference toxicant should have a definite threshold of toxicity for commonly tested species of fish and that there should be minimum change in its toxicity at different levels of hardness and pH. They considered that as a reference toxicant, sodium pentachlorophenate was difficult to analyze and also not easily available in its pure form; dodecyl sodium sulfate lost its toxicity upon being left on the shelf for some time and had no definite threshold of toxicity to rainbow trout. Only phenol met all the requirements of a standard reference toxicant. On the other hand, the usefulness of standard reference toxicants as a means of promoting standardization of toxicity test procedures and detecting differences in the sensitivity of groups of fish, was questioned.[194] Strains of rainbow trout may differ in their sensitivity to the same compound, and starvation, temperature, crowding stress, etc., may affect the sensitivity of rainbow trout to the reference toxicants. Out of five chemicals tested, viz., phenol, dodecyl sodium sulfate, sodium azide, sodium pentachlorophenate, and copper sulfate, only phenol could detect differences among strains and also could detect the effect of starvation, temperatures, and preexposure to chlorine. It could not detect the effect of three brands of food and failed to bring out differences due to loading density. Alexander and Clarke[194] contended that phenol is of limited use as a reference toxicant. They also questioned the very idea of a reference toxicant because differences among different strains or stocks of fish brought out by a reference toxicant may not necessarily affect the results of tests with other chemicals. They concluded that a series of physiological and behavioral tests may be more useful than reference toxicants in bringing out the differences in the sensitivity of test fish at different times of the year in the same laboratory or among different strains of the same species of test fish at the same time, or also between different laboratories. While noting variation in the data generated by seven laboratories in British Columbia, it was suggested that such reference toxicants may be useful in detecting only large differences in the sensitivity of test fish.[189] Marking[195] evaluated p,p'-DDT as a reference toxicant and found it to be of limited use for this purpose.

V. TYPES OF TOXICITY TESTS

The acute toxicity test is one of the most commonly used tests in the evaluation of the environmental impact of chemicals. According to Lloyd,[196] for any new chemical, the primary information in the process of aquatic hazard evaluation is obtained from the short-term or acute toxicity test. He was of the opinion that detailed statistical analysis of the LC 50 value to obtain the confidence limits and slope is of dubious value. He suggested that more meaningful information can be gathered from the slope of the concentration response curve (CRC) with little extra effort, if the concentration of the toxicant is held as constant as possible. As per the standard fish toxicity test protocol of the International Standard Organisation, the report of the test results should include both the 96-h LC 50 and the CRC, which can be constructed from a series of fixed period LC 50s, i.e., 3, 6, 24, 48, and 96 hr.[196] Although the CRCs can be very useful in drawing meaningful conclusions about further test requirements, false inflection of the curve may be caused by a decrease in the concentration of the pollutant during the test. Hence, the toxicant concentration must be kept as close to the desired concentration as possible during the test. In general, there are very few significant differences in the CRCs obtained with a toxicant and several species of test fish, even though the position of the curve, with respect to time and concentration axes, will be changed.

Apart from the 96-hr acute toxicity tests, the following tests are conducted to assess the environmental hazard of pollutants: chronic or life cycle tests, partial life cycle tests, embryo-larval tests, behavioral tests, biochemical-physiological tests, histological-histochemical tests, cell culture tests, algal culture tests, the residue (bioconcentration/bioaccumulation) tests and the organoleptic or flavor impairment tests.

Branson et al.[197] explained the different levels of toxicity testing and hazard evaluation. The short-term test is only one of the means of hazard assessment of pesticides. Brungs and Mount[135] underlined that no single class of tests provides all the information. Different approaches to toxicity testing serve different purposes and a single unified approach for the evaluation of the hazard of chemicals is not possible and does not give meaningful information.

In chronic or life cycle tests, all life stages are exposed to the toxic agent; to ensure this, the test is begun with eggs or fry, and they are exposed through maturity and spawning. The test is continued until the offspring of these fish are 30 days old. A partial chronic test is similar to a chronic test, is conducted with species that take a long time to attain maturity, begins with immature fish that are several months old, and continues until the offspring are 30 days old. Based on the chronic or partial life cycle tests, the highest concentration that does not affect growth, reproduction, survival of test fish, hatching success of the embryos, and the growth of the resultant fry, and the lowest concentration of the toxicant that affects one or more of these factors, are identified. The range between these two concentrations is termed the Maximum Acceptable Toxicant Concentration (MATC) (see Chapter 5).[198,199] McKim and Benoit[200] found that exposure to sublethal concentrations of copper, from yearlings, through spawning, to 3-month old juveniles, was sufficient to calculate the MATC.

The chronic and partial life cycle tests are time-consuming and expensive. Toxicity tests with embryos and larvae can provide data as useful as those obtained in complete or partial life cycle tests. McKim[201] analyzed the data on 56 life cycle toxicity tests completed between 1957 and 1977 with four species of fish and 34 different organic and inorganic chemicals and concluded that embryo-larval and early juvenile stage tests were more sensitive or at least as sensitive as the life cycle tests. In 82% of the cases, the MATC estimated by the embryo-larval test was identical to the MATC calculated by the longer, more involved, and expensive chronic (whole-life cycle) toxicity test. Water quality, species, type of toxicant, and parental exposure had little effect on this conclusion and hence McKim[201] considered that time, effort, and money can be saved by resorting to embryo-larval tests. This viewpoint was confirmed by Holcombe et al.[202] on the basis of their studies with four phenolic compounds and fathead minnow as the test fish. A fish reproduction test combined with embryo-larva test was proposed by Bresch[203] as a means of gaining more information.

Since the entire life cycle, partial life cycle, or embryo-larval tests take a few weeks to a few months, Maki[204] developed a method to continuously monitor the ventilation frequency of bluegills under flow-through exposure. Bluegills were exposed to surfactants and the ventilation rate was recorded over a period of 48 hr. The no-effect concentration, i.e., the concentration at which there was no significant difference between the control and test fish ventilation rates, was determined. There was a good agreement between the no-effect concentration derived from a 5-day ventilation frequency test and a costlier and time-consuming chronic, partial life cycle or embryo-larval test. Maki[205] found a high positive correlation ($r = 0.98$) between 21-day *Daphnia* chronic tests and 1 year fish chronic tests and suggested that the former is an attractive alternative to the longer fish chronic test.

Behavioral tests sometimes can be very useful in evaluating the effect on a whole population. Small changes in learning, dominance, parental behavior, orientation in the school, schooling and feeding behavior, food selection, migration, etc., induced by a toxicant, were suggested as excellent tools and also as a quick screening procedure for understanding the toxic effects of pesticides, but the usefulness of behavioral tests is rather limited because they are subjective and depend on the judgment of the investigator. It is also difficult to quantify the results of many behavioral tests.

Physiological and biochemical tests and also histological/histochemical studies have not achieved importance in pollution studies because of the lack of experimental evidence for their biological significance. Although it can easily be shown that change occurs under given, specified conditions of an altered environment, it is difficult to show the significance of this change. In nature, changes by themselves are normal and are not unwelcome. Hence, all changes by themselves are not detrimental. Also, the normal range of activity or normal range of expression of many physiological, biochemical, or histological factors is not well-understood. In the absence of such basic information, it would be difficult to evaluate the significance of the observed change. Further, every organism is capable of adjusting itself to a certain amount of change, induced either environmentally or otherwise. To what extent this inherent ability to cope with change helps the aquatic organism to tolerate and overcome the pollutant induced stress is not yet understood.

Residue tests, especially the bioconcentration/bioaccumulation tests, are a very good means of assessing the uptake of the toxicant which ultimately influences the toxic effect under chronic conditions. The Quantitative Structure-Activity Relationship (QSAR) studies are not actually a test procedure but are useful in evaluating and predicting the possible extent of bioaccumulation and bioconcentration of a chemical, as well as its environmental behavior.

According to Brungs and Mount,[135] algal assays have not been well used in hazard evaluation but have potential in hazard assessment, especially because the relative sensitivity of mixed phytoplanktonic cultures can throw light on community changes.

The organoleptic or residue and flavor tests assess the tainting of the fish flesh which often causes a great problem to the consumer rather than to the fish population itself. From the human point of view, such tests are useful in assessing the adverse effects of pesticides and other xenobiotic chemicals.

The in vitro tests involving cell culture may in the near future serve as a quick screening test. Cultured fish cells had a slow and decreased mitotic rate at concentrations of zinc much lower than those to which whole animals were sensitive.[206]

It would be interesting to speculate on the relative usefulness of the various tests described. The participants at a workshop on aquatic toxicology held at Pellston, Mich., were asked to rate the relative utility of 11 toxicity tests using the criteria of ecological significance, scientific and legal defensibility, availability of acceptable methods, and utility of test results, in predicting the effects in the aquatic environment.[207] In terms of utility for assessing the hazard in aquatic environments, acute lethality test was rated highest followed by embryo-larval test, chronic toxicity test measuring reproductive effects, and residue accumulation studies, in that order. "Histological tests ranked 9th, and physiological and biochemical tests 10th, . . . because of the inability to relate the results of these tests to adverse environmental impacts." Mehrle and Mayer[207] also stressed that biochemical and physiological tests have low utility in the case of aquatic organisms, although they are rated high in the realms of mammalian toxicology, because it is not understood to what extent the chemical-induced change impairs the ability of the organism to survive in its natural habitat. This problem of interpreting the toxic significance of biochemical change, the authors pointed out, stems from the fact that our knowledge of the physiological and biochemical regulatory mechanisms in fish is limited. Furthermore, the deviations from the physiological norms which the fish can tolerate are not very well understood. This problem is accentuated by the fact that many factors unrelated to pollutant-induced stress, like diet, age, season, reproductive stage, strain of handling, etc., are known to cause some biochemical or physiological changes.

In traditional toxicity testing, the effect of the toxicant on a single species of organism has been highlighted, but in nature an organism is part of a larger community. One of the major criticisms against single-species toxicity testing (acute, chronic, sublethal, etc.) is that unfortunately the accuracy of estimates based on laboratory toxicity tests has rarely been directly verified in either laboratory microcosms or in field situations. The usefulness of laboratory experiments for extrapolation to the field is limited, as the laboratory experiments are usually conducted with filtered water or reconstituted and deionized water. One problem with such tests is that the toxicant, to the extent it is made homogenous in the test medium, is uniformly available for absorption and uptake by the test species. On the other hand, in nature, the toxicant may be associated with the particulate matter, especially the lipid material, and hence may not be directly available for absorption and uptake by the test organism or by other species.[208] Although it has been suggested that laboratory and field investigations on the 96-h LC 50 value of the herbicide Roundup® gave identical values,[209] Hooper and Fukano[210] found that the toxicity values obtained in the laboratory varied from the actual toxicity under natural conditions. Cairns[211] questioned whether laboratory tests on an array of single species can be an adequate surrogate for natural ecosystems. At times, single-species test systems have been replaced by three-species assemblage (i.e., an alga, daphnid, and a fish) in order to evaluate the effect of the toxicant at three trophic levels. Even such an approach does not adequately reflect the diversity of the organisms in nature. Even an attempt to expand the species array to include as many as seven trophic level representatives may not adequately represent all trophic levels and functional systems found in nature.

With a view to deriving maximum amount of information with minimum toxicity testing and at the least expense, Kenaga[212] studied the possible correlation between the LD 50 and LC 50 values of 75 chemicals with eight species of test organisms (rat and mallard duck, oral LD 50, bobwhite dietary LD 50, rainbow trout, salt water fish, *Daphnia* and shrimp LC 50, and honey bee LD 50). On the basis of these comparisons, Kenaga concluded that for acute toxicity testing the most useful predictive indicative organisms and method of testing appear to be the rat oral LD 50, fish LC 50, and *Daphnia* LC 50. In a recent attempt, Daniels and Allan[213] studied the intrinsic rate of population increase as a bioassay statistic to understand the sublethal stress of toxicants. They found that the lifetable estimates of "r" appears to be an ecologically realistic measure of sublethal stress and that it requires a shorter time than the conventional long-term test. By subjecting the test organisms to conditions of stress in toxicity tests using very small and sensitive species and increasing the carrier solvent concentration, Bowman et al.[214] concluded that it is possible to perform toxicity tests in small containers and in less time, resulting in considerable saving of money, space, time, and effort.

Another test which has not received the wide attention that it deserves is the residual oxygen test in which every test organism contributes to the final result, whereas in the routine toxicity test only those that show the desired effect would contribute to the final calculation.[215] In the residual oxygen test, animals are held in sealed containers with graded concentration of the test material and the final level of the oxygen at the time of the death of the test fish is used as a measure of the toxicity of the material. Stressed fish die quicker than the controls and hence consume less oxygen before death.[197] When variables that may lead to inconsistent results, like size of the test fish, temperature, etc., are controlled, the test results are comparable to routine toxicity tests. While routine toxicity tests gave a 24-h LC 50 value of 2.54 mg/ℓ of mercuric chloride and 12.91 of phenol, the average LTC with the residual oxygen method was 2.88 mg/ℓ of mercuric chloride in 6 experiments; 3.63 mg/ℓ in 10 experiments; and 5.37 mg/ℓ in 9 other experiments. In one set of 10 experiments with phenol, the average LTC was a 11.41 mg/ℓ; in another set of experiments it was 6.71 mg/ℓ. Thus the values obtained with the residual oxygen method are very much of the same magnitude as those of a routine toxicity test. The method takes only 8 hr and hence is cost- and time-efficient.

After intensive experimentation with different numbers, biomass loading, and volume, the use of five test fish in 500 mℓ of water with 170 mℓ/g wet weight loading was recommended.[215] Temperature had no effect on the toxicity threshold of mercuric chloride but with phenol at 15°C the toxicity threshold was one third that of the value at 45°C. At the lower temperature, the exposure time was doubled. Because of its cost-efficient nature, the residual oxygen method deserves to be considered and tried on a

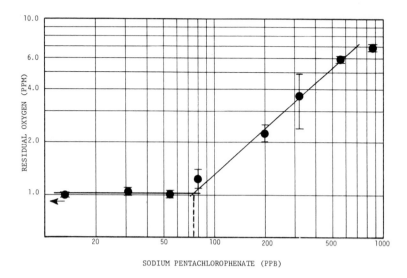

A

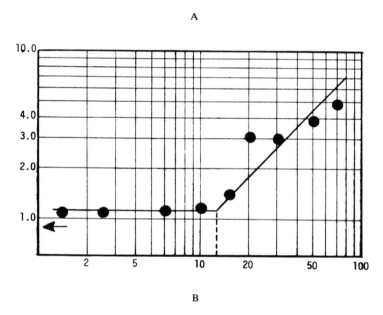

B

FIGURE 3.   A log-log plot of toxicant concentration vs. residual dissolved oxygen.
(A) Threshold value for sodium pentachlorophenate. Bars indicate the range in observations; (B), (C), (D), threshold value for three samples of kraft mill bleach plant
effluents. (B) Threshold value 13%, (C) threshold value 11.5%, and (D) threshold
value 13%. (Reprinted with permission from Vigers, G. A. and Maynard, A. W.,
Water Res., 11, 343, 1977. Copyright 1977, Pergamon Press.)

wider scale. While earlier the residual dissolved oxygen at the time of the death of the
test fish was plotted against the toxicant concentration as a continuous curve using a
semi-log paper, Vigers and Maynard[216] plotted the data on log-log scale which provided
a distinct threshold level (Figure 3). The threshold level thus calculated, for example,
with sodium PCP was 75.3 $\mu g/\ell$. (with 95% confident limits of 90.3 and 60.4 $\mu g/\ell$).
The calculated 96-h LC 50 value was 90 $\mu g/\ell$. The difference in the values obtained by
the different tests was not statistically significant. Thus the residual oxygen test appears
to be rapid, sensitive, and cost-efficient.

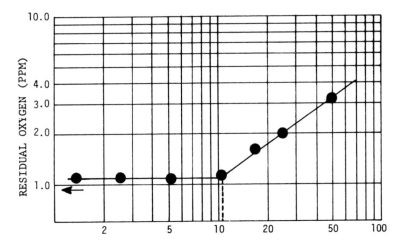

FIGURE 3C.

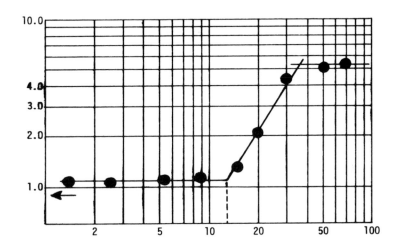

EFFLUENT CONCENTRATION (%V/V)

FIGURE 3D.

VI. CONCLUSIONS

The first attempts to test the toxicity of the synthetic organic pesticides to fish were made at about the same time large-scale application of synthetic pesticides began. Such attempts were very few in the beginning, but once it was realized that pesticides are in general highly toxic to the nontarget organisms, much work on the evaluation of their toxicity to the aquatic organisms followed. The need for standardizing toxicity test procedures was soon realized and culminated in the publication of the recommendations of Doudoroff et al., APHA standard methods, Recommendations of the Committee on Methods for Toxicity Tests with Aquatic Organisms, the ASTM Subcommittee on Pesticide Safety, and the OECD Guidelines.

It is necessary to distinguish between toxicity tests, which evaluate the adverse effect of a toxicant, and bioassay tests, which measure the concentration or amount of a chemical or effluent, using the known response of a test organism. The latter depend on the principle of parallelism and hence on the comparability of dose-response curves.

To ensure reproducibility of the tests, not only should the test fish be of uniform size and unstressed, but the physicochemical and biological conditions of the test should be as uniform and optimal as possible. Flow-through tests ensure such uniform conditions, but static tests, too, are useful in toxicity testing. Several types of dosing apparatus are in use to ensure constant toxicant concentration. Prolongation of the short-term test beyond 96 hr seems rarely necessary and seldom justifies the additional expenditure. LC 50, the concentraion that kills 50% of the test population in a given period of time, is used as a measure of toxicity in short-term tests. A number of methods are available for calculating this value and test results with one or no partial kills need not be discarded. Writing the LC 50 with a subscript (as LC_{50}) is not historically justified. Methods for assessing the toxicity of aged solutions or to compare the relative toxicity of two or more compounds have been described.

The use of a standard test fish and reference toxicants has been recommended for comparing test results of the same laboratory at different times or those of different laboratories, but such a practice is not yet standard and its utility has been questioned. The different types of toxicity tests in vogue and their relative usefulness have been reviewed.

REFERENCES

1. Ellis, M. M., Westfall, B. A., and Ellis, M. D., Toxicity of dichloro-diphenyl-trichloroethane (DDT goldfish and frogs, *Science*, 11, 477, 1944.
2. Ginsburg, J. M., *J. Econ. Entomol.*, 38, 274, 1945, in Odum, E. P. and Sumerford, W. T., Comparative toxicity of DDT and four analogues to goldfish, *Gambusia,* and *Culex* larvae, *Science,* 104, 480, 1946.
3. Odum, E. P. and Sumerford, W. T., Comparative toxicity of DDT and four analogues to goldfish, Gambusia, and culex larvae, *Science,* 104, 480, 1946.
4. Cairns, J., Jr., Coping with point source discharges, *Fisheries,* 5, 5, 1980.
5. Anon., Aquatic toxicology comes of age. ASTM conference heard the recent developments in this emerging discipline, *Environ. Sci. Technol.,* 12, 23, 1978.
6. Stephan, C. E., Methods for calculating an LC_{50}, *Aquatic Toxicology and Hazard Evaluation,* ASTM STP 634, Mayer, F. L. and Hamelink, J. L., Eds., American Society for Testing and Materials, Philadelphia, 1977, 65.
7. Brown, V. M., in *Bioassay Techniques and Environmental Chemistry,* Vol. 2, Glass, G. E., Ed., Ann Arbor Science, Ann Arbor, Mich., 1973, 73.
8. Mount, D. I., Present approaches to toxicity testing—a perspective, *Aquatic Toxicology and Hazard Evaluation,* ASTM STP 634, Mayer, F. L. and Hamelink, J. L., Eds., American Society for Testing and Materials, Philadelphia, 1977, 5.
9. Doudoroff, P., Anderson, B. G., Burdick, G. E., Galsoff, P. S., Hart, W. B., Patrick, R., Strong, E. R., Surber, E. W., and Horn, W. M. V., Bio-assay methods for the evaluation of acute toxicity of industrial wastes to fish, *Sewage Ind. Wastes,* 23, 1380, 1951.
10. APHA Standard Methods, For the examination of water and wastewater, 14th ed., American Public Health Association, Washington, D.C., 1975, 1193.
11. Sprague, J. B., Measurement of pollutant toxicity to fish. I. Bioassay methods for acute toxicity, *Water Res.,* 3, 793, 1969.
12. Sprague, J. B., Measurement of pollutant toxicity to fish. II. Utilizing and applying bioassay results, *Water Res.,* 4, 3, 1970.
13. Sprague, J. B., Measurement of pollutant toxicity to fish. III. Sublethal effects and "SAFE" concentrations, *Water Res.,* 5, 245, 1971.
14. Anon., Methods for acute toxicity tests with fish, macroinvertebrates and amphibians, US EPA-660/3-75-00, U.S. Environmental Protection Agency, Washington, D.C., 1975, 61.

15. *Standard Practice for Conducting Acute Toxicity Tests with Fishes, Macroinvertebrates, and Amphibians,* American Society for Testing and Materials, Philadelphia, 1980, 1.
16. *OECD Guidelines for Testing Chemicals,* OECD 1981 Draft, Paris, 1981, 1.
17. Pielou, D. P., Lethal effects of DDT on young fish, *Nature,* 15, 378, 1946.
18. Cottam, E. and Higgins, E., DDT: its effect on fish and wildlife, *Circ. Fish Wildl. Serv.,* Fish and Wildlife Service, U.S. Department of the Interior, Washington, D.C., 1946, 11.
19. Langford, R. R., The effect of DDT on freshwater fishes, in forest spraying and some effects of DDT, *Div. Res. Biol. Bull.,* Dept. Lands Forests, Ontario, Canada, 2, 19, 1949.
20. Hughes, J. S. and Davis, J. T., Variations in toxicity to bluegill sunfish of phenoxy herbicides, *Weeds,* 11, 50, 1963.
21. Burkett, R. D., The influence of temperature on uptake of methylmercury-203 by bluntnose minnows, *Pimephales notatus* (Rafinesque), *Bull. Environ. Contam. Toxicol.,* 12, 703, 1974.
22. Branson, D. R., Blau, G. E., Alexander, H. C., and Peters, T. L., Taint threshold of dephenyl oxide in rainbow trout, *Aquatic Toxicology,* ASTM STP 667, Marking, L. L. and Kimerle, R. A., Eds., American Society for Testing and Materials, Philadelphia, 1979, 107.
23. Hughes, D. N., Boyer, M. G., Papst, M. H., Fowle, C. D., Rees, G. A. V., and Baulu, P., Persistence of three organophosphorus insecticides in artificial ponds and some biological implications, *Arch. Environ. Contam. Toxicol.,* 9, 269, 1980.
24. Giam, C. S., Trace analyses of phthalates (and chlorinated hydrocarbons) in marine samples, in *Marine Pollution Monitoring,* Goldberg, E. D., Ed., John Wiley & Sons, New York, 1976, 61.
25. Giam, C. S., Chan, H. S., and Neff, G. S., Sensitive method for determination of phthalate ester plasticizers in open-ocean biota samples, *Anal. Chem.,* 47, 2225, 1975.
26. Anon., Water quality criteria, *Environ. Sci. Technol.,* 2, 662, 1968.
27. DeFoe, D. L., Temperature safety device for aquatic laboratory systems, *Prog. Fish-Culturist,* 39, 131, 1977.
28. Drummond, R. A. and Dawson, W. F., An inexpensive method for simulating diel patterns of lighting in the laboratory, *Trans. Am. Fish. Soc.,* 99, 434, 1970.
29. Lee, G. F., Review paper: chemical aspects of bioassay techniques for establishing water quality criteria, *Water Res.,* 7, 1525, 1973.
30. Sanders, H. O. and Walsh, D. F., Toxicity and residue dynamics of the lampricide 3-trifluoromethyl-4-nitrophenol (TFM) in aquatic invertebrates, Investigations in Fish Control 59, Fish and Wildlife Service, U.S. Department of the Interior, Washington, D.C., 1975.
31. Bass, M. L., Cardiovascular and respiratory changes in rainbow trout, *Salmo gairdneri,* exposed intermittently to chlorine, *Water Res.,* 11, 497, 1977.
32. Cherry, D. S., Larrick, S. R., Giattina, J. D., Cairns, J., Jr., and Hassel, J. V., Influence of temperature selection upon the chlorine avoidance of cold-water and warmwater fishes, *Can. J. Fish. Aquat. Sci.,* 39, 162, 1982.
33. Fandrei, G. and Collins, H. L., Total residual chlorine: the effect of short-term exposure on the emerald shiner *Notropis atherinoides* (Rafinesque), *Bull. Environ. Contam. Toxicol.,* 23, 262, 1979.
34. Zillich, J. A., Toxicity of combined chlorine residuals to freshwater fish, *J. Water Pollut. Control Fed.,* 44, 212, 1972.
35. Suzuki, M., Yamato, Y., and Watanabe, T., Analysis of environmental samples for organochlorine insecticides and related compounds by high-resolution electron capture gas chromatography with glass capillary columns, *Environ. Sci. Technol.,* 11, 1109, 1977.
36. Katz, B., Relationship of the physiology of aquatic organisms to the lethality of toxicants: a broad overview with emphasis on membrane permeability, in *Aquatic Toxicology,* ASTM STP 667, Marking, L. L. and Kimerle, R. A., Eds., American Society for Testing and Materials, Philadelphia, 1979, 62.
37. Henderson, C. and Pickering, Q. H., Use of fish in the detection of contaminants in water supplies, *J. Am. Water Works Assoc.,* 55, 715, 1963.
38. Armstrong, F. A. J. and Scott, D. P., Photochemical dechlorination of water supply for fish tanks, with commercial water stabilisers, *J. Fish. Res. Board Can.,* 31, 1881, 1974.
39. Brungs, W. A., Continuous-flow bioassays with aquatic organisms: procedures and applications, in *Biological Methods for the Assessment of Water Quality,* ASTM STP 528, American Society for Testing and Materials, Philadelphia, 1973, 117.
40. Alabaster, J. S., Survival of fish in 164 herbicides, insecticides, fungicides, wetting agents and miscellaneous substances, *Int. Pest Control,* 2, 29, 1969.
41. Birge, W. J., Black, J. A., Hudson, J. E., and Bruser, D. M., Embryo-Larval toxicity tests with organic compounds, in *Aquatic Toxicology,* ASTM STP 667, Marking, L. L. and Kimerle, R. A., Eds., American Society for Testing and Materials, Philadelphia, 1979, 131.
42. Cairns, J., Jr. and Loos, J. J., Changed feeding rate of *Brachydanio rerio* (Hamilton-Buchanan) resulting from exposure to sublethal concentrations of zinc, potassium dichromate, and alkyl benzene sulfonate detergent, *Proc. Pa. Acad. Sci.,* 11, 47, 1967.

43. Trama, F. B. and Benoit, R. J., Toxicity of hexavalent chromium to bluegills, *J. Water Pollut. Control Fed.*, 32, 868, 1960.
44. Lennon, R. E. and Walker, C. R., Laboratories and methods for screening fish-control chemicals, *Investigations in Fish Control 1,* Bureau of Sport Fisheries and Wildlife Circular 185, Fish and Wildlife Service, U.S. Department of the Interior, Washington, D.C., 1964.
45. Freeman, L., A standardized method for determining toxicity of pure compounds to fish, *Sewage Ind. Wastes,* 25, 845, 1953.
46. Marking, L. L., Toxicological assays with fish, *Bull. Wildl. Dis. Assoc.,* 5, 291, 1969.
47. Courtright, R. C., Breese, W. P., and Krueger, H., Formulation of a synthetic sea water for bioassays with *Mytilus edulis* embryos, *Water Res.,* 5, 877, 1971.
48. Lillie, W. R. and Klaverkamp, J. F., A system for regulating and recording pH of solutions in aquatic flow-through toxicity tests, Tech. Rep. No. 710, Department of the Environment Research and Development Directorate Freshwater Institute, Winnipeg, Manitoba, 1977.
49. Statham, C. N., Melancon, M. J., Jr., and Lech, J. J., Bioconcentration of xenobiotics in trout bile: a proposed monitoring aid for some waterborne chemicals, *Science,* 193, 680, 1976.
50. McLeese, D. W., Metcalfe, C. D., and Zitko, V., Lethality of permethrin, cypermethrin and fenvalerate to salmon, lobster and shrimp, *Bull. Environ. Contam. Toxicol.,* 25, 950, 1980.
51. Lorio, W. J., Jenkins, J. H., and Huish, M. T., Deposition of dieldrin in four components of two artificial aquatic systems and a farm pond, *Trans. Am. Fish. Soc.,* 105, 695, 1976.
52. Mount, D. I., Additional information on a system for controlling the dissolved oxygen content of water, *Trans. Am. Fish. Soc.,* 93, 100, 1964.
53. Buikema, A. L., Jr., Niederlehner, B. R., and Cairns, J., Jr., Biological monitoring. IV. Toxicity testing, *Water Res.,* 16, 239, 1982.
54. Fujiwara, K., Japanese law on new chemicals and the methods to test the biodegradability and bioaccumulation of chemical substances, in *Analyzing the Hazard Evaluation Process,* Dickson, K. L., Maki, A. W., and Cairns, J., Jr., Eds., American Fisheries Society, Washington, D.C., 1979, 50.
55. Herzel, F. and Murty, A. S., Do carrier solvents enhance the water solubility of hydrophobic compounds?, *Bull. Environ. Contam. Toxicol.,* 32, 53, 1984.
56. Buccafusco, R. J., Ells, S. J., and LeBlanc, G. A., Acute toxicity of priority pollutants to bluegill *(Lepomis macrochirus), Bull. Environ. Contam. Toxicol.,* 26, 446, 1981.
57. Heitmuller, P. T., Hollister, T. A., and Parrish, P. R., Acute toxicity of 54 industrial chemicals to sheepshead minnows *(Cyprinodon variegatus), Bull. Environ. Contam. Toxicol.,* 27, 596, 1981.
58. Hylin, J. W., Pesticide residue analysis of water and sediments: potential problems and some philosophy, *Residue Rev.,* 76, 203, 1980.
59. Brungs, W. A. and Bailey, G. W., Influence of suspended solids on the acute toxicity of endrin to fathead minnows, Proc. 21st Purdue Industrial Waste Conf., *Eng. Bull. Purdue Univ.,* 50, 4, 1967.
60. Sugiura, K., Hattori, M., Washino, T., Goto, M., Leimgruber, R., and Batzer, H., Effects of surface-active agents on the amount and rate of accumulation of tris (2,4,-di-*ter*-butylphenyl) phosphite in fish, *Chemosphere,* 9, 743, 1978.
61. Mac, M. J. and Seelye, J. G., Potential influence of acetone in aquatic bioassays testing the dynamics and effects of PCBs, *Bull. Environ. Contam. Toxicol.,* 27, 359, 1981.
62. Majewski, H. S., Klaverkamp, J. F., and Scott, D. P., Acute lethality, and sub-lethal effects of acetone, ethanol, and propylene glycol on the cardiovascular and respiratory systems of rainbow trout *(Salmo gairdneri), Water Res.,* 13, 217, 1978.
63. Roesijadi, G., Petrocelli, S. R., Anderson, J. W., Giam, C. S., and Neff, G. E., Toxicity of polychlorinated biphenyls (Aroclor 1254) to adult, juvenile, and larval stages of the shrimp *Palaemonetes pugio, Bull. Environ. Contam. Toxicol.,* 15, 297, 1976.
64. Shubat, P. J., Poirier, S. H., Knuth, M. L., and Brooks, L. T., Acute toxicity of tetrachloroethylene and tetrachloroethylene with dimethylformamide to rainbow trout *(Salmo gairdneri), Bull. Environ. Contam. Toxicol.,* 28, 7, 1982.
65. Murty, A. S. and Hansen, P. D., Influence of the carrier solvent on aquatic toxicity tests, in Proc. Int. Symp. Chemicals in the Environment, Copenhagen, October 1982, Christiansen, K., Koch, B., and Rasmussen, F. B., Eds., Technical University of Denmark, Lyngby, 1983, 334.
66. Chadwick, G. G. and Kiigemagi, U., Toxicity evaluation of a technique for introducing dieldrin into water, *J. Water Pollut. Control Fed.,* 40, 76, 1968.
67. Gingerich, W. H., Seim, W. K., and Schonbrod, R. D., An apparatus for the continuous generation of stock solution of hydrophobic chemicals, *Bull. Environ. Contam. Toxicol.,* 23, 685, 1979.
68. Borthwick, P. W., Tagatz, M. E., and Forester, J., A gravity-flow column to provide pesticide-laden water for aquatic bioassays, *Bull. Environ. Contam. Toxicol.,* 13, 183, 1975.
69. Veith, G. D. and Comstock, V. M., Apparatus for continuously saturating water with hydrophobic organic chemicals, *J. Fish. Res. Board Can.,* 32, 1849, 1975.

70. Cope, O. B., Wood, E. M., and Wallen, G. H., Some chronic effects of 2,4-D on the bluegill *(Lepomis macrochirus), Trans. Am. Fish. Soc.,* 99, 1, 1970.
71. Hamburger, B., German experience with the Japanese fish accumulation test, *Ecotoxicol. Environ. Saf.,* 4, 17, 1980.
72. Brauhn, J. L. and Schoettger, R. A., Acquisition and culture of research fish: rainbow trout, fathead minnows, channel catfish, and bluegills, EPA-600/3-75-011, U.S. Environmental Protection Agency, Corvallis, Ore., 1975.
73. Hunn, J. B., Schoettger, R. A., and Whealdon, E. W., Observations on the handling and maintenance of experimental fish, *Prog. Fish-Culturist,* 30, 164, 1968.
74. Hesselberg, R. J. and Burress, R. M., Labor-saving devices for bioassay laboratories, Fish and Wildlife Service, U.S. Dept. of the Interior, Washington, D.C., 1967.
75. Fabacher, D. L., Davis, J. D., and Fabacher, D. A., Apparent potentiation of the cotton defoliant DEF by methyl parathion in mosquitofish, *Bull. Environ. Contam. Toxicol.,* 16, 716, 1976.
76. Linden, E., Bengteson, B. E., Svanberg, D., and Sundstrom, G., The acute toxicity of 78 chemicals and pesticide formulations against two brackish water organisms, the bleak *(Alburnus alburnus)* and the harpacticoid *Nitocra spinipes, Chemosphere,* 45, 843, 1979.
77. Adelman, I. R., Smith, L. L., Jr., and Siesennop, G. D., Effect of size or age of goldfish and fathead minnows on use of pentachlorophenol as a reference toxicant, *Water Res.,* 10, 685, 1976.
78. Wedemeyer, G., Some physiological consequences of handling stress in the juvenile coho salmon *(Oncorhynchus kisutch)* and steelhead trout *(Salmo gairdneri), J. Fish. Res. Board Can.,* 29, 1980, 1972.
79. Grant, B. F. and Mehrle, P. M., Endrin toxicosis in rainbow trout *(Salmo gairdneri), J. Fish. Res. Board Can.,* 30, 31, 1973.
80. McCann, J. A. and Jasper, R. L., Vertebral damage to bluegills exposed to acutely toxic levels of pesticides, *Trans. Am. Fish. Soc.,* 101, 317, 1972.
81. Fabacher, D. L., Hepatic microsomes from freshwater fish. II. Reduction of benzo(a)pyrene metabolism by the fish anesthetics quinaldine sulfate and tricaine, *Comp. Biochem. Physiol.,* 73, 285, 1982.
82. Wedemeyer, G., Stress of anesthesia with M.S. 222 and benzocaine in rainbow trout *(Salmo gairdneri), J. Fish. Res. Board Can.,* 27, 909, 1970.
83. Cooke, A. S., The influence of rearing density on the subsequent response to DDT dosing for tadpoles of the frog *Rana temporaria, Bull. Environ. Contam. Toxicol.,* 7, 837, 1979.
84. French, M. C. and Jefferies, D. J., The preservation of biological tissue for organochlorine insecticide analysis, *Bull. Environ. Contam. Toxicol.,* 6, 460, 1971.
85. Chadwick, G. G. and Brocksen, R. W., Accumulation of dieldrin by fish and selected fish-food organisms, *J. Wildl. Manage.,* 33, 693, 1969.
86. Mehrle, P. M., Johnson, W. W., and Mayer, F. L., Jr., Nutritional effects on chlordane toxicity in rainbow trout, *Bull. Environ. Contam. Toxicol.,* 12, 513, 1974.
87. Boyd, E. M. and Krijnen, C. J., Dietary protein and DDT toxicity, *Bull. Environ. Contam. Toxicol.,* 4, 256, 1969.
88. Mehrle, P. M., Mayer, F. L., and Johnson, W. W., Diet quality in fish toxicology: effects on acute and chronic toxicity, *Aquatic Toxicology and Hazard Evaluation,* ASTM STP 634, Mayer, F. L. and Hamelink, J. L., Eds., American Society for Testing and Materials, Philadelphia, 1977, 269.
89. Elson, P. F., Meister, A. L., Saunders, J. W., Saunders, R. L., Sprague, J. B., and Zitko, V., Impact of chemical pollution on Atlantic salmon in North America, Int. Atlantic Salmon Symp., International Atlantic Salmon Foundation, St. Andrews, New Brunswick, Canada, 1973, 83.
90. Cuerrier, J. P., Keith, J. A., and Stone, E., Problems with DDT in fish culture operations, *Nat. Can.,* 94, 315, 1967.
91. Crockett, A. B., Wiersma, G. B., Tai, H., and Mitchell, W., Pesticide and mercury residues in commercially grown catfish, *Pestic. Monit. J.,* 8, 235, 1975.
92. Laska, A. L., Bartell, C. K., Condie, B. D., Brown, J. W., Evans, R. L., and Laseter, J. L., *Toxicol. Appl. Pharmacol.,* 43, 1, 1978.
93. Parejko, R. and Wu, C. J., Chlorohydrocarbons in Marquette fish hatchery lake trout *(Salvelinus namaycush), Bull. Environ. Contam. Toxicol.,* 17, 90, 1977.
94. Niimi, A. J. and Cho, C. Y., Uptake of hexachlorobenzene (HCB) from feed by rainbow trout *(Salmo gairdneri), Bull. Environ. Contam. Toxicol.,* 24, 834, 1980.
95. Stober, Q. J. and Payne, W. R., Jr., A method for preparation of pesticide-free fish food from commercial fish food pellets, *Trans. Am. Fish. Soc.,* 95, 212, 1966.
96. Cairns, J., Jr., van der Schalie, W. H., and Westlake, G. F., The effect of lapsed time since feeding upon the toxicity of zinc to fish, *Bull. Environ. Contam. Toxicol.,* 13, 269, 1975.
97. Phillips, G. R. and Buhler, D. R., Influence of dieldrin on the growth and body composition of fingerling rainbow trout *(Salmo gairdneri)* fed Oregon moist pellets or tubificid worms (*Tubifex* sp.), *J. Fish. Res. Board Can.,* 36, 77, 1979.

98. Sastry, K. V. and Sharma, S. K., In vivo effect of endrin on three phosphatases in kidney and liver of the fish *Ophiocephalus punctatus, Bull. Environ. Contam. Toxicol.*, 21, 185, 1979.
99. Sastry, K. V. and Sharma, S. K., The effect of *in vivo* exposure of endrin on the activities of acid, alkaline and glucose-6-phosphatases in liver and kidney of *Ophiocephalus (Channa) punctatus, Bull. Environ. Contam. Toxicol.*, 20, 456, 1978.
100. Sharma, S. K. and Sastry, K. V., Alteration in enzyme activities in liver and kidney of *Channa punctatus* exposed to endrin, *Bull. Environ. Contam. Toxicol.*, 22, 17, 1979.
101. Iwama, G. K. and Greer, G. L., Toxicity of sodium pentachlorophenate to juvenile chinook salmon under conditions of high loading density and continuous-flow exposure, *Bull. Environ. Contam. Toxicol.*, 25, 711, 1979.
102. Jensen, A. L., Standard error of LC_{50} and sample size in fish bioassays, *Water Res.*, 6, 85, 1972.
103. Arunachalam, S., Jeyalakshmi, K., and Aboobucker, S., Toxic and sublethal effects of carbaryl on a freshwater catfish, *Mystus vittatus* (Bloch), *Arch. Environ. Contam. Toxicol.*, 9, 307, 1980.
104. Palawski, D., Buckler, D. R., and Mayer, F. L., Survival and condition of rainbow trout *(Salmo gairdneri)* after acute exposures to methyl parathion, tri-phenyl phosphate and DEF, *Bull. Environ. Contam. Toxicol.*, 30, 614, 1983.
105. Fogels, A. and Sprague, J. B., Comparative short-term tolerance of zebrafish, flagfish, and rainbow trout to five poisons including potential reference toxicants, *Water Res.*, 11, 811, 1977.
106. Kaila, K. and Saarikoski, J., Toxicity of pentachlorophenol and 2,3,6-trichlorophenol to the crayfish *(Astacus fluviatilis* L.), *Environ. Pollut.*, 12, 119, 1977.
107. Phipps, G. L., Holcombe, G. W., and Fiandt, J. T., Acute toxicity of phenol and substituted phenols to the fathead minnow, *Bull. Environ. Contam. Toxicol.*, 26, 585, 1981.
108. Alexander, H. C., Bodner, K. M., and Mayes, M. A., Evaluation of the OECD "Fish prolonged toxicity study at least 14 days", *Chemosphere*, 12, 415, 1983.
109. McLeese, D. W., Burridge, L. E., and Dinter, J. V., Toxicities of five organochlorine compounds in water and sediment to *Neries virens, Bull. Environ. Contam. Toxicol.*, 28, 216, 1982.
110. Singh, H. and Singh, T. P., Short-term effect of two pesticides on the survival, ovarian ^{32}P uptake and gonadotrophic potency in a freshwater catfish, *Heteropneustes fossilis* (Bloch), *J. Endrocrinol.*, 85, 193, 1980.
111. Macek, K. J., Hutchinson, C., and Cope, C. B., The effects of temperature on the susceptibility of bluegills and rainbow trout to selected pesticides, *Bull. Environ. Contam. Toxicol.*, 4, 174, 1969.
112. Pickering, Q. H., Henderson, C., and Lemke, A. E., The toxicity of organic phosphorus insecticides to different species of warm water fishes, *Trans. Am. Fish. Soc.*, 91, 175, 1962.
113. Nevins, M. J. and Johnson, W. W., Acute toxicity of phosphate ester mixtures to invertebrates and fish, *Bull. Environ. Contam. Toxicol.*, 19, 250, 1978.
114. Buckler, D. R., Witt, A., Jr., Mayer, F. L., and Huckins, J. N., Acute and chronic effects of Kepone and mirex on the fathead minnow, *Trans. Am. Fish. Soc.*, 110, 270, 1981.
115. Lincer, J., Solon, J. M., and Nair, J. H., DDT and endrin fish toxicity under static versus dynamic bioassay conditions, *Trans. Am. Fish. Soc.*, 99, 13, 1970.
116. Applegate, V. C., Howell, J., and Smith, M. A., Use of mononitrophenols containing halogens as selective sea lamprey larvicides, *Science*, 127, 336, 1958.
117. Marking, L. L., Bills, T. D., and Chandler, J. H., Toxicity of the lampricide 3-trifluoromethyl-4-nitrophenol (TFM) to nontarget fish in flow-through tests, Fish and Wildlife Service, U.S. Department of the Interior, Washington, D.C., 1975.
118. Adelman, I. R. and Smith, L. L., Jr., Fathead minnows *(Pimephales promelas)* and goldfish *(Carassius auratus)* as standard fish in bioassays and their reaction to potential reference toxicants, *J. Fish. Res. Board Can.*, 33, 209, 1976.
119. Alexander, H. C., McCarty, W. M., and Bartlett, E. A., Toxicity of perchloroethylene, trichloroethylene, 1,1,1-trichloroethane, and methylene chloride to fathead minnows, *Bull. Environ. Contam. Toxicol.*, 20, 344, 1978.
120. USEPA, Ambient Water Quality Criteria for endosulfan, EPA 440/5-80-046, U.S. Environmental Protection Agency, Office of Water Regulations and Standards Criteria and Standards Division, Washington, D.C., 1980.
121. Holden, A. V., A study of the absorption of ^{14}C-labelled DDT from water by fish, *Ann. Appl. Biol.*, 50, 467, 1962.
122. Mauck, W. I., Olson, L. E., and Marking, L. L., Toxicity of natural pyrethrins and five pyrethroids to fish, *Arch. Environ. Contam. Toxicol.*, 4, 18, 1976.
123. Kobylinski, G. J. and Livingston, R. J., Movement of mirex from sediment and uptake by the hogchoker, *Trinectes maculatus, Bull. Environ. Contam. Toxicol.*, 14, 692, 1975.
124. Schreck, C. B. and Brouha, P., Dissolved oxygen depletion in static bioassay systems, *Bull. Environ. Contam. Toxicol.*, 14, 149, 1975.

125. Thurston, R. V., Phillips, G. R., Russo, R. C., and Hinkins, S. M., Increased toxicity of ammonia to rainbow trout *(Salmo gairdneri)* resulting from reduced concentrations of dissolved oxygen, *Can. J. Fish. Aquat. Sci.*, 38, 983, 1981.

126. Becker, C. D. and Crass, D. W., Examination of procedures for acute toxicity tests with the fathead minnow and coal synfuel blends, *Arch. Environ. Contam. Toxicol.*, 11, 33, 1982.

127. Sasaki, K., Takeda, M., and Uchiyama, M., Toxicity absorption and elimination of phosphoric acid triesters by killifish and goldfish, *Bull. Environ. Contam. Toxicol.*, 27, 775, 1981.

128. Schaefer, C. H., Dupras, E. F., Jr., Stewart, R. J., Davidson, L. W., and Colwell, A. E., The accumulation and elimination of diflubenzuron by fish, *Bull. Environ. Contam. Toxicol.*, 21, 249, 1979.

129. Merna, J. W., Bender, M. E., and Novy, J. R., The effects of methoxychlor on fishes. I. Acute toxicity and breakdown studies, *Trans. Am. Fish. Soc.*, 101, 298, 1972.

130. Feroz, M. and Khan, M. A. Q., Fate of ^{14}C-cis-chlordane in goldfish, *Carassius auratus* (L.), *Bull. Environ. Contam. Toxicol.*, 23, 64, 1979.

131. Ferguson, D. E., Ludke, J. L., and Murphy, G. G., Dynamics of endrin uptake and release by resistant and susceptible strains of mosquitofish, *Trans. Am. Fish. Soc.*, 95, 335, 1966.

132. Sprague, J. B., The ABC's of pollutant bioassay using fish, *Biological Methods for the Assessment of Water Quality*, ASTM STP 528, American Society for Testing and Materials, Philadelphia, 1973, 6.

133. Mount, D. I., Adequacy of laboratory data for protecting aquatic communities, in *Analyzing the Hazard Evaluation Process*, Dickson, K. L., Maki, A. W., and Cairns, J. Jr., Eds., *American Fisheries Society*, Washington, D.C., 1979, 112.

134. Cairns, J. Jr. and Gruber, D., Coupling mini and microcomputers to biological early warning systems, *Bioscience*, 29, 665, 1979.

135. Brungs, W. A. and Mount, D. I., Introduction to a discussion of the use of aquatic toxicity tests for evaluation of the effects of toxic substances, *Estimating the Hazard of Chemical Substances to Aquatic Life*, ASTM STP 657, Cairns, J. Jr., Dickson, K. L., and Maki, A. W., Eds., American Society for Testing and Materials, Philadelphia, 1978, 15.

136. Sprague, J. B. and Fogels, A., Watch the Y in bioassay, Proc. 3rd Aquatic Toxicity Workshop, Halifax, Nova Scotia, November 2 to 3, 1976. Environmental Protection Service Tech. Rep. No. EPS-5-AR-77-1, Halifax, Canada, 1977, 107.

137. Mount, D. I. and Warner, R. E., A serial-dilution apparatus for continuous delivery of various concentrations of materials in water, Public Health Service Division of Water Supply and Pollution Control, U.S. Department of Health, Education, and Welfare, Cincinnati, Ohio, 1965.

138. Mount, D. I. and Brungs, W. A., A simplified dosing apparatus for fish toxicology studies, *Water Res.*, 1, 21, 1967.

139. Brungs, W. A. and Mount, D. I., A water delivery system for small fish-holding tanks, *Trans. Am. Fish. Soc.*, 99, 799, 1970.

140. Brungs, W. A. and Mount, D. I., A device for continuous treatment of fish in holding chambers, *Trans. Am. Fish. Soc.*, 96, 55, 1967.

141. McAllister, W. A., Jr., Mauck, W. L., and Mayer, F. L., Jr., A simplified device for metering chemicals in intermittent-flow bioassays, *Trans. Am. Fish. Soc.*, 101, 555, 1972.

142. Abram, F. S. H., Apparatus for control of poison concentration in toxicity studies with fish, *Water Res.*, 7, 1875, 1973.

143. Granmo, A. and Kollberg, S. O., A new simple water flow system for accurate continuous flow tests, *Water Res.*, 6, 1597, 1972.

144. Benoit, D. A. and Puglisi, F. A., A simplified flow-splitting chamber and siphon for proportional diluters, *Water Res.*, 7, 1915, 1973.

145. Chandler, J. H., Jr., Sanders, H. O., and Walsh, D. F., An improved chemical delivery apparatus for use in intermittent-flow bioassays, *Bull. Environ. Contam. Toxicol.*, 12, 123, 1974.

146. DeFoe, D. L., Multichannel toxicant injection system for flow-through bioassays, *J. Fish. Res. Board Can.*, 32, 544, 1975.

147. Solon, J. M., Lincer, J. L., and Nair, J. H., III, A continuous flow, automatic device for short-term toxicity experiments, *Trans. Am. Fish. Soc.*, 97, 501, 1968.

148. Smith, A. D., Butler, J. R., and Ozburn, G. W., A pneumatic dosing apparatus for flow-through bioassays, *Water Res.*, 11, 347, 1977.

149. Burke, W. D. and Ferguson, D. E., A simplified flow-through apparatus for maintaining fixed concentrations of toxicants in water, *Trans. Am. Fish. Soc.*, 97, 498, 1968.

150. Boling, R. H., Jr., A technique for computer-controlled toxicant injection, *Bull. Environ. Contam. Toxicol.*, 27, 773, 1981.

151. Benoit, D. A., Matison, V. R., and Olson, D. L., A continuous-flow mini-diluter system for toxicity testing, *Water Res.*, 16, 457, 1982.

152. Novak, A. J., Berry, D. F., Walters, B. S., and Passino, D. R. M., New continuous-flow bioassay technique using small crustaceans, *Bull. Environ. Contam. Toxicol.,* 29, 253, 1982.

153. Smith, R. L. and Hargreaves, B. R., A simple toxicity apparatus for continuous flow with small volumes: demonstration with mysids and naphthalene, *Bull. Environ. Contam. Toxicol.,* 30, 406, 1983.

154. Brenniman, G., Hartung, R., and Weber, W. J., Jr., A continuous flow bioassay method to evaluate the effects of outboard motor exhausts and selected aromatic toxicants on fish, *Water Res.,* 10, 165, 1976.

155. Schimmel, S. C., Patrick, J. M., Jr., and Forester, J., Toxicity and bioconcentration of BHC and lindane in selected estuarine animals, *Arch. Environ. Contam. Toxicol.,* 6, 355, 1977.

156. Marking, L. L. and Olson, L. E., Toxicity of the lampricide 3-trifluoromethyl-4-nitrophenol (TFM) to nontarget fish in static tests, Investigations in Fish Control 60, Fish and Wildlife Service, U.S. Department of the Interior, Washington, D.C., 1975.

157. Mauck, W. L., Olson, L. E., and Hogan, J. W., Effects of water quality on deactivation and toxicity of mexacarbate (Zectran®) to fish, *Arch. Environ. Contam. Toxicol.,* 6, 385, 1977.

158. Jarvinen, A. W. and Tanner, D. K., Toxicity of selected controlled release and corresponding unformulated technical grade pesticides to the fathead minnow *Pimephales promelas, Environ. Pollut.,* 27, 179, 1982.

159. Johnson, W. W. and Julin, A. M., Acute toxicity of toxaphene to fathead minnows, channel catfish, and bluegills, EPA-600/3-80-005, U.S. Environmental Protection Agency, Duluth, Minn., 1980.

160. Galassi, S. and Vighi, M., Testing toxicity of volatile substances with algae, *Chemosphere,* 10, 1123, 1981.

161. Zitko, V., Carson, W. G., and Metcalfe, C. D., Toxicity of pyrethroids to juvenile Atlantic salmon, *Bull. Environ. Contam. Toxicol.,* 18, 35, 1977.

162. Gillespie, D. M., Eldredge, J. D., and Thompson, C. K., A kinetic model for static bioassay of insecticides, *Water Res.,* 9, 817, 1975.

163. Spencer, W. F., Distribution of pesticides between soil, water and air, in *Pesticides in the Soil: Ecology, Degradation, and Movement,* Michigan State University, East Lansing, 1970.

164. Mackay, D. and Leinonen, P. J., Rate of evaporation of low-solubility contaminants from water bodies to atmosphere, *Environ. Sci. Technol.,* 9, 1178, 1975.

165. Mackay, D. and Wolkoff, A. W., Rate of evaporation of low-solubility contaminants from water bodies to atmosphere, *Environ. Sci. Technol.,* 7, 611, 1973.

166. Ernst, W., Determination of the bioconcentration potential of marine organisms — a steady state approach. I. Bioconcentration data for seven chlorinated pesticides in mussels *(Mytilus edulis)* and their relation to solubility data, *Chemosphere,* 11, 731, 1977.

167. Södergren, A., Composition and properties of lipid surface films produced by *Chlorella pyrenoidosa, Mitt. Int. Verein Limnol.,* 21, 248, 1978.

168. Södergren, A., Significance of interfaces in the distribution and metabolism of di-2-ethylhexyl phthalate in an aquatic laboratory model ecosystem, *Environ. Pollut.,* 27, 263, 1982.

169. Sharom, M. S. and Solomon, K. R., The influence of adsorption on glass, pH and temperature on the disappearance of permethrin in aqueous system, *Environ. Pollut.,* 4, 249, 1982.

170. Pepe, M. G. and Byrne, J. J., Adhesion-binding of 2,2',4,4',5,5'-hexachlorobiphenyl to glass and plastic: a possible source of error for PCB analysis, *Bull. Environ. Contam. Toxicol.,* 25, 936, 1980.

171. Fabacher, D. L., Toxicity of endrin and an endrin-methyl parathion formulation to largemouth bass fingerlings, *Bull. Environ. Contam. Toxicol.,* 16, 376, 1976.

172. Murphy, P. G. and Murphy, J. V., Correlations between respiration and direct uptake of DDT in the mosquitofish *Gambusia affinis, Bull. Environ. Contam. Toxicol.,* 6, 581, 1971.

173. Holden, A. V., The possible effects on fish of chemicals used in agriculture, *J. Proc. Inst. Sewage Purif., Part 4,* 4, 361, 1964.

174. Cairns, J., Jr., Heath, A. G., and Parker, B. C., Temperature influence on chemical toxicity to aquatic organisms, *J. Water Pollut. Control Fed.,* 47, 267, 1975.

175. Lloyd, R. and Tooby, T. E., New terminology required for short-term static fish bioassays: LC(I) 50, *Bull. Environ. Contam. Toxicol.,* 22, 1, 1979.

176. Litchfield, J. T., Jr. and Wilcoxon, F., A simplified method of evaluating dose-effect experiments, *J. Pharmacol. Exp. Ther.,* 96, 99, 1949.

177. Hamilton, M. A., Russo, R. C., and Thurston, R. V., Trimmed Spearman-Karber method for estimating median lethal concentrations in toxicity bioassays, *Environ. Sci. Technol.,* 11, 715, 1977.

178. Finney, D. J., *Probit Analysis,* 3rd ed., Cambridge University Press, Cambridge, 1971, 1.

179. Lee, J. H., Sylvester, J. R., and Nash, C. E., Effects of mirex and methoxychlor on juvenile and adult striped mullet, *Mugil cephalus* L., *Bull. Environ. Contam. Toxicol.,* 14, 180, 1975.

180. Valin, C. C. V., Andrews, A. K., and Eller, L. L., Some effects of mirex on two warm-water fishes, *Trans. Am. Fish. Soc.,* 97, 185, 1968.

181. Henderson, C., Pickering, Q. H., and Tarzwell, C. M., Relative toxicity of ten chlorinated hydrocarbon insecticides to four species of fish, *Trans. Am. Fish. Soc.*, 88, 23, 1959.

182. Macek, K. J. and Sanders, H. O., Biological variation in the susceptibility of fish and aquatic invertebrates to DDT, *Trans. Am. Fish. Soc.*, 99, 89, 1970.

183. Solon, J. M., Lincer, J. L., and Nair, J. H., III, The effect of sublethal concentration of LAS on the acute toxicity of various insecticides to the fathead minnow (*Pimephales promelas* Rafinesque), *Water Res.*, 3, 767, 1969.

184. Brown, V. M., The calculation of the acute toxicity of mixtures of poisons to rainbow trout, *Water Res.*, 2, 723, 1968.

185. Grant, B. F. and Mehrle, P. M., Chronic endrin poisoning in goldfish, *Carassius auratus, J. Fish. Res. Board Can.*, 27, 2225, 1970.

186. Singh, B. B. and Narain, A. S., Acute toxicity of Thiodan to catfish *(Heteropneustes fossilis), Bull. Environ. Contam. Toxicol.*, 28, 122, 1982.

187. Adelman, I. R. and Smith, L. L., Jr., Toxicity of hydrogen sulfide to goldfish *(Carassius auratus)* as influenced by temperature, oxygen, and bioassay techniques, *J. Fish. Res. Board Can.*, 29, 1309, 1972.

188. Smith, W. E., A cyprinodontid fish, *Jordanella floridae,* as a laboratory animal for rapid chronic bioassays, *J. Fish. Res. Board Can.*, 30, 329, 1973.

189. Davis, J. C. and Hoos, R. A. W., Use of sodium pentachlorophenate and dehydroabietic acid as reference toxicants for salmonid bioassays, *J. Fish. Res. Board Can.*, 32, 411, 1975.

190. Cairns, J., Jr., Developing a toxicity testing capability for Australia, *Water,* 7, 14, 1980.

191. Newsome, C. S., A multigeneration fish toxicity test as an aid in the hazard evaluation of aquatic pollutants, *Ecotoxicol. Environ. Saf.*, 4, 362, 1980.

192. Schimmel, S. C. and Hansen, D. J., Sheepshead minnow *(Cyprinodon variegatus):* an estuarine fish suitable for chronic (entire life-cycle) bioassays, Proc. 28th Annu. Conf. Southeast. Assoc. Game and Fish Commissioners, 1975.

193. Klaverkamp, J. F., Kennedy, A., Harrison, S. E., and Danell, R., An evaluation of phenol and sodium azide as reference toxicants in rainbow trout. 2nd Annu. Aquatic Toxicity Workshop: 1975 Proc., Ontario Ministry of the Environment, Toronto, Ontario.

194. Alexander, D. G. and Clarke, R. Mc. V., The selection and limitations of phenol as a reference toxicant to detect differences in sensitivity among groups of rainbow trout *(Salmo gairdneri), Water Res.*, 12, 1085, 1978.

195. Marking, L. L., Evaluation of *p,p'*-DDT as a reference toxicant in bioassays, Investigations in Fish Control 10, Fish and Wildlife Service, U.S. Department of the Interior, Washington, D.C., 1966.

196. Lloyd, R., The use of the concentration-response relationship in assessing acute fish toxicity data, in *Analyzing the Hazard Evaluation Process,* Dickson, K. L., Maki, A. W., and Cairns, J., Jr., Eds., American Fisheries Society, Washington, D.C., 1979, 58.

197. Branson, D. R., Armentrout, D. N., Parker, W. M., Hall, C. V., and Bone, L. I., Effluent monitoring step by step, *Environ. Sci. Technol.*, 15, 513, 1981.

198. Mount, D. I. and Stephan, C. E., A method for establishing acceptable toxicant limits for fish — malathion and the butoxyethanol ester of 2,4-D, *Trans. Am. Fish. Soc.*, 96, 185, 1967.

199. Eaton, J. G., Recent developments in the use of laboratory bioassays to determine "SAFE" levels of toxicants for fish, in *Bioassay Techniques and Environmental Chemistry,* Ann Arbor Science, Ann Arbor, Mich., 1973, 107.

200. McKim, J. M. and Benoit, D. A., Duration of toxicity tests for establishing "No Effect" concentrations for copper with brook trout *(Salvelinus fontinalis), J. Fish. Res. Board Can.*, 31, 449, 1974.

201. McKim, J. M., Evaluation of tests with early life stages of fish for predicting long-term toxicity, *J. Fish. Res. Board Can.*, 34, 1148, 1977.

202. Holcombe, G. W., Phipps, G. L., and Fiandt, J. T., Effects of phenol, 2,4-dimethylphenol, 2,4-dichlorophenol, and pentachlorophenol on embryo, larval, and early-juvenile fathead minnows *(Pimephales promelas), Arch. Environ. Contam. Toxicol.*, 11, 73, 1982.

203. Bresch, H., Investigation of the long-term action of xenobiotics on fish with special regard to reproduction, *Ecotoxicol. Environ. Saf.*, 6, 102, 1982.

204. Maki, A. W., Respiratory activity of fish as a predictor of chronic fish toxicity values for Surfactants, *Aquatic Toxicology,* ASTM STP 667, Marking, L. L. and Kimerle, R. A., Eds., American Society for Testing and Materials, Philadelphia, 1979, 77.

205. Maki, A. W., Correlations between *Daphnia magna* and fathead minnow *(Pimephales promelas)* chronic toxicity values for several classes of test substances, *J. Fish. Res. Board Can.*, 36, 411, 1979.

206. Rachlin, J. W. and Perlmutter, A., Fish cells in culture for study of aquatic toxicants, *Water Res.*, 2, 409, 1968.

207. Mehrle, P. M. and Mayer, F. L., Clinical tests in aquatic toxicology: state of the art, *Environ. Health Perspect.*, 34, 139, 1980.

208. Dagani, R., Aquatic toxicology matures, gains importance, *Chem. Eng. News.*, 58, 18, 1980.
209. Hildebrand, L. D., Sullivan, D. S., and Sullivan, T. P., Experimental studies of rainbow trout populations exposed to field applications of Roundup® herbicide, *Arch. Environ. Contam. Toxicol.*, 11, 93, 1982.
210. Hooper, F. F. and Fukano, K. G., Summary of experimental lake treatment with toxaphene 1954—1958. Mich. *Dept. Cons., Inst. Fish. Res.*, Rep. No. 1584, 1.
211. Cairns, J., Jr., Beyond single species toxicity testing, *Environ. Res.*, 3, 157, 1980.
212. Kenaga, E. E., Test organisms and methods useful for early assessment of acute toxicity of chemicals, *Environ. Sci. Technol.*, 12, 1322, 1978.
213. Daniels, R. E. and Allan, J. D., Life table evaluation of chronic exposure to a pesticide, *Can. J. Fish. Aquat. Sci.*, 38, 485, 1981.
214. Bowman, M. C., Oller, W. L., Cairns, T., Gosnell, A. B., and Oliver, K. H., Stressed bioassay systems for rapid screening of pesticide residues. I. Evaluation of bioassay system, *Arch. Environ. Contam. Toxicol.*, 10, 9, 1981.
215. Ballard, J. A. and Oliff, W. D., A rapid method for measuring the acute toxicity of dissolved materials to marine fishes, *Water Res.*, 3, 313, 1969.
216. Vigers, G. A. and Maynard, A. W., The residual oxygen bioassay: a rapid procedure to predict effluent toxicity to rainbow trout, *Water Res.*, 11, 343, 1977.

Appendix I

INDEX OF COMPOUNDS MENTIONED IN THE TEXT AND THEIR CHEMICAL NAMES

Abate®	See Temephos
ABS	Alkylbenzene sulfonate
Acephate	*O,S*-Dimethyl *N*-acetylphosphoramidothioate
Akton®	*O,O*-Diethyl *O*-(2-chloro-1-[2,5-dichlorophenyl])vinyl-phosphorothioate
Aldrin	1,2,3,4,10,10-Hexachloro-1,4,4a,5,8,8a-hexahydro-1,4-endo-exo-5,8-dimethanonaphthalene
Allethrin	dl-2-Allyl-4-hydroxy-3-methyl-2-cyclopenten-1-one ester of dl cis/trans-2,2-dimethyl-3-(2-methylpropenyl)-cyclopropanecarboxylic acid
Aminocarb	4-(Dimethylamino)-*m*-tolyl methylcarbamate
Anilazine	4,6-Dichloro-*N*-(2-chlorophenyl)-1,3,5-triazin-2-amine
Aquathol® K 40	Formulation of endothall, see endothall
Aroclors®	Commercial formulations of polychlorinated biphenyls and terphenyls of differing chlorine content, marketed by Monsanto Co.
Asulam®	Methyl(4-aminobenzenesulfonyl)carbamate
Atrazine	2-Chloro-4-ethylamino-6-isopropylamino-1,3,5-triazine
Azinophos ethyl	*O,O*-Diethyl *S*-([4-oxo-1,2,3-benzotriazin-3(4H)-yl]methyl) phosphorodithioate
Azinophos methyl	*O,O*-Dimethyl *S*-([4-oxo-1,2,3-benzotriazin-3-(4H)-yl]methyl) phosphorodithioate
Azodrin®	Dimethyl phosphate of 3-hydroxy-*N*-methyl-cis-crotonamide
Bayer® 73	See Bayluscide®
Baygon®	See propoxur
Bayluscide®	2′,5-Dichloro-4′-nitrosalicylamide, 2-aminoethanol salt
Bensulide	*O,O*-Diisopropyl phosphorodithioate *S*-ester of *N*-(2-mercaptoethyl) benzenesulfonamide
Benzo(a)pyrene	
Bioallethrin®	See Allethrin
Bioethanomethrin	
Bis(tributyltin) oxide	
Bolero®	See thiobencarb
Bromoxynil	3,5-Dibromo-4-hydroxybenzonitrile
Bromobiphenyls, di, tri, tetra	See polybrominated biphenyls
Butoxy ethyl ester of 2,4-D	See 2,4-D
Captan	*N*-(Trichloromethylthio)-4-cyclohexene-1,2-dicarboximide
Carbaryl	1-Napthyl *N*-methyl carbamate
Carbofuran	2,3-Dihydro-2,2-dimethyl-7-benzofuranyl methyl carbamate
Carbophenothion	*S*-(*p*-Chlorophenyl methylthio) *O,O*-diethyl phosphorodithioate
Chlordane, cis- and trans-	1,2,4,5,6,7,8,8-Octachloro-2,3,3a,4,7,7a-hexahydro-4,7-methanoindene

Chlordecone	Decachlorooctahydro-1,3,4-metheno-2H-cyclobuta (cd)-pentalen-2-one
Chlorobiphenylols	Hydroxylated polychlorinated biphenyls
2-Chlorophenol	
Chlorpyrifos	*O,O*-Diethyl *O*-(3,5,6-trichloro-2-pyridyl) phosphoro-thioate
Chlorinated dibenzodioxins	
Chlorinated dioxins	
Chlorinated terphenyls	See polychlorinated terphenyls
Clophen	See polychlorinated biphenyls
CNP	1,3,5-Trichloro-2-(4-nitrophenoxy) benzene
Coumaphos	*O,O*-Diethyl *O*-(3-chloro-4-methyl-2-oxy[2H]-1-benzo-pyran-7-yl)phosphorothioate
CPDPP	Cumylphenyl diphenyl phosphate
Cypermethrin®	(±)*a*-Cyano-3-phenoxybenzyl(±)*cis,trans*-3-(2,2-dichloro-vinyl)-2,2-dimethyl cyclopropane carboxylate
2,4-D	2,4-Dichlorophenoxyacetic acid
2,4-D esters	Alkonalamine, butoxy ethanol, dimethyl amine, dodecyl amine, isopropyl butyl, polyethylene glycol butyl ether, tetradodecyl amine esters of 2,4-D
p,p'-DBH	bis-*p*-Chlorophenyl methanol
DBNP	Butyl ester of 2,4-D
p,p'-DBP	4-4'-Dichlorobenzophenone
DCPA	Dimethyl tetrachlorotetraphthalate
p,p'-DDA	2,2-bis-(*p*-Chlorophenyl) acetic acid
DDD	2,2-bis(*p*-Chlorophenyl)-1,1-dichloroethane
DDE	2,2-bis(*p*-Chlorophenyl)-1,1-dichloroethylene
p,p'-DDMS	2,2-bis(*p*-Chlorophenyl)-1-chloroethane
p,p'-DDMU	2,2-bis(*p*-Chlorophenyl)-1-chloroethylene
p,p'-DDNU	1,1-bis(*p*-Chlorophenyl)ethylene
p,p'-DDOH	2,2-bis(*p*-Chlorophenyl)ethanol
p,p'-Cl DDT	1,1,1-Trichloro-2-chloro-2,2-bis(*p*-chlorophenyl)ethane
p,p'-DDT	2,2-bis (*p*-Chlorophenyl)-1,1,1-trichloroethane
Σ DDT	Total DDT, i.e., *p,p'*-DDT+*p,p'*-DDE+*p,p'*-DDD
DDVP	See dichlorvos
Decachlorodiphenyl	See polychlorinated biphenyls
DEF®	*S,S,S*-Tributyl phorophorotrithioate
DEHP	di-2-Ethylhexyl phthalate
Delnav®	See dioxathion
Demeton	*O,O*-Diethyl *O*-[2-(ethylthio)ethyl] phosphorothioate and *O,O*-diethyl *S*-[2-(ethylthio) ethyl] phosphorothioate
Demeton-*S*-methyl	*S*-2-Ethylthioetnyl *O,O*-dimethyl phosphorothioate
Dianisyl neopentane	1,1-bis(*p*-Methoxyphenyl)-2,2-dimethyl propane
Diazinon	*O,O*-Diethyl *O*-(2-isopropyl-6-methyl-4-pyrimidinyl) phos-phorothioate
Dibenzofurans	
Dicamba®	2-Methoxy-3,6-dichlorobenzoic acid
Dicapthon	*O,O*-Dimethyl *O*-2-chloro-4-nitrophenyl phosphoro-thioate
Dichlobenil	2,6-Dichlorobenzonitrile
Dichlofenthion	*O,O*-Diethyl *O*-(2,4-dichlorophenyl)phosphorothioate

Dichlone	2,3-Dichloro-1,4-naphthoquinone
Dichlorobenzophenone	See DBP
Dichlorvos	2,2-Dichlorovinyl dimethyl phosphate
Dicofol	1,1-bis(4-Chlorophenyl)-2,2,2-trichlorethanol
Dieldrin	1,2,3,4,10,10-Hexachloro-exo-6,7-epoxy-1,4,4a,5,6,7,8,8a-octahydro-1,4-endo-exo-5,8-dimethanonaphthalene
Diflubenzuron	N-{[(4-Chlorophenyl)amino]carbonyl}-2,6-difluorobenzamide
Dimetilan	1-Dimethylcarbamoyl-5-methylpyrazol-3-yl-dimethylcarbamate
Dimethoate	O,O-Dimethyl S-(N-methylcarbamoylmethyl) phosphorodithioate
Dimethrin	2,4-Dimethylbenzyl-2,2-dimethyl-3-(2-methylpropenyl) cyclopropanecarboxylate
Dimilin®	See diflubenzuron
Dinitramine	N^3,N^3-Diethyl-2,4-dinitro-6-(trifluoromethyl)-1,3-phenylenediamine
Dinitrophenol	
Dinoseb	2-(sec-Butyl)-4,6-dinitrophenol
Dioxathion	2,3-p-Dioxanedithiol S,S-bis(O,O-diethyl phosphorodithioate)
Diquat	6,7-Dihydrodipyrido (1,2-a:2′,1′-c) pyrazinediium dibromide, monohydrate
Disulfoton	O,O-Diethyl S-(2-[ethylthio]ethyl) phosphorodithioate
Disyston®	See disulfoton
Diuron	3-(3,4-Dichlorophenyl)-1,1-dimethylurea
DNP	Dinitrophenol
Dursban®	See chlorpyrifos
Dylox®	See trichlorfon
Dyrene®	See anilazine
EDP	Ethyl diphenyl phosphate
EHDP	2-Ethylhexyl diphenyl phosphate
Enchlor®	See polychlorinated biphenyls
Endosulfan	6,7,8,9,10,10-Hexachloro-1,5,5a,6,9,9a-hexahydro-6,9-methano-2,4,3-benzodioxathiepin-3-oxide
Endothall	7-Oxabicyclo[2.2.1] heptane-2,3-dicarboxylic acid
Endrin	1,2,3,4,10,10-Hexachloro-6,7-epoxy-1,4,4a,5,6,7,8,8a-octahydro-1,4-endo, endo-5, 8-dimethanonaphthalene
EPN	O-Ethyl-O-(p-nitrophenyl) phenyl phosphonothioate
S-ethyl N,N′-dipropyl thiocarbamate	
Ethyl parathion	See parathion ethyl
Fenitrothion	O,O-dimethyl O-(4-nitro-m-tolyl) phosphorothioate
Fenoprop	2-(2,4,5-Trichlorophenoxy) propionic acid
Fenpropanate	α-Cyano-3-phenoxybenzyl-2,2,3,3-tetramethyl-cyclopropanecarboxylate
Fenvalerate	α-Cyano-3-phenoxybenzyl 2(4-chlorophenyl)-3-methyl butyrate
Fluridone	1-Methyl-3-phenyl-5-(3-trifluoromethylphenyl)-4 (1H)-pyridinone
Furadan®	See carbofuran

GD-174   2-(Digeranylamino) ethanol
Glyphosate   N-(Phosphonomethyl) glycine
Glyphosate   Isopropyl amine salt
Guthion®   See azinophos methyl
HBB   Hexabromobenzene
HCB   See hexachlorobenzene
HCH   See hexachlorocyclohexane
HCP   Hexachlorophene
HEOD   See dieldrin
Heptachlor   1,4,5,6,7,8,8-Heptachloro-3a,4,7,7a-tetrahydro-4,7-meth-
                                   anoindene
Heptachlor epoxide
Heptachlorobornane
Hexachlorobenzene
Hexachlorobiphenyl   See polychlorinated biphenyls
Hexachlorocyclohexane $\alpha,\beta,\gamma,\delta,\varepsilon$ Isomers of 1,2,3,4,5,6-hexachlorocyclohexane;
                                   formerly called benzene hexachloride or BHC
Hydrothal and   See endothall
Hydrothal 191
Isodrin
Isopropyl PCBs   Isopropyl polychlorinated biphenyls
Kelevan   (Ethyl)-(-5-hydroxyl-1,2,3,4,6,7,8,9,10,10-dicachloro-pen-
                                   tacyclo- $5.3.0.0^{26}.0^{39}.0^{48}$ decyl) levulinate
Kepone®   See chlordecone
Knox out® 2FM   Formulation of diazinon, see diazinon
Leptophos   O-(4-Bromo-2,5-dichlorophenyl) O-methylphenylphos-
                                   phonothioate
Lindane γ-Isomer of hexachlorocyclohexane
Malathion   O,O-Dimethyl S-(1,2-dicarbethoxyethyl) phosphorodi-
                                   thioate
MCPA   4-Chloro-2-methylphenoxy acetic acid
Merphos   Tributyl phosphorotrithioite
Metasystox®   See demeton-S-methyl
Methamidophos   See methazole
Methazole   2-(3,4-Dichlorophenyl)-4-methyl-1,2,4-oxadiazolidine-3,5-
                                   dione
Methoprene   Isopropyl(2E,4E)-11-methoxy-3,7,11-trimethyl-2,4-dode-
                                   cadienoate
Methoxychlor   2,2-bis(p-Methoxyphenyl)-1,1-trichloroethane
Methylmercury
Methyl parathion   See parathion methyl
Mevinphos   Dimethyl phosphate of methyl-3-hydroxy-cis-crotonate
Mexacarbate   4-(dimethylamino)-3,5-xylyl methylcarbamate
Mirex   Dodecachloroctahydro-1,3,4-methano-2H-cyclo-
                                   buta(cd)pentalene
Molinate   S-Ethyl hexahydro-1 H-azepine-1-carbothioate
MSMA   Monosodium methanearsonate
Nabam   Disodium ethylene bis-dithiocarbamate
Naled   1,2-Dibromo-2,2-dichloroethyl dimethyl phosphate
Nitrofen   2,4-dichlorophenyl-p-nitrophenyl ether
Nitrosalicylinides   3'-Chloro-3-nitrosalicylanilide

Nonachlor

Nonylphenol

NPDPP   Nonylphenyl diphenyl phosphate

Octachlorostyrene

Oxychlordane

Parathion ethyl   *O,O*-Diethyl *O*-*p*-nitrophenyl phosphorothioate

Parathion methyl   *O,O*-dimethyl-*O*-*p*-nitrophenyl phosphorothioate

PBBs   See polybrominated biphenyls

PCA   See pyrazon

PCBs   See polychlorinated biphenyls

PCDF   Polychlorinated dibenzofuran

PCP   See pentachlorophenol

Penncap-M®   Formulation of methyl parathion; see parathion methyl

Pentachlorobenzene

Pentachlorobiphenyl   See polychlorinated biphenyls

Permethrin   3-(Phenoxyphenyl)methyl(I)-cis,trans-3-(2,2-dichloro-
                                        ethenyl)-2,2-dimethyl-cyclopropanecarboxylate

Phenochlor   See polychlorinated biphenyls

Phorate   *O,O*-Diethyl *S*-([ethylthio]methyl) phosphorodithioate

Phosalone   *O,O*-Diethyl *S*-(6-chloro-3-[mercaptomethyl]-2-benzoxa-
                                        zolinone) phosphorodithioate

Phosmet   *N*-(Mercaptomethyl)phthalimide *S*-(*O,O*-dimethyl phos-
                                        phorodithioate)

Phosphamidon   2-Chloro-*N,N*-diethyl-3-(dimethyloxyphosphinyloxy)cro-
                                        tonamide

Phosphoric acid triesters   See pydraul

Phthalate esters   See phthalic acid esters

Photoaldrin

Photochlordane

Photodieldrin

Photoheptachlor

Picloram   4-Amino-3,5,6-trichloropicolinic acid

Piscicide GD-174   See GD-174

Polybrominated biphenyls   PBBs

Polychlorinated biphenyls

Polychlorinated terphen-   Aroclors® with 54% chlorine
  yls

Profenofos   *O*-(4-Bromo-2-chlorophenyl) *O*-ethyl *S*-propyl phosphoro-
                                        thioate

Propanil   3′,4′-Dichlorophenylpropionanilide

Propoxur   *O*-Isopropoxyphenyl *N*-methylcarbamate

Pydraul   Mixture of tri-aryl phosphate esters

Pyralene   See polychlorinated biphenyls

Pyrazon   5-Amino-4-chloro-2-phenyl-3(2*H*)-Pyridazinone

Pyrethrum   Mixture of natural pyrethrins

Quinalphos   *O,O*-Diethyl-*O*-(2-quinoxalinyl)-phosphorothioate

Reglone®   See diquat

Reldan®   *O,O*-Dimethyl *O*-(3,5,6-trichloro-2-pyridyl) phosphoro-
                                        thioate

Resmethrin   (5-Benzyl-3-furyl)methyl 2,2-dimethyl-3-(2-methylpro-
                                        penyl) cyclopropane-carboxylate

Rogor®	See dimethoate
Ronnel	*O,O*-Dimethyl *O*-(2,4,5-trichlorophenyl) phosphoro-thioate
Rotenone	1,2,12,12a-Tetrahydro-2-isopropenyl-8-9-dimethyoxy (1)benzopyrano (3,4-b)furo(2,3-b) (1)benzopyran-6(6aH)-one
Roundup®	See glyphosate
Rovral®	3-(3,5-Dichlorophenyl)- *N*-(1-methylethyl)-2,4-dioxo-1-imidazoline carbamide
Santotherm®	See polychlorinated biphenyls
SBP-1382	See resmethrin
Sesamex	5-{1-(2-[2-Ethoxyethoxy]ethoxy)ethoxy}-1,3-benzodioxole
Silvex®	See 2,4,5-T
Simazine	2-Chloro-4,6-bis(ethylamino)-s-triazine
SKF-525A	
Sodium arsenite	
Strobane®	Polychlorinates of camphene, pinene, and related terpenes
Systox®	See demeton
2,4,5-T	2,4,5-Trichlorophenoxy acetic acid
TBTO	See bis(tributyltin oxide)
TCA	See trichloroacetic acid
TCDD	See tetrachloro dibenzo dioxin
TCDF	See tetrachloro dibenzo furan
TCP	Tricresyl phosphate
TDCPP	Tris (1,3-Dichloroisopropyl) phosphate
Telodrin	
Temephos	*O,O,O′,O′*-Tetramethyl *O,O′*-(thiodi-*p*-phenylene) diphosphorothioate
TEPA	Tris (1-Aziridinyl) phosphine oxide
TEPP	Tetraethyl diphosphate; tetraethyl pyrophosphate
Terbutryn	2-(tert-Butylamino)-4-(ethylamino)-6-(methylthio)-*s*-triazine
Tetrachlorobiphenyl	See polychlorinated biphenyls
Tetradifon	4-Chlorophenyl 2,4,5-trichlorophenyl sulfone; (2,4,5,4′-tetrachlorodiphenyl sulfone)
TFM	3-Trifluoromethyl-4-nitrophenol, sodium salt
Therminal	See polychlorinated biphenyls
Thidiazuron	*N*-Phenyl- *N′*-(1,2,3-thiadiazol-5-yl)urea
Thimet®	See phorate
Thiobencarb	*S*-(4-Chlorobenzyl) *N,N*-diethylthiocarbamate
Toxaphene	Chlorinated camphene (67—69% chlorine) mixture
TPP	Triphenyl phosphate
Trichlorfon	Dimethyl(2,2,2-trichloro-1-hydroxyethyl)phosphonate
Trichloro biphenyl	See polychlorinated biphenyls
2,4,6-trichlorophenyl	*p*-Nitrophenyl ether
Trichlorophenol	
Trichloropyridinol	
Trifluralin	*a,a,a*-Trifluoro-2,6-dinitro-*N,N*-dipropoyl-*p*-toludine
Tris phosphate	tris (2,4-di-*ter*-Butylphenyl)phosphate
Trithion®	See carbophenothion
Zolone®	See phosalone

Appendix II

COMMON NAMES OF FISH MENTIONED IN THE TEXT AND THEIR SCIENTIFIC NAMES

African lakefish	*Tilapia* sp.
Alewife	*Alosa pseudoharengus* (Wilson)
American shad	*Alosa sapidissima* (Wilson)
American smelt	*Osmerus mordax*
Arctic char	*Salvelinus alpinus* (Linn.)
Atlantic cod	*Gadus* sp.
Atlantic croakers	*Micropogon* sp.
Atlantic salmon	*Salmo salar* Linn
Atlantic silverside	*Menidia menidia*
Baltic flounder	*Platichthys flesus*
Barbus sp.	
Bass	See white bass and yellow bass
Bigmouth buffalo	*Ictiobus cyprinellus* (Valenciennes)
Black bullheads	*Ictalurus melas* (Rafinesque)
Black crappie	*Pomoxis nigromaculatus* (LeSueur)
Black surfperch	*Embiotoca jacksoni*
Bluegills	*Lepomis macrochirus* Rafinesque
Bluntnose minnows	*Pimephales notatus* (Rafinesque)
Brook trout	*Salvelinus fontinalis* (Mitchill)
Brown bullheads	*Ictalurus nebulosus* (LeSueur)
Brown trout	*Salmo trutta*
Bullheads	See brown bullheads
Burbot	*Lota lota* (Linn.)
Carp	*Cyprinus carpio* Linn.
Channa	*Channa punctata*
Channel catfish	*Ictalurus punctatus* (Rafinesque)
Char	See Arctic char
Chinook salmon	*Oncorhynchus tschawytscha* (Walbaum)
Chub	*Coregonus alpenae*
Cirrhinus mrigala	
Cisco	*Coregonus artedii* Le Sueur
Cod	*Gadus morrhua*
Coho salmon	*Oncorhynchus kisutch* (Walbaum)
Common shiner	*Notropis cornutus* (Mitchill)
Convict cichlid	*Cyclosoma nigrofasciatum*
Creek chub	*Semotilus atromaculatus* (Mitchill)
Crucian carp	*Carassius carassius*
Cutthroat trout	*Salmo clarki* Richardson
Cynoglossus	
Dogfish	*Squalus* sp.
English sole	*Parophrys vetulus*
Fathead minnow	*Pimephales promelas*
Flagfish	*Jordanella floridae*
Flounder	*Platichthys* sp.
Gizzard shad	*Dorosoma crepedianum* (LeSueur)
Glyphocephalus	
Gobi fish	*Gobius* sp.

Goldenshiners	*Notemigonus crysoleucas* (Mitchill)
Goldfish	*Carassius* sp.
Goldorfe	*Leusescus ides*
Green sunfish	*Lepomis cyanellus* Rafinesque
Guppy	*Poecilia* sp.
Harlequin fish	*Rosbora heteromorpha*
Herring	*Clupea harengus*
Johnny darter	*Etheostoma nigrum* Rafinesque
Killifish	*Oryzeas latipes*
King salmon	*Oncorhynchus tshawytscha*
Labeo rohita	
Landlocked salmon	*Salmo salar* Linn.
Lake herring	See cisco
Lake trout	*Salvelinus namaycush* (Walbaum)
Lamprey	*Petromyzon* sp.
Largemouth bass	*Micropterus salmoides* (Lacépède)
Leucaspius dileneatus	
Limnothrissa	
Longear sunfish	*Lepomis megalotis*
Longnose killifish	*Fundulus similis*
Longnose sucker	*Catostomus catostomus*
Medaka	*Oryzias latipes*
Menhaden	*Brevoortia* sp.
Minnow	*Phoxinus phoxinus*
Mosquitofish	*Gambusia affinis* (Baird and Girard)
Motsugo fish	*Pseudorasbora parva*
Mullet	*Mugil* sp.
Mystus cavasius	
Northern anchovy	*Engraulis modax*
Northern puffers	*Sphaeroides maculatus*
Paddlefish	*Polyodon spathula* (Walbaum)
Perch	*Perca fluviatilis*
Pike	*Esox lucius* Linn.
Pinfish	*Lagodon rhomboides*
Pumpkin seed	*Lepomis gibbosus* (Linn.)
Rainbow trout	*Salmo gairdneri* Richardson
Redear sunfish	*Lepomis microlophus* (Gunther)
Redhorse suckers	*Moxostoma macrolepidotum* (LeSueur)
Reticulate sculpins	*Cottus perplexus*
Riogrande perch	*Cichlasoma cyanoguttatum*
Rivercarp sucker	*Capiodes carpio*
Roach	*Rutilus rutilus*
Sailfin mollies	*Poecilia latipinna*
Salmon	*Salmo* sp.
Sand trout	
Sardine	*Sardina* sp.
Sea trout	*Cynoscion* sp.
Sheepshead minnow	*Cyprinodon variegatus*
Shiners	See golden shiners
Smallmouth bass	*Micropterus dolomieui* Lacépède
Sockeye salmon	*Oncorhynchus nerka* (Walbaum)
Speckled trout	

Spot	*Leiostomus xanthurus*
Statothrissa	
Steelhead trout	Sea running phase of the rainbow trout *Salmo gairdneri*
Stickleback	*Gasterosteus* sp.
Striped bass	*Morone saxatilis*
Suckers	*Catostomus* sp.
Swordfish	*Xiphias gladias*
Therapon jarbua	
Thorny skate	*Raja radiata*
Tilapia	
Topmouth gudgeon	*Pseudorasbora parva*
Varichorhinus	
Wall eye	*Stizostedion vitreum vitreum* (Mitchill)
White bass	*Roccus chrysops* (Rafinesque)
White crappie	*Pomoxis annularis* Rafinesque
White fish	*Coregonus clupeaformis* (Mitchill)
White perch	*Roccus americanus* (Gmelin)
White suckers	*Catostomus commersoni* (Lacépède)
Winter flounder	*Pseudopleuronectes americanus*
Xiphias gladias	
Yellow bass	*Roccus mississippiensis* (Jordan and Eigenmarine)
Yellow bullheads	*Ictalurus natalis* (LeSueur)
Yellow perch	*Perca flavescens* (Mitchill)
Zebra danio	*Brachydanio rario*

INDEX

I

J

K

atmospheric residues of, 9
BCF of, 70
in bioaccumulation model, 74
bioaccumulation of, 73, 88
in biomagnification studies, 76
metabolism of, 90, 91
nonpesticide sources of, 5
persistence of, 5, 25
residue levels of in Great Lakes, 44
residue leves of in U.S., 41
seasonal variation in residue levels of, 57
in static vs. flow-through tests, 130
variability of data of in toxicity tests, 137
Mixed function oxidase (MFO), 57, 92—96
Mixostoma macrolepidotum, see Redhorse suckers
Molecular structure
    bioconcentration and, 71—72
    persistence and, 5, 27
Molinate, 6
Monitoring, 58—59
Monochlorobiphenyls, 104
Mononitrophenols, 130
Monosodium methanearsonate, see MSMA
Mosquitofish, 41, 42, 56
MSMA (monosodium methanearsonate), 13
Mullet, 42

N

Naphthalene, solubility of, 98
1-Nathphyl *N*-methyl carbamate, see Carbaryl
National Pesticide Monitoring Program (NPMP), 58
Nematicides, spills of, 18
Neustonic organisms, bioconcentration by, 20
para-Nitroanisole, 94
Nitrobenzene, 98
Nitro compounds, history of use of, 2
Nitrofen, 6, 122
p-Nitrophenyl ether, see 2,4,6-Trichlorophenyl
Nonachlor, 16, 39, 48
Nonylphenyl diphenyl phosphate (NPDPP), 97
Northern anchovy, 83
Northern pike, 43, 53
NPDPP, see Nonylphenyl diphenyl phosphate
NPMP, see National Pesticide Monitoring Program (NPMP)

O

OC, see Organochlorines (OC)
OCS (octachlorostyrene)
    bioaccumulation pathways of, 84—85
    residue levels of in Europe, 45
1,2,4,5,6,7,8,8-Octachloro-2,3,3a,4,7,7a-hexahydro-4,7-methanoindene, see Chlordane
Octachlorosytrene, see OCS
OP, see Organophosphates
Orange-red killifish, 123
Organic matter

bioconcentration and, 71, 73
    soil adsorption and, 14, 23—24
Organization for Economic Cooperation and Development (OECD), monitoring programs of, 58—59
Organochlorines (OC), see also specific organochlorines
    adsorption of, 13—14, 22
    adverse effects of, 2, 3
    atmospheric residues of, 10
    BCF and, 99, 101
    bioaccumulation of, 86—88
    calculation of BCF of, 100
    degradation of, 25, 26
    diet and toxicity, 125
    in drinking water, 20
    environmental monitoring of, 58
    history of use of, 1, 2
    in identification of contamination source, 18
    lipid content and, 55
    metabolism and elimination of, 90, 91
    metabolites of, 86, 87
    MFO in detoxification of, 94
    mobility of in soil, 12—14
    molecular structure of and BCF, 99
    persistence of, 5, 6, 25
    in precipitation, 10—11
    in predator mortality, 2
    range of residues of, 48—50
    residue levels of in Europe, 45
    residue levels of in Great Lakes, 44
    residues of in precipitation, 11
    in sewage effluent, 16
    size of fish and, 51
    soil mobility of, 12
    in surface microlayers, 19
    tissue extraction of, 38
    trends in residue levels of, 41—50
    from urban sewage, 15
    volatilization of, 8
    wind transport of, 10
Organoleptic tests, see also Toxicity tests, 142
Organophosphates (OP), see also specific organophosphates
    adsorption of, 13, 14
    adverse effects of, 2
    analytical errors with, 39
    BCF and, 99—101
    bioaccumulation of, 88
    bioconcentration of, 48
    calculation of BCF of, 100
    in coastal waters, 20
    degradation of, 25, 26, 94—95
    history of use of, 1—2, 6
    MFO in detoxification of, 94—95
    mobility of in soil, 12—14
    molecular structure of and BCF, 99—100
    persistence of, 6, 25
    QSAR descriptors of, 102
    resistance to by pests, 2
    in sediments, 22—23

White sucker, 54, 71
Wind erosion, in pesticide transport, 9—10
Winter flounder, 43

X

Xiphias gladias, see Swordfish
XMC, 88

Y

Yellow perch, 54, 55

Z

Zebra danio, 139
Zebrafish, 123, 138